Pregnancy

from preconception to birth

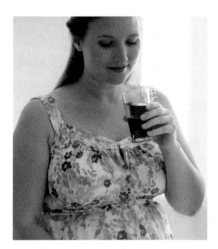

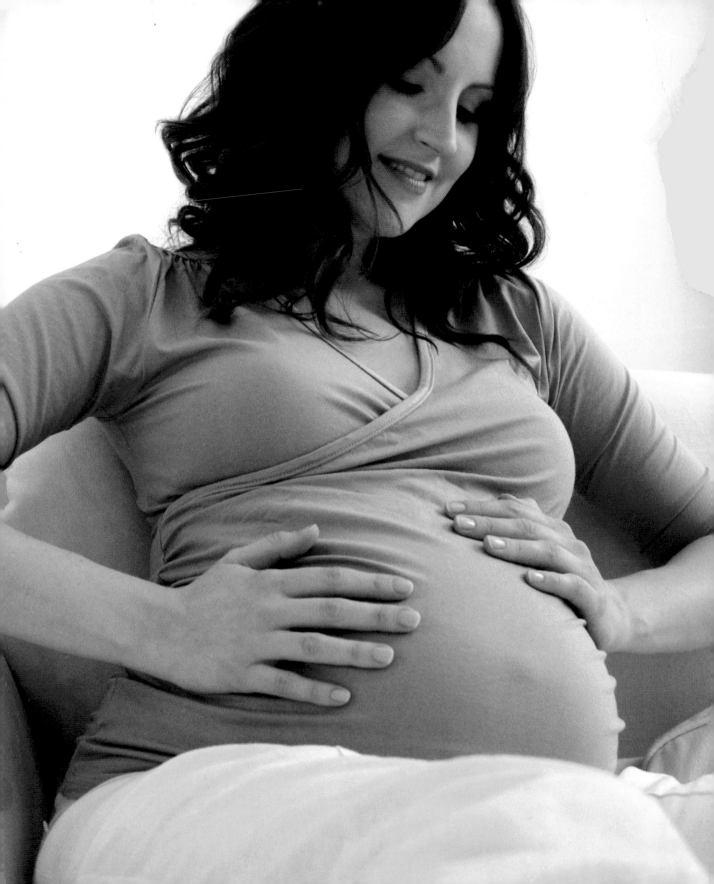

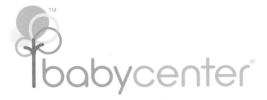

Pregnancy

from preconception to birth

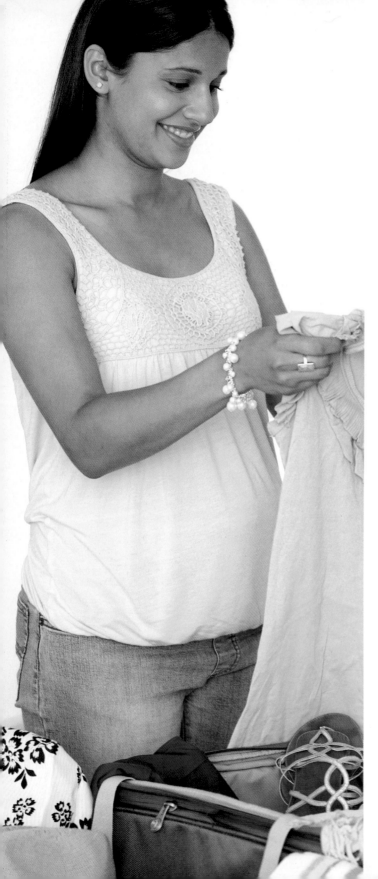

London • New York • Munich Melbourne • Delhi

For BabyCenter
Editor Linda Murray
Project editor Victoria Farrimond
Contributing editor Darienne Hosley Stewart

For DK
Project editor Hilary Mandleberg
Project designers Hannah Moore and Kevin Smith
Senior editor Emma Maule
Senior art editor Isabel de Cordova
US editors Shannon Beatty and Jane Perlmutter
US medical consultant Mary Jane Minkin, MD
Designer Saskia Janssen
Photographer Ruth Jenkinson
Photography art direction Isabel de Cordova
Production editor Maria Elia
Senior production editor Jennifer Murray
Production controller Seyhan Esen
Creative technical support Sonia Charbonnier
Managing editor Penny Warren
Managing art editors Glenda Fisher and Marianne Markham
Category publisher Peggy Vance

Every effort has been made to ensure that the information contained in this book is complete and accurate. However, neither the publisher nor the author are engaged in rendering professional advice or services to the individual reader. The ideas, procedures, and suggestions contained in the book are not intended as a substitute for consultation with your health-care provider. All matters regarding the health of you and your child require medical supervision. Neither the publisher nor the author accept any legal responsibility for any personal injury or other damage or loss arising from the use or misuse of the information and advice in this book.

First American Edition, 2010
Published in the United States by
DK Publishing, 375 Hudson Street
New York, New York 10014

11 12 10 9 8 7 6 5 4 3 2
004-BD694-August 2010

Published in Great Britain by Dorling Kindersley Limited.

A catalog record for this book is available from the Library of Congress
ISBN 978-0-7566-5040-7

DK books are available at special discounts when purchased in bulk for sales promotions, premiums, fund-raising, or educational use. For details, contact: DK Publishing Special Markets, 375 Hudson Street, New York, New York 10014 or SpecialSales@dk.com.

Color reproduction by Colourscan, Singapore
Printed and bound in Singapore by Tien Wah Press

Discover more at
www.dk.com

Contents

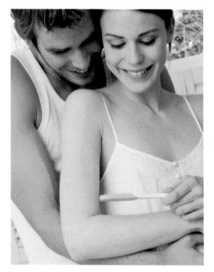
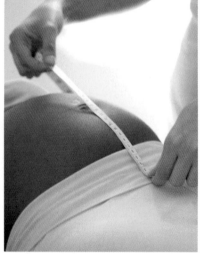
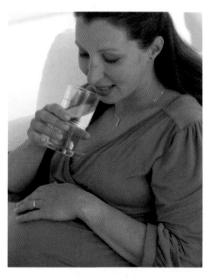

Birth and beyond
Becoming a parent

Life with your new baby

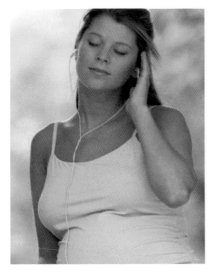
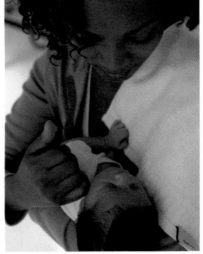
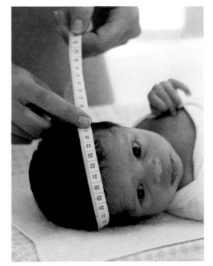

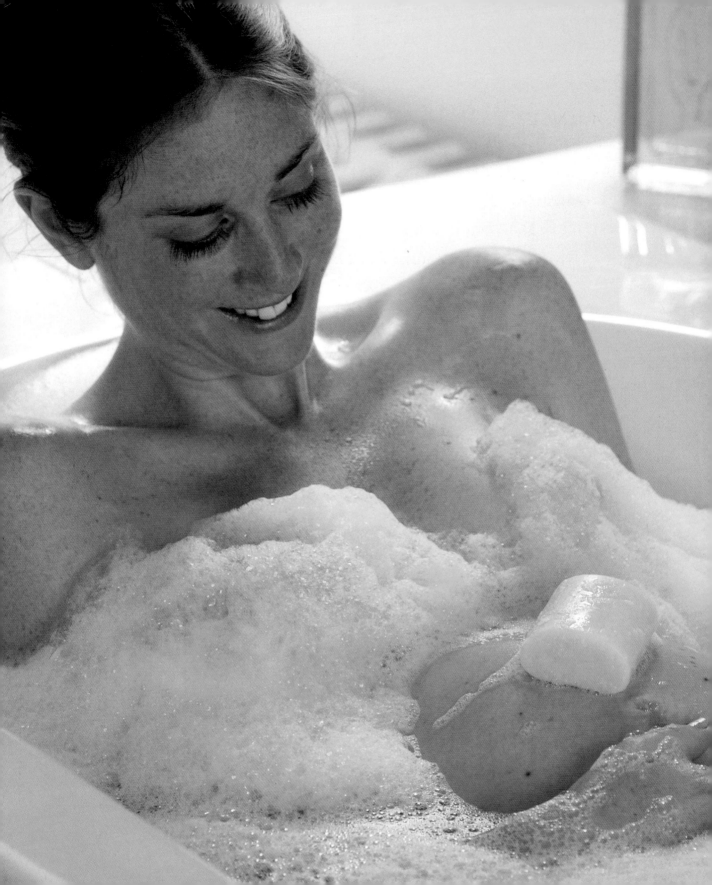

Foreword

Having a baby will be the most extraordinary and joyous thing you'll ever do. It will also be worrying, and at times overwhelming and exhausting. When you become pregnant, your life—and your body—changes forever and although it makes for an exciting journey, it's not without its challenges.

As a mom myself, I know the best way to cope with these changes is to arm yourself with the best information you can find—and some good friends to back you up! The moment you find out you're pregnant your mind is filled with questions: Is my baby developing normally? Why am I feeling like this? Can I eat this? Can I do that? You have to make a lot of decisions, too. Which prenatal tests do you want? Which doctor or midwife is right for you? What do need to buy for your newborn? And, of course, what will you name your baby?

That's where BabyCenter comes in. We can answer your most pressing questions and help you make the right decisions for your family. For over 10 years we've been the number one resource for pregnant women and new parents. Our trusted expert advice —backed up by a team of medical advisors—and our open, supportive community have helped well over 100 million people make the transition to parenthood.

This book, with its in-depth information and beautiful photographs, is an exciting new venture for us. We're thrilled to be working with Dorling Kindersley to create such a fantastic publication. It brings together BabyCenter's expert content and the voices of real moms and dads from our online community in a gorgeous book that takes you from the miracle of conception to those first precious weeks with your newborn baby. So sit back, put your feet up (go on, it's good for you!) and enjoy the journey.
Have a happy, healthy pregnancy!

Linda

Linda Murray, Editor
www.babycenter.com

Introduction

BabyCenter Pregnancy is designed to accompany you all the way along your incredible journey into parenthood, from the moment when you make the decision to start a family through to those first precious weeks with your newborn.

Your pregnancy guide

This book is packed with all the information you'll need throughout your pregnancy, including a week-by-week pregnancy diary, helpful hints and checklists, and tips and advice from moms and dads who've all been there, done it, and have the milk-stained T-shirt to prove it.

We at BabyCenter want to be your most trusted parenting resource—that's why we offer practical advice from expert sources, such as doctors, midwives, and fellow parents. We've divided the book into the four following sections:

Getting ready for pregnancy

Deciding to have a baby is one of the most momentous decisions you're ever likely to make. It requires a lifetime commitment of love and care, not to mention financial support, both in the early years and for many years afterward.

In this chapter, we'll give you all the information you need to build the right foundations for a happy and healthy pregnancy and baby, whether it's your first baby or a new addition to your family. We'll also give you the low-down on preparing your body for pregnancy, from eating the right foods and cutting out vices such as smoking and drinking, to managing any preexisting medical conditions.

Dads take note too—your health and lifestyle can affect your fertility. We'll help you protect your potency and prepare yourself for parenthood.

So, what happens next? There are all sorts of fascinating biological events that take place behind the scenes, from ovulation to conception. We cover them all and help to give you a better understanding of your own fertility.

Staying safe and healthy

Once you're pregnant, you'll have many questions about how best to take care of yourself and your baby. What should—and shouldn't—you be eating? How can you stay fit and active without getting hurt? What medicines are safe and which should you avoid? Are there any hazards at work or at home you should be concerned about? Being pregnant can seem like a minefield at times. In this chapter, we'll let you know what is safe and what isn't, and give you advice on how you can protect yourself and your baby.

Being pregnant isn't just about your physical well-being. You'll find yourself on an emotional roller coaster over the next nine months; elated one day, anxious about how your life will change the next. We'll help you deal with these feelings and offer some practical tips, from making the decision to return to work and avoiding isolation after your baby is born, to how your relationship is about to change.

Although you might not feel it in those first nauseous months, being pregnant makes you beautiful. We'll outline all the changes that your body will go through and what beauty treatments will enhance your pregnancy glow, and we'll give tips on how you can update your wardrobe to accommodate your growing belly.

Nine months may seem like a long time, but before you know it you'll be holding your tiny newborn. We'll explain how you and your partner can bond with your baby before he arrives. We'll also help you prepare your home for his arrival.

Your pregnancy diary

At the heart of the book is a week-by-week pregnancy diary. Here you can find the information you need, right when you need it. You'll find out about how your baby is developing and the remarkable changes your body is going through. You'll find out about common health concerns, your prenatal care options, exercise for each stage of pregnancy, and information on dealing with pregnancy while you're at work.

This section is divided into the three trimesters of pregnancy, each of which is made up of around 13 weeks. Here you'll find stage-based tips on healthy eating and how to get a good night's sleep. You'll also discover what scans and prenatal tests are available and, as you enter the third trimester, you'll find plenty of advice on preparing for the birth. This chapter also includes a comprehensive health section, covering all the common medical pregnancy concerns.

Birth and beyond

Every birth is different but our labor and birth information will help you plan and prepare for the big day. We will guide you through the different stages of childbirth and look at all the options available to you—whether you are planning to have your baby at home, in a hospital, or at a birthing center. We'll take you through the process of labor and birth stage by stage, from the first signs of labor, to the moment you hold your newborn.

In this section you'll find out about natural and medical pain relief and positions for labor and birth. You'll also find out all about assisted births, breech births, and cesarean sections, and what happens when you're overdue. And in the unlikely event that your labor happens very quickly, we'll let you know how to deal with an emergency home birth.

The first few weeks with your baby can be wonderful, challenging, and tiring all at the same time. Here you'll find lots of practical advice on caring for your newborn, including "how tos" on feeding, bathing, holding him, and changing his diaper. We'll also help you adapt to your new life as a parent, with information on coping with fatigue and understanding your emotions in these wearying early weeks.

"This **book is packed** with all the **information** needed **to guide you** through **pregnancy**."

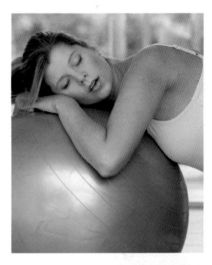

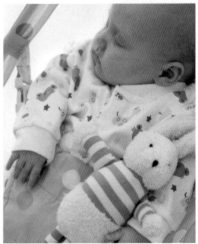

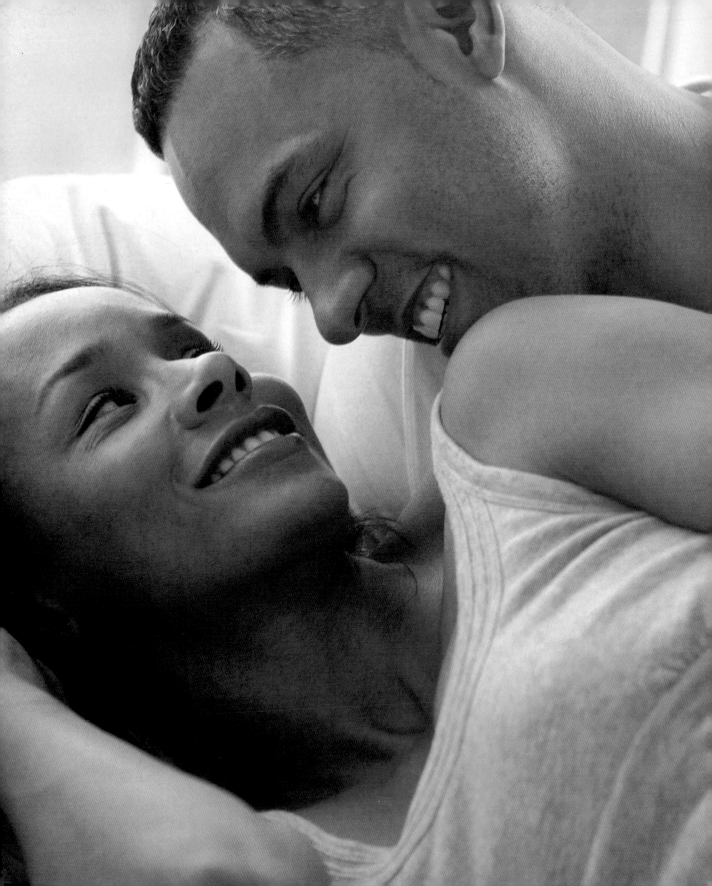

Getting ready for pregnancy

Before you start

A child demands a lifetime commitment to provide love, nurturing, nourishment, shelter, education, and attention. So before you decide to have a baby, it's important that you and your partner consider your decision carefully. This is a decision that will change your lives forever.

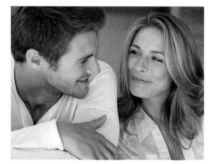

Becoming parents will have a major impact on many aspects of your lives. You and your partner should discuss it carefully.

Thinking your decision through

Having a baby won't have just a small impact on your life; it's going to shift the entire center of your universe. Think about how you'll feel, how you usually deal with change, and how you can prepare yourselves properly.

Some key questions to consider include:

- Are you both truly committed to becoming parents?
- Have you thought through how you'll handle balancing work and family?
- Are you prepared for the possibility that you may have twins or more?
- Are you ready to give up sleeping in on Sundays or to line up a babysitter every single time you want to go out?
- If you have religious differences, have the two of you discussed how these will affect your child?
- Have you considered how becoming parents may change you and your close relationships with others?

Start early

Giving your baby the best possible start means getting your own life sorted out well before you get pregnant. Plan a few months ahead if you can, so that changes to your diet and lifestyle (see pp.16–17) have time to take effect. If you have an existing medical condition, such as epilepsy, asthma, or diabetes (see pp.22–3) you may need to make some changes to your treatment before you conceive. Most doctors are happy to give you a general pre-pregnancy health checkup to make sure you're in the best possible health for pregnancy.

Stopping contraception

For some people, stopping contraception is as easy as shoving the condoms or diaphragm to the back of a drawer. If you've been on the pill, the usual advice is to start trying once you've had one normal period. If you've been having contraceptive injections, it may take a while for the effect to wear off (about 12 weeks, according to manufacturers).

To have an intrauterine device (IUD or coil) or intrauterine system (IUS) removed, you'll need to make an appointment with your doctor or your family planning clinic. Your normal fertility will return as soon as you have the IUD removed, but it may take a month or so if you use an IUS because of the effects of hormones in your system.

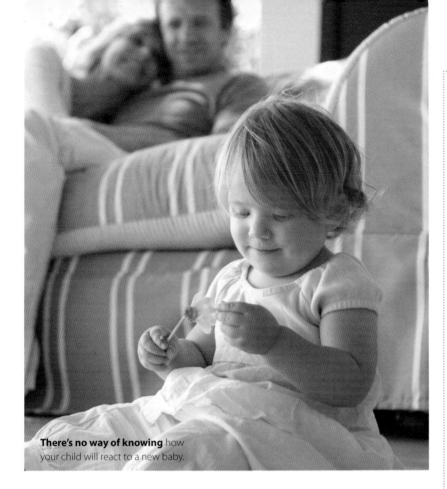
There's no way of knowing how your child will react to a new baby.

Another baby?

When it comes to deciding when the right time is to have another baby, there are no right or wrong answers. Most doctors recommend waiting at least six months after the birth of one child before trying again, and research suggests that leaving a gap of 18 to 23 months before conceiving again is the optimum timing for a healthy baby.

Having said that, there are other factors you'll need to take into account. Sometimes one partner is ready and the other isn't. This is a tough one but the first step is to start talking about your differences. You may not solve anything but at least you'll have a better understanding of the issues involved.

Think about your lifestyle. Do you have good child-care arrangements in place? Are your other children sleeping through the night? Maybe you've gone back to work and you love it. Money isn't everything, but if you're thinking of another baby, you may well need a little extra in your monthly budget before conceiving again.

At the end of the day, you can mull over the pros and cons of having another child forever. This is one of those decisions that's best led by the heart, so go ahead and follow yours. If you want another baby, and your partner is happy with that, then there may be no time like the present.

Dad's **Diary**

I'm going to be a dad

"It's a week since we discovered we're pregnant. A week since finding out I'm going to be a father. A dad. Daddy, Pop, Pa. I'm so excited. I'm walking around with the biggest grin on my face. I—okay we—made a baby! I'm scared too, for many reasons.

But mostly I'm daunted. It will be my responsibility to teach our child life skills, to guide him, and show him right from wrong. What's my opinion on computer games versus outdoor activities? Should I let him play with guns and toy soldiers?

'Is any of this really worth worrying about right now?' my wife asks, as I consider the cost of buying and owning a pony. Yes. It is. The problem is that I can't help but look at the bigger picture, even if it has yet to be drawn.

'You're going to make a great dad!' she reassures me. But what do I know about being a dad? The only point of reference I have is taking care of Paddy my dog. And of course my own father. I suppose he did a good job.

And now it's my time to live up to and pass on the example that he set me. It's my turn to be Dad."

Parents**Ask...**

When's a good time to add to my family?

There's no absolute "right" time. If you're worried about your fertility, took a long time to conceive before, or you're over 35, you might want to get moving. On the other hand, if you're in your twenties and have toddler twins, it might make sense delaying a third baby! Every age gap between children has its pros and cons, and personality factors mean that what works well in one family isn't as successful in another.

Health and lifestyle checks for you

You've decided it's time to start your family. But are you ready? Perhaps you're concerned that you're a little overweight. Or maybe your diet needs a bit of an overhaul. One thing's for sure: by making a few lifestyle changes now, you'll be getting your baby off to the best start.

Organized mom

If you like to do things by the book, you may want a checkup before trying to conceive.

"I drive my husband and family crazy with the way I always want to prepare properly for everything. They say I'm a control freak. Well, maybe I am, but I decided it was worth it when it came to checking out what I could do to improve my chances of having a healthy pregnancy *before* I conceived.

First of all I checked that I'd had a recent pap smear and I had a urine analysis done, too. I've had urinary tract infections in the past and I certainly didn't want to have one now. I also got checked out for anemia, with a blood test, and while he was at it, my doctor took my blood pressure, too. My vaccinations were up to date, so no problems there, but my doctor did suggest I get tested for any sexually transmitted diseases, as well as for viral infections like the potentially dangerous toxoplasmosis.

I don't take any medications regularly, but if I did, one thing I'd definitely think about would be to check with my doctor they were safe to take during pregnancy. And last but not least, I've started taking folic acid."

Getting your health on track

Now more than ever, proper nutrition is essential. Forget all those fad diets, and learn to eat real food. That means a balanced diet of at least three meals a day, including at least five portions of fruit and vegetables.

Three of the most important nutrients you will need for a healthy pregnancy are calcium, iron, and folic acid, so be sure to drink plenty of milk and eat citrus fruits and juices, dark green leafy vegetables, nuts, whole grains, and fortified breads and cereals.

You may also want to cut back on your caffeine. Research linking a woman's caffeine consumption with a lower chance of conception is contradictory but, in general, low levels of caffeine consumption are recommended. By contrast, dads-to-be should feel free to drink an extra cup: caffeine may help to increase male fertility by stimulating sperm motility.

Prenatal supplements

While it's no substitute for a healthy, balanced diet, taking a prenatal supplement ensures that you're getting enough of several important vitamins and minerals. At the top of that list is folic acid, which is a B vitamin that helps prevent neural tube defects in developing babies. Ask your doctor or midwife to recommend a vitamin supplement for you.

Think about your weight

Being underweight or overweight can affect your fertility and pose significant risks to your pregnancy. Now's the time to try to hit a healthy weight if you want to increase your chances both of conception and a healthy pregnancy.

If you're overweight or obese, do it steadily. Crash dieting can deplete your body's nutritional reserves. Nor is it a good idea to diet while you're pregnant because you may limit your baby's access to important nutrients. The best route to success is to combine a balanced diet with an exercise program before you get pregnant. Aim for a safe weight loss of up to 2 pounds a week.

If you're underweight, get some meat on you! Your risk of miscarriage is higher if you conceive while underweight. And while skinny women can and do have healthy babies, studies show that underweight mothers are more likely to have low-birthweight babies. Gorging yourself on chocolate won't give you the important vitamins and minerals you need, so try to get your extra calories from a healthy, balanced diet.

Getting your lifestyle on track

A balanced exercise program is a great place to start when you're preparing for pregnancy. Exercise will give you stamina, strength, and flexibility. You'll need all three to lift and carry a baby, run after a small child, and deal with the day-to-day challenges of motherhood. Plus, getting in shape at least three months before you conceive may make it easier to maintain an active lifestyle during pregnancy, not to mention helping you get through labor. Great exercises to help you get into shape for pregnancy include running and jogging, walking, swimming, bicycling, and aerobics.

Stop drinking, smoking, and taking drugs

It doesn't take a rocket scientist to figure out that smoking, taking drugs, and drinking alcohol during pregnancy can harm your baby. Study after study has shown that all three of these are connected to miscarriage, low-birthweight babies, and premature birth. Smoking in pregnancy can increase your baby's risk of SIDS (sudden infant death syndrome), and drinking during pregnancy can seriously affect your baby's development. If you're still partying, now's the time to clean up your lifestyle.

Eliminate environmental dangers

There are certain jobs that can be hazardous to you and your unborn baby. If you stand all day, fly a lot, or are exposed to chemicals or radiation regularly, you may need to make changes before you conceive. Talk to your doctor about it and see if you can come up with ways to avoid or eliminate hazards in your workplace. The Occupational Health and Safety Administration also has useful information on how you can make your work environment safer.

Get your finances in order

You may never feel you *really* have enough money to have a baby, but that doesn't mean you shouldn't try to save a little before you get pregnant. After all, having a baby is expensive, and that expense goes on for 18 years or more! Some other financial issues you may want to consider include taking out life insurance and making a will.

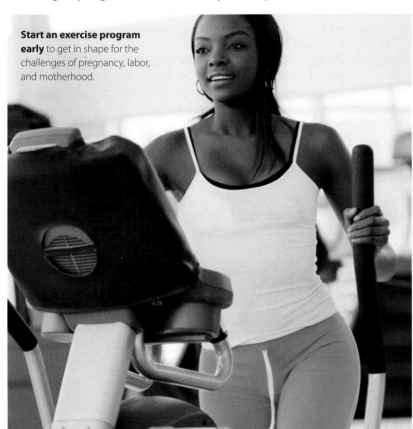

Start an exercise program early to get in shape for the challenges of pregnancy, labor, and motherhood.

Lifestyle readiness

Follow the points in this handy checklist to ensure you get your pregnancy off to a good start:
- Improve your diet.
- Achieve a healthy weight.
- Create (and follow!) an exercise plan.
- If you drink, smoke, or take drugs, then stop as soon as you can.
- Start taking folic acid.
- Get your finances in order.
- Start taking a special pregnancy multivitamin.
- Stop using contraception.
- Eliminate environmental dangers.
- Be sure parenthood is really for you.

Getting ready for pregnancy

Staying safe and healthy

Your pregnancy diary

Birth and beyond

Partners take note

Taking care of your health as a prospective father is very important since there is a host of lifestyle factors that can affect your potency. The good news is, once you become aware of these often hidden threats to fertility, they are fairly easy to avoid.

Father's health and lifestyle

Dads-to-be should aim to maintain a healthy body mass index (BMI) of 20 to 25 while trying to conceive, as having a low or high BMI is associated with a reduction in sperm. It also helps if your diet includes zinc (found in ground beef and baked beans), folates (eat green, leafy vegetables), and vitamin C (citrus fruit is a good source), since all of these help your body to make healthy sperm.

Keep drinking coffee if you like it—studies show that caffeine may improve sperm motility—but you should cut back on alcohol. An occasional drink (of one drink—one ounce—a day) is considered safe, but experts agree that drinking too much will harm the quality of your sperm.

Lifestyle and fertility

Besides food, there are other lifestyle factors that can affect your fertility:

- **Stress** This can sometimes affect men's sperm counts, so simply relaxing may increase your fertility.
- **Medicines** Whether prescription or over the counter, certain medications, such as the antihistamine cimetidine, can affect semen quality. Check with your doctor if you are concerned.
- **Cancer treatment and X-rays** Chemotherapy treatment can induce a permanent loss of fertility, but the jury is still out on whether X-rays have any effect on sperm.
- **Injury to your genitals** This could impair your ability to produce sperm or to ejaculate. If you play contact sports, wear protective gear.
- **Smoking** Men who smoke damage the quantity and quality of their sperm (yet another reason to quit!). Most doctors' offices have smoking cessation information and there are lots of support services to help you succeed.
- **Recreational drugs** Cocaine, marijuana, and anabolic steroids have all been linked with reduced sperm quality.

Dad's **Diary**

Right from the start: counting down to healthy fatherhood

"Claire has given my diet an overhaul since we've been trying for a baby. I thought I was healthy enough, but apparently what you put in your body can really affect the strength of your little swimmers. So, takeout and fast-food snacks are out, and green vegetables and whole grains are in. She's even making me eat the skin on my baked potatoes—horror of horrors! The good news is that lean red meat is on the good list, so at least I get a decent steak once a week. And I haven't had to reduce my coffee consumption, but the bad news is that I've had to cut down on alcohol—apparently it impairs the quality of your sperm. I'm sure my co-workers will laugh. However, a couple of drinks a week shouldn't hurt. Everything in moderation, as they say. I guess a few months of good, clean living will do the trick."

A healthy dad makes healthy sperm, so it pays prospective dads to watch their lifestyle.

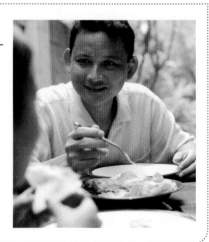

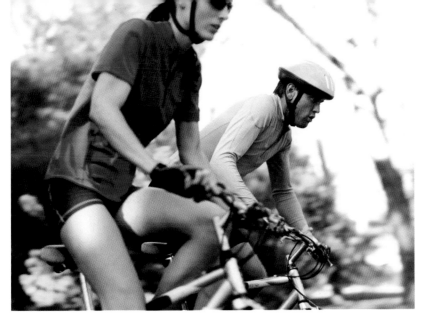

Cycling can protect against impotence but limit your cycling to less than three hours a week and invest in a wide, well-padded seat.

Sperm safety

One thing scientists do know is that testicles produce the best-quality sperm when they keep their cool. "The boys" are happiest at or 94 to 96° F (34.5 to 36° C), which is a couple of degrees cooler than normal body temperature. Working in a hot environment or sitting for long periods of time have been linked to an abnormal sperm count or semen quality. Using a laptop on your lap and driving for long periods can also cause overheating, while heated waterbeds and electric blankets are bigger culprits for raising scrotal temperature than hot baths and hot tubs.

One study showed that men and their sperm are better off wearing loose-fitting boxer shorts than tighter fitting briefs. Another showed no difference in scrotal temperature between men wearing briefs and men wearing boxer shorts, although both types of underwear increased the scrotal temperature compared to wearing no underwear at all. However, this is not an invitation to go commando—more research is needed before you can use this as an excuse.

Cycling rules

Erectile dysfuntion can also be a side effect of too much cycling. A study from the University of Southern California School of Medicine found that while cycling for less than three hours a week has a protective effect against impotence, cycling for three hours or more significantly increases the risk.

Having said that, there are many health benefits from leading an active lifestyle, including preventing heart disease. Besides, impotence can also be developed through inactivity. To avoid developing a problem while cycling, periodically lift yourself off the seat when riding long distances. Better still, invest in a wider, padded bicycle seat, which will spread the load. See a doctor if you feel any numbness or pain or have erection problems after cycling.

You're in this together

Deciding to have a baby is one of the biggest decisions you'll ever make. A new baby will bring huge changes to both you and your partner's lives, not to mention your relationship. That's why it's so important to make this decision together.

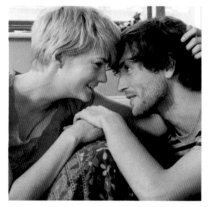

It's important to discuss how the two of you will deal with the transition from being a couple to being a family.

Working mom

If you've decided to return to work after the birth, it's never too soon to start thinking about child care.

"I knew that I'd be in for a bit of a juggling act. My husband couldn't stay home with our baby so we had to plan carefully to get dependable child care. That meant finding a caregiver that we could both trust. We needed to feel 100 percent happy that we would be leaving our baby in the hands of the right person, so we put lots of effort into setting things up. The reward? Having peace of mind once we were both back at work."

Are you both committed?

The decision to have a baby is a milestone in any relationship. It can be exciting but also sometimes scary to imagine yourselves as parents. However, you shouldn't forget that, in addition to being parents, you will still a couple. Pregnancy and having a baby can bring you closer than you've ever been before. But it can also put pressure on your relationship as you move from being a couple to becoming a family.

So before you take this big step, it's definitely worth both of you thinking about some of the problems that may lie ahead. If you're lucky, you may not encounter any of these problems, but talking them through now, before you embark on parenthood, will mean that you are well prepared in case you do.

The highs and lows

The high excitement of a positive pregnancy test can be quickly followed by a low as you struggle through what can be a difficult first trimester. You'll probably feel tired as you never have before, your hormones will send you on an emotional roller coaster, and you may suffer from pregnancy sickness that can strike at any time of the day or night. If it's difficult to deal with the symptoms of early pregnancy, living with someone who's experiencing them can be equally hard. Your partner may be wondering what has happened to the woman he loves. He may also feel that he simply doesn't know what he can do to help. If both of you understand why you feel the way you do it will really help you manage as a couple, so read up now on pregnancy symptoms and talk about ways in which you might relieve them.

Pregnancy can also have a dramatic effect on your sex life, though just what this effect will be can be hard to predict. For some couples pregnancy is a time of heightened sensuality when love making becomes more meaningful and intense. Others find that desire diminishes or disappears altogether. Unfortunately, the two of you won't always feel the same way, so one of you may feel more passionate than ever, while the other only wants to snuggle.

Keep talking

Talking about sex can be difficult but it's much better to discuss these potential problems now than when you are dealing with them for real. You may need to find other ways to express your love and affection during your pregnancy and beyond. If it's difficult to find the energy or desire for sex while you're pregnant, it doesn't get much easier in those early, sleep-deprived weeks with a new baby.

Have you thought about whether one of you will stop working after you've had your baby? If that's the case, will the one at home feel trapped? It's easy to become resentful if you miss the mental stimulation of working. Equally, the working partner may feel resentful that they have to go out to work while the other one gets to stay home with the baby. That doesn't mean life will be harmonious if you both go back to work.

Finding good child care can be difficult and expensive and even the best plans can go wrong. If your child care falls apart, perhaps because either your baby, or her caregiver, is sick, who's going to take a day off work to cover? All these are difficult issues that can put a strain on your relationship. At this stage it can be hard to make plans—after all, you may feel very differently after your baby is born. Exploring your options, and all their pros and cons, will put you in a strong position to make these decisions as a couple when the time comes.

Having a family: the financial cost

A new baby brings many things: love, joy, a sense of family—and a large dent in your budget. If you're going to manage financially once your baby is born, it's wise to start thinking about your finances now.

The word budget might fill you with horror. But the financial freedom it could give you can't be sniffed at. Start by reviewing your spending, organizing it into categories, and deciding what you can give up without changing your lifestyle too much.

Stay on the case

For a budget to work you'll need to sit down once a week or month with pen and paper or a computer program to budget and track your money. The more time you spend on this, the better you'll understand your financial situation. Try to save as much money as possible

before your baby is born. It's sensible advice for everyone to have three months' emergency money up their sleeve and, if you haven't got that amount already, now is a good time to build it up.

Don't forget to tell friends and family you're tightening your belt. This will reinforce it in your own mind and may even encourage them to do the same!

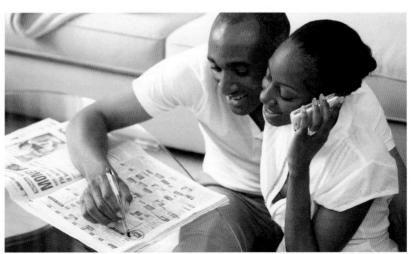

Part of your financial planning can mean shopping around before making a large purchase rather than impulse buying.

Preexisting medical conditions

Try not to be too concerned if you are trying to have a baby and have an ongoing medical condition. Most conditions can now be effectively managed so that you have a safe pregnancy and a healthy baby. Just make sure you see your obstetrician early on to talk through your options.

Will I have a safe pregnancy?

When you have a preexisting medical condition, planning your pregnancy can be a little more complicated. If you're on medication, your dosage may need to be altered or you may need to change medicines before you conceive. You'll need to be carefully monitored once you are pregnant. Don't worry too much: your doctor will be there to give you expert care from the word go.

Underactive thyroid

If your thyroid levels are low you may not ovulate normally, which can make it difficult to get pregnant. Taking the right dose of thyroxine, which is the hormone you lack, can get ovulation back on track and restore your fertility.

A trip to your doctor to get your thyroid levels checked *before* you conceive is very important. If your thyroid levels are low, your doctor will probably suggest that you establish the right level of thyroxine treatment before you start trying to get pregnant.

As long as you manage it well, having an underactive thyroid does not have a significant effect on pregnancy. By having regular blood tests every four to six weeks, you can make sure that your thyroxine is at the correct level.

Asthma

Most drugs used to treat asthma are considered safe in pregnancy (including terbutaline, albuterol, prednisone, and theophylline) and many women continue their usual medication. However, if you are trying to have a baby, it's a good idea to review your treatment with your doctor or asthma specialist, since your particular medication or dosage may need to be adjusted. If you're one of those women

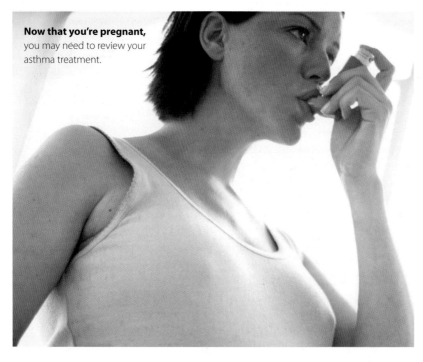

Now that you're pregnant, you may need to review your asthma treatment.

33%

of pregnant women with asthma

experience an improvement in their asthma, according to studies, while for another 33 percent, their asthma worsened.

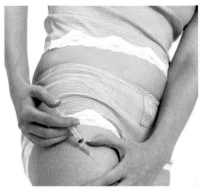

Diabetes is manageable in pregnancy but your doctor may suggest changing from oral medication to insulin injection.

whose asthma improves in pregnancy, you may be able to reduce your dosage, but only under your doctor's supervision.

Diabetes

Whether you have Type 1 or Type 2 diabetes, you are at a higher risk of having a miscarriage or a baby born with a congenital abnormality. You can lower these risks considerably by seeing your doctor or your diabetes specialist and getting your diabetes under control before you start trying to conceive.

Your doctor may recommend that you need to change your diabetes treatment, for example from oral medication to insulin. Babies born to diabetic mothers have a higher-than-average risk of birth defects, so it is especially important to take folic acid during your pregnancy. Your doctor will probably advise you to take about 10 times the usual dose of 400 micrograms (mcg). Diet is key, too. Eating a healthy diet and monitoring your glucose levels carefully and frequently will help maximize your chances of having a healthy pregnancy.

Epilepsy

If you have epilepsy and are thinking of having a baby, you should see your epilepsy specialist or obstetrician first.

Epilepsy and its medication carry some risks in pregnancy, but there are ways to minimize them. Your doctor may advise you to change your medication before trying for a baby. The goal will be to reduce your medication to as few anti-epileptic drugs (AEDs) as possible. Your doctors will probably also advise you to take a higher dose of folic acid than usual because AEDs affect your body's ability to absorb it. Most mothers on anti-epileptic medication give birth to normal, healthy babies.

Irritable bowel syndrome (IBS)

If you are on medication for your IBS, you should see your doctor before you start trying for a baby so that any adjustments to your treatment can be made before you conceive. Certain IBS drugs are not recommended in pregnancy. Loperamide, polycarbophil, and methylcellulose are considered generally safe. You might want to use natural remedies containing psyllium, which is in Metamucil.

Lupus

Lupus erythematosus (LE) takes three forms: systemic LE (SLE); discoid LE; and drug-induced LE. SLE is the most common and, when severe, the symptoms (high fever, chest pain, kidney problems)— and some of the treatments —can seriously complicate pregnancy. Women with uncomplicated, mild lupus often have no problems. If you are pregnant and have lupus, your obstetrician may decide to refer you to a specialist.

Migraines

If you're taking migraine or anti-nausea medication, your doctor may adjust your regimen before you get pregnant. If you use injectable drugs, you will have to stop using them since there's

not enough evidence regarding their safety during pregnancy. Under your doctor's supervision, you should also stop taking preventative drugs. Acetaminophen is the painkiller of choice. Check with your obstetrician before taking ibuprofen if acetaminophen isn't working, but don't take it after 30 weeks of pregnancy.

Getting ready for pregnancy

Staying safe and healthy

Your pregnancy diary

Birth and beyond

Age and fertility

More of us are waiting longer to start a family than ever before. There are many reasons for this, including financial pressures to work and improved contraception. Don't let it go too long, though, since female fertility starts to decline rapidly after the age of 35.

What happens as we get older

Many more of us are having babies later in life these days—you're likely to know at least one thirty-something first-time mom. But putting off starting a family can have its problems. Fertility falls more sharply for women than for men. As you can see from the chart below, women are most fertile between the ages of 20 and 24. As they grow older the likelihood of getting pregnant falls steeply.

According to the British Human Fertilization and Embryology Authority: "At 35 you're half as fertile as when you were 25; at 40 you're half as fertile as when you were 35." This means it can take a great deal longer to get pregnant when you hit your late thirties and you may have problems conceiving at all. Six percent of women who are 35 years old and 23 percent of those who are 38 years old will not have conceived after three years of regular unprotected sex.

"**At 35** you're **half as fertile as** you were **when you were 25**."

Fertility factors that change as we grow older include:

- **Fewer eggs** As you get older you have fewer viable eggs left.
- **Menstrual cycle** As women approach menopause their menstrual cycles can become irregular.
- **Lining of the uterus** The lining (endometrium) may become thinner and less hospitable to a fertilized egg.
- **Mucus secretions** Vaginal secretions can become less fluid and more hostile to sperm.
- **Diseases affecting the reproductive system** Some conditions can damage the reproductive organs as time passes, including endometriosis and chlamydia.
- **Chronic illnesses** Some illnesses can have a negative impact on fertility.
- **Weight problems** Being overweight or obese can make it more difficult to become pregnant.

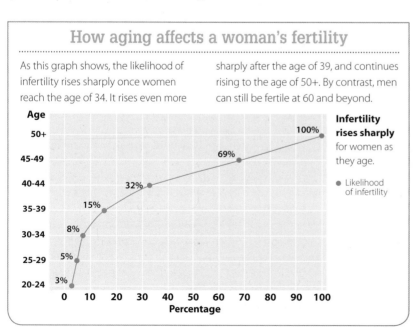

How aging affects a woman's fertility

As this graph shows, the likelihood of infertility rises sharply once women reach the age of 34. It rises even more sharply after the age of 39, and continues rising to the age of 50+. By contrast, men can still be fertile at 60 and beyond.

Age

50+	100%
45-49	69%
40-44	32%
35-39	15%
30-34	8%
25-29	5%
20-24	3%

Percentage: 0 10 20 30 40 50 60 70 80 90 100

Infertility rises sharply for women as they age.

● Likelihood of infertility

Effects of age on male fertility

We now know that men have a biological clock ticking away their reproductive years, too. It's thought that the odds on conceiving within a year of trying decrease by three percent for every year over the age of 24.

As men age, their testes become smaller and softer and the volume, morphology (shape) and motility (ability to move) of their sperm declines. This makes it more difficult for the sperm to fertilize an egg. What's more, there's also growing evidence that the offspring of older fathers run an increased risk of having genetic abnormalities and other long-term health problems.

Improving your fertility

There is plenty you can do to keep your potency in tip-top condition. To begin with, you can put yourself on that diet you've been meaning to start. A man's waist size is directly proportional to his testosterone level (a bigger waist means less testosterone). A waist size of 40 inches or more is also a risk factor for heart disease in men, which slows blood flow, and that includes the blood flow in your penis.

You may also want to go over other aspects of your lifestyle that could impact your fertility—consider scheduling an appointment with your doctor for an exam and to discuss your fertility. Common causes of male infertility include clogged ejaculatory ducts and enlarged veins—called varicoceles—in the scrotum. But do not worry: both conditions are treatable.

Finally, comfort yourself with the fact that, while male fertility may gradually decline with the years, most men are still fertile and functioning at 60 and beyond. Compare that with women's

Lead a healthy lifestyle, keep your weight in check and ask your doctor for a checkup to maximize your potency.

fertility freefall after the age of 35. In fact, men in their 70s and 80s can, and do, father children, but a man this age is more likely to take years rather than months to get his partner pregnant.

ParentsTalk...

"I thought I'd be a lean, mean baby-making machine for as long as I wanted—I've already got two kids from a previous relationship, and now I want a baby with my new wife. She's 15 years younger than me, and I thought that even though I'm in my late forties we wouldn't have any trouble conceiving. We've been trying for over a year, and it turns out it's me, not her, that's the problem."
Mike, 48, dad to teenagers Chris and Samantha

"I'm 44 and my wife's 36. We're trying to start a family but I'm worried that we've waited too long. At first, I thought my wife's age would be a bigger issue than mine. But my age might mean that I'd have trouble getting her pregnant even if she were 25 years old!"
Nick, 44, hoping to be a dad for the first time

"After two failed marriages, I found love again. She's 34 and I'm 55. I've got kids from my previous marriages, but I wanted to start a new family with her. It took several months to conceive, which our doctor said was because I'm an older dad. And the fact I'm an older dad may also have played a part in our baby having Down syndrome— so it turns out it's not just the mother's biological clock we need to listen to."
Graeme, 55, dad to Eliott, 13, Stephen, 10, and year-old Jamie

"My partner and I are both 36 and we've been trying to get pregnant for a year. After various tests our doctor told us that the reason we're having trouble conceiving is a ticking biological clock—and that applies to me as well as her."
Alexander, 36

Getting ready for pregnancy

Staying safe and healthy

Your pregnancy diary

Birth and beyond

The beginnings of life

We all know how babies are made: man meets woman, they make love and nine months later out pops a baby! But do you know what's really happening when sperm meets egg? Read on to discover the fascinating biological facts behind getting pregnant.

How babies are made

Each month, usually during the middle of your menstrual cycle, between one and three eggs start maturing in one of your ovaries. The ripest egg is released and sucked up by the nearest fallopian tube. This is known as ovulation. The egg lives for about 12 to 24 hours after release, so it has to meet up with a sperm soon if a baby is to be conceived.

Men's bodies, meanwhile, are constantly at work producing millions of microscopic sperm. It takes about 64 to 72 days to create a new sperm cell. Since the average sperm lives only a few weeks, and as many as 300 million are set free with each ejaculation, this sperm factory is kept pretty busy.

The quest to find the egg

When you and your partner make love, your bodies build up tension that you hope will end in orgasm. In men, their orgasm propels sperm-rich semen into the vagina and up toward the cervix at roughly 10 miles per hour. A woman's climax also aids conception: research shows that the wavelike contractions associated with "the big O" help pull the sperm farther into the cervix. While you and your partner are enjoying a relaxing post romp cuddle, those millions of sperm have begun their quest to find your egg. The fastest swimmers may find it in as little as 45 minutes. If they do not find an egg in the fallopian tubes, the sperm can wait there for another

Female organs

Male organs

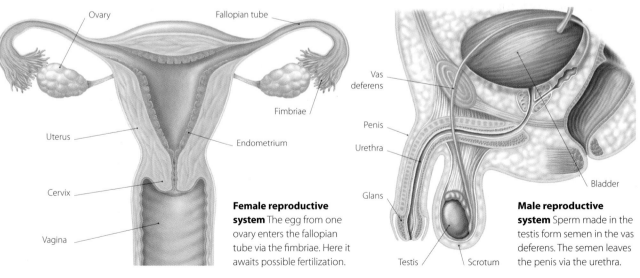

Female reproductive system The egg from one ovary enters the fallopian tube via the fimbriae. Here it awaits possible fertilization.

Ovary
Fallopian tube
Fimbriae
Uterus
Endometrium
Cervix
Vagina

Vas deferens
Penis
Urethra
Glans
Bladder
Testis
Scrotum

Male reproductive system Sperm made in the testis form semen in the vas deferens. The semen leaves the penis via the urethra.

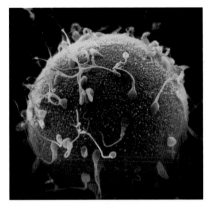

Sperm swarm over the egg in their attempt to penetrate the egg's outer layer.

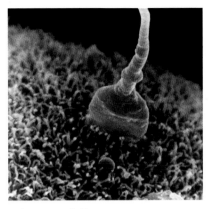

The successful human sperm manages to penetrate and fertilize the egg.

12 to 24 hours, so there is still a chance of conception if you should ovulate within this time.

The mortality rate for sperm is so high that only a few dozen make it to the egg. The rest get trapped or lost, or die. The lucky few who get near the egg then have to work frantically to penetrate its outer shell. When the hardiest makes it through, the outer layer of the egg immediately changes so that no other sperm can get in.

What happens during fertilization

An egg will usually be fertilized within about 24 hours of its release from the ovary. The genetic material from the sperm combines with that in the egg to create a new cell that rapidly starts dividing. But you are not actually pregnant until that bundle of new cells, known as the embryo, travels the rest of the way down the fallopian tube and attaches itself to the wall of your uterus.

Occasionally the embryo implants somewhere other than the uterus, usually in the fallopian tube. This is known as an ectopic pregnancy (see pp.44–5). An ectopic pregnancy cannot grow into a baby, and the embryo has to be surgically removed to prevent

the fallopian tube from rupturing and causing internal bleeding.

The final leg of the trip, from fallopian tube to uterus, takes about three days, but it will be a couple of weeks until you miss a period and suspect that you're going to have a baby.

Once you have missed your period or noticed one of the other signs of pregnancy (see p.36), if you choose to, you can then use a home pregnancy test to find out for sure if you've got a little one on the way. If so, congratulations, and welcome to the start of another incredible journey.

(see pp.44–5) ... (see p.36)

🛋 Laid-back mom

You'll try most lovemaking options—within reason!—for a better chance of conception.

"We're now on number three and we've found that the best position for conceiving is that old favorite—the missionary position, with him on top. It allows for really deep penetration so the sperm ends up right next to the opening of your uterus.

Another position that's good is with him entering you from behind. He can get closer to your cervix so the sperm is right where it needs to be. Many of my girlfriends tell me they find it easier to orgasm in this position, too, and it turns out that the contractions of orgasm help carry the sperm farther into the uterus.

I've also tried lying on my back after sex for at least half an hour with my hips raised on a pillow. I've heard this stops the sperm from having to swim against gravity. I sometimes lie on my back and bicycle my legs in the air too. That always gives my husband a laugh!"

Parents**Talk...**

"I had no idea that sperm could find an egg in just 45 minutes, or wait in the fallopian tubes for up to 24 hours for one to come along. I guess that means I could get pregnant a whole day after having sex if I ovulate during that time!"
Catherine, 23

"I always knew it. My body is amazing. Each little guy can take up to 72 days to make, and every

time I ejaculate, as many as 300 million of them are set free. That's definitely something to boast about!"
Ben, 24

"Now I know that the contractions during orgasm pull the sperm farther into my cervix, I've got a really good reason to make sure my partner understands the importance for me of having an orgasm."
Linda, 28

Getting ready for pregnancy

Staying safe and healthy

Your pregnancy diary

Birth and beyond

Your menstrual cycle

If you're trying to get pregnant, now is a great time to learn a little more about how your body works. Your menstrual cycle indicates when you are fertile, so understanding the changes your body goes through each month can help you to spot any possible problems early on.

Periods and how they happen

Your menstrual cycle is under the control of an array of hormones, and the whole process starts in the brain. The hypothalamus produces gonadotropin-releasing hormone (GnRh), which travels to the pituitary gland and signals it to release follicle-stimulating hormone (FSH). FSH is carried round the body in the bloodstream and stimulates the ovaries to start ripening eggs. Between 15 and 20 egg-containing sacs, called follicles, then start to mature in the ovaries. One follicle (or, occasionally, two or more) grows faster than all the others.

The role of estrogen

FSH also stimulates the ovaries to produce estrogen. This encourages the eggs to mature and starts to thicken the lining of the uterus so that it is ready to support a pregnancy. As estrogen levels rise, levels of FSH fall temporarily and then rise again, accompanied by a huge surge of luteinizing hormone (LH) from the pituitary gland. It is this hormone that triggers ovulation—the moment that the most mature egg in the ovaries bursts out of its sac and away on its journey.

The journey continues

In the ovary, the now-empty follicle collapses and becomes a "corpus luteum." This small yellow mass of cells starts to produce the hormone progesterone. Progesterone acts on the lining of the uterus, which becomes thick and spongy, ready to receive a fertilized egg. As the levels of progesterone rise in your body, your breasts may start to feel stretched and tingly. The pituitary gland stops producing FSH so that no more eggs mature in your ovaries.

Parents**Talk...**

"Premenstrual syndrome (PMS) is something so many women experience—and unfortunately I get it really bad. My mood swings take me through a range of emotions which are provoked by the tiniest things. I burst into tears when I spill my coffee, I forget to do simple things like take the garbage out, I get depressed and tired one minute and then angry and irritable the next. And I become very unreasonable—the other day I saw red when my sister popped the foil on my new can of coffee before I could (it's a little obsession of mine). And all this is just the emotional side of PMS—I also get sore boobs, headaches, stomach ache, and sometimes nausea, too."
Hannah, 36, mom to William and Tess

"When it's the 'time of the month' I just want to curl up into a ball and hug a hot water bottle for a few days. My cramps are probably fairly normal for most women—not so mild they're barely there or so painful I can't move. I just have a continuous back and stomach ache which makes me feel sluggish and uncomfortable."
Hilary, 37, mom to Joel and Natasha

"I'm now back on the pill (though a different pill than before) so I'm hoping my period cramps will calm down now or stop entirely. It was so nice not having any periods while I was pregnant."
Vicky, 27, mom to month-old Nathan

What happens if fertilization doesn't occur

Early in your menstrual cycle, FSH (see opposite) is released by the pituitary gland and travels in the bloodstream. It stimulates the ovaries so they start to ripen eggs. Ovulation happens when one (occasionally two) of the 15 to 20 egg-containing sacs, or follicles, ruptures and releases its egg. This happens about halfway through the menstrual cycle. The empty follicle then turns into a corpus luteum.

The endometrium

Meanwhile, influenced by estrogen and progesterone, the lining of the uterus (endometrium) gets thicker and more spongy, ready to receive a fertilized egg. If the egg isn't fertilized, it disintegrates and the corpus luteum shrinks. The thickened endometrium is shed next time you have a period.

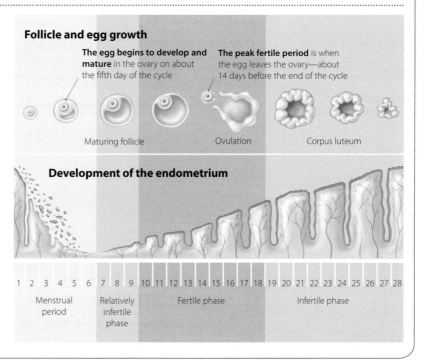

Follicle and egg growth

The egg begins to develop and mature in the ovary on about the fifth day of the cycle

The peak fertile period is when the egg leaves the ovary—about 14 days before the end of the cycle

Maturing follicle | Ovulation | Corpus luteum

Development of the endometrium

1 2 3 4 5 6 7 8 9 10 11 12 13 14 15 16 17 18 19 20 21 22 23 24 25 26 27 28

Menstrual period | Relatively infertile phase | Fertile phase | Infertile phase

---

If fertilization occurs, the egg continues to travel to the uterus, where it beds down in the lining. Your progesterone levels will stay high and you may start to feel the very early signs of pregnancy.

If fertilization doesn't occur, or the egg doesn't successfully implant, it starts to disintegrate and the corpus luteum shrinks. Your estrogen and progesterone levels drop and the lining of your uterus starts to produce prostaglandins (the hormones that can cause cramps). These cause changes in the blood supply to your uterus, breaking up the lining, and stimulating the uterus to contract. The lining of

your uterus is shed along with the unfertilized egg, and your menstrual cycle starts again.

Your menstrual cycle's length

An average menstrual cycle lasts 28 days—that's counting from the first day of one period to the day before the next. Some women have much shorter cycles, possibly lasting only 23 days, and some have much longer ones, lasting up to 35 days. Cycles that are shorter or longer than this are probably not normal, and you should see your doctor. You should also see your doctor if you bleed between periods or after sex.

"The **fertilized egg** beds down in the **lining of the uterus**."

Signs of a normal cycle

If your menstrual cycle tallies with these three signs, chances are that everything's normal.

Signs of a normal menstrual cycle include:

● A cycle that lasts 23 to 35 days. So, for example, a woman with a 28-day cycle starts a period every four weeks while a woman with a 23-day cycle starts hers every three weeks or so. The length of the cycle includes the days of the period.

● Regular periods—if yours are very irregular you may be not be ovulating at all or infrequently.

● No spotting between periods—bleeding between periods should always be reported to your doctor.

Getting ready for pregnancy

Staying safe and healthy

Your pregnancy diary

Birth and beyond

Ovulation calendars

Ovulation is the magical moment that occurs each month when one of your ovaries releases an egg ready for fertilization. Knowing the signs of ovulation can help you pinpoint those days when you're most likely to conceive and give you a better understanding of your fertility.

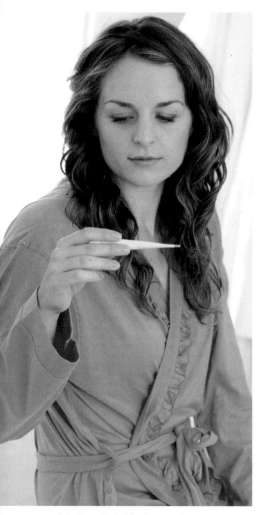

Using a basal body temperature thermometer each morning helps predict when you ovulate. You're most fertile a few days before your temperature rises.

What is ovulation?

Ovulation is when one, or occasionally more, eggs are released from one of your ovaries, and it's the most fertile time of your menstrual cycle. It usually takes place 12 to 16 days before the start of your next period. So, for a woman with a 28-day menstrual cycle, ovulation takes place sometime around day 13 to 15.

Possible signs that ovulation is imminent include:

● **Changes in cervical mucus** As your cycle progresses, rising estrogen levels mean your cervical mucus increases in volume and changes texture. You are your most fertile when the mucus becomes clear, slippery and stretchy, somewhat like raw egg white. The position and feel of your cervix also changes around this time, from hard, low, closed, and dry, to soft, high, open and wet.

● **Lower abdominal pain** About one fifth of women actually feel it when they ovulate. The sensation can range from mild achiness to twinges of pain, and may last anywhere from a few minutes to a few hours.

Other possible signs include:

● **Feeling sexy and flirty** Having an increased libido, being in a better mood, and feeling more social may all be signs that you're at your most fertile.

● **Looking more attractive** Studies have been carried out showing that both how attractive you feel and how attractive you look to others increases when you near ovulation. You may choose clothes that flatter you and take more care accessorizing and grooming.

● **Smelling good** It's been found that women smell more attractive to men just before ovulation. All these signs must be nature's way of helping ensure you mate at the right time!

Following ovulation, your temperature can increase by 0.5 to 1.6 degrees. You won't feel the shift but you may be able to detect it by using a basal body temperature (BBT) thermometer. You can buy one at your pharmacy.

You're most fertile in the two to three days before your temperature rises. That's why some experts recommend you chart your temperature (taken each morning) for a few months to pinpoint your likely ovulation date. Then you can plan to have sex during the two to three days before your temperature normally rises. However, most fertility experts recommend regular sex throughout your cycle in order to conceive. Regular tends to be defined as at least twice a week.

Ovulation predictor kits

Experts recommend regular sex throughout your cycle as the best way to maximize your chances of conception. Having said that, for various reasons, some couples prefer to identify when they're most likely to conceive and ovulation predictor kits, or OPKs, can help. They give you a quick result and are easy to use. They're available at most pharmacies and supermarkets without a prescription, and you can also buy them online.

There are two sorts of OPKs:

● A urine-based OPK detects the increase, or surge, of the luteinizing hormone (LH) that occurs approximately one to two days before ovulation.

at home. Unfortunately, they are not foolproof. They can measure LH, but since LH can surge with or without the release of an egg, they can't indicate whether you have definitely ovulated after a positive response.

● Saliva-based OPKs test for rising estrogen levels as you near ovulation, not the hormone that triggers it. A saliva-based OPK is basically a pocket-sized microscope that shows if "salivary ferning" has occurred when your saliva dries on a glass slide. Ferning is more likely to occur in the few days leading up to ovulation. Salivary ferning OPKs can be more economical than urine-based ones, but some experts say they are not as accurate and that ferning

"Ovulation **predictor kits,** or OPKs, give you a **quick result** and are **easy to use**."

Depending on the type of urine-based OPK, you'll either collect your urine in a cup or hold a stick in your urine stream. Colored bands will appear on the test card or stick to indicate whether or not the LH surge is occurring. Urine-based OPKs generally provide five to nine days' worth of tests. They are generally seen as the best method of ovulation prediction available for women to use

15-20 eggs will mature each month inside a woman's ovaries but only the ripest egg will be released into the fallopian tube ready for fertilization.

can sometimes be seen at other times of the menstrual cycle. Also, if your vision is poor these kits may not be the best method for you.

With either type of OPK, it helps to figure out when your fertile period is likely to start. It's usually the length of your usual cycle minus 17 days. So, if you have a 28-day cycle, start testing on day 11 and continue for six days.

Acetaminophen and other common drugs don't affect the tests, but contact your doctor if you're taking hormonal medication. Drugs containing human chorionic gonadotropin (hCG; see p.74) or LH (see p.28) can affect the results, and the fertility drug clomiphene can affect the salivary ferning test.

Organized mom

If you are trying to get pregnant, it might want to keep track of when you are ovulating.

"When I was trying to get pregnant, I really appreciated the fact that there were things I could buy that would help me to keep track of when I was ovulating and most fertile.

The first thing I invested in was an ovulation predictor kit—they look and work the same way as a home pregnancy test but can predict ovulation 24 to 36 hours in advance. I also monitored my basal body temperature—when you've ovulated, your temperature can increase very slightly, which you'd never be able to feel, but I could check it using a special basal body temperature thermometer. My pharmacist ordered one for me.

I even bought a salivary ferning kit—there's something in your saliva that helps you predict when you're going to ovulate. I found this quite fascinating, actually—apparently when you're ovulating, you produce more salt, which causes your saliva to crystallize into frostlike ferns when dried and viewed on a slide.

I know that these things aren't for everyone. Some couples might get too stressed using them, and may feel pressured to have sex only when the gadgets tell them to, but they suited us."

A urine-based ovulation predictor kit detects the very slight increase in LH (see p.28) that occurs just before you ovulate.

Getting ready for pregnancy

Staying safe and healthy

Your pregnancy diary

Birth and beyond

Boy or girl?

For most couples, not knowing whether you're having a boy or girl is one of the most exciting parts of having a baby. Here's how your baby's sex is determined and, just for fun, some traditional ways to bump up your chances of having either a boy or a girl.

X and Y chromosomes

Is it a boy or girl? It's the question we all want to know the answer to. The sex of your baby is actually determined at the moment of conception.

The sex chromosomes are called X and Y. Eggs always contain an X chromosome. If the sperm that fertilizes the egg contains an X chromosome as well, then the resulting XX combination equals a girl. If the sperm contains a Y chromosome, the resulting XY combination equals a boy.

You may have heard the old wives' tales: if you carry in front it's a boy, if you crave sweet foods it's a girl. You may have tried sex predictor methods that involved odd and even days and the numbers of the year. They are fun but none have any facts to back them up.

Scientific studies

Some scientific studies have shown, however, that certain circumstances may influence the sex of the baby.

● **How old are you and your partner?** There is some evidence that the older you are when you have your first baby, the more likely you are to have a girl. Some experts believe that sex of the baby is partly controlled by the level of the hormone gonadotropin, and this declines with age. Likewise, it seems that the older a dad is, the less likely the male sperm are to fertilize the egg and the female sperm win the race. The latest evidence is that older men produce fewer male sperm.

● **Were you newlyweds when you conceived?** If so, you may be more likely to have a boy. The theory is the longer you have been married, the less sex you have, thus the later in the cycle conception is likely to occur and the more likely you are to have a girl. But it could simply be a matter of age.

● **Do you eat a high-calorie diet including breakfast?** If you do, you are more likely to have a boy. In a study of 740 British women, 56 percent of those with the highest caloric intake had boys. In women with the lowest caloric intake, the proportion who had boys dropped to 45 percent. It has been suggested that our bodies only invest in boys (who are more fragile and statistically less likely to survive) when food is abundant. In times of famine, we "play safe" with more robust girls. However, these studies are small-scale and show only minor changes in the likelihood of having a boy or girl.

X and Y chromosomes

Women have two X chromosomes (XX) and men have one X and one Y chromosome (XY). A man can pass on an X or a Y chromosome. The woman's egg always contains an X chromosome.

Dad decides

If the sperm that fertilizes your egg contains an X chromosome, that gives the egg two X chromosomes and means your baby is a girl. If the sperm contains a Y chromosome, the egg will have an X and a Y—and it's a boy!

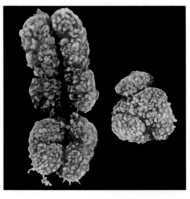

X and Y On the left is the larger X chromosome, with the Y on the right.

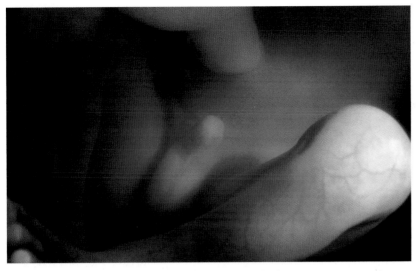

The legs and genitals of this 22-week old male fetus are clearly visible, as is the umbilical cord at the center top of the scan.

> ### Laid-back mom
>
> *For most parents-to-be, knowing the sex of their unborn baby is less important than its health.*
>
> "I have two fabulous sons and, although everyone says 'Ooh, might be a girl this time', I can honestly say I would be as delighted with another son as with a daughter. Why wouldn't I be? I love both my sons to bits and they love their mom. The relationship you have with your children is what you make of it, whether it's a boy or a girl. As long the baby's healthy, that's all that matters. My partner wants another boy, my mom thinks it's going to be a girl this time. I don't care as long as it's healthy. I will honestly be happy with what ever I get."

Science and sex selection

Choosing your child's sex is technically possible now, thanks to the many advances there have been in fertility treatments in recent years. But the options available today are not always effective, affordable, or available, and some are unregulated.

Preimplantation genetic diagnosis (PGD)

This is an in vitro fertilization technique in which embryos are created outside the uterus and can then be tested for genetic disorders and gender.

Effectiveness Almost 100 percent effective.

Cost IVF cycles cost an average of $12,400, not including the costs of the consultations, tests, and drugs. PGD adds about $3,000 per treatment cycle.

Availability Most clinics that provide PGD only allow it for a medical reason, such as a family history of genetic diseases.

Ericsson method

This sperm-sorting technique was developed by Dr. Ronald Ericsson in the mid-1970s. Sperm of the desired gender are inserted into your uterus via artificial insemination (AI).

Effectiveness Claimed to be 78 to 85 percent effective for choosing boys and 73 to 75 percent effective for girls.

Cost The cost is approximately $600 per insemination.

Availability This is available to anyone who wants it at clinics in California, Michigan, Texas, Connecticut, Montana, Washington, Florida, New Mexico, Maine, and New York.

Shettles method

This advocates timed intercourse on specific days of your cycle.

Effectiveness It is claimed that the technique is 75 percent effective.

Cost None.

Availability Anyone can try it.

Whelan method

This also advocates timed intercourse on specific days of your cycle.

Effectiveness Elizabeth Whelan claims her technique is 68 percent effective for boys and 56 percent effective for girls, but many experts dispute this.

Cost None.

Availability Anyone can try it.

Sex-selection kits

These are based on the Shettles theory. Separate girl and boy kits include a thermometer, ovulation predictor test sticks, vitamins, herbal extracts, and douches.

Effectiveness Kit makers claim a 96 percent success rate, but the American Society for Reproductive Medicine disputes this.

Cost $199 for a 30-day kit.

Availability These kits are available in the United States through the GenSelect company.

Conception

You probably won't know you have conceived yet, but inside your body there's lots of frantic activity going on. Within days of conceiving, the embryo that will grow to become your baby implants in the lining of your uterus where it rapidly starts to grow and develop.

What happens during the first days?

As soon as your egg is fertilized, it goes into action. While it's being wafted gently down your fallopian tube toward your uterus, it begins dividing into a microscopic ball of cells. By the time it reaches the uterus, about three to four days after conception, it has already divided into about 16 cells and looks a bit like a miniscule blackberry.

Around day four, this bundle of cells starts to hollow out in the middle and to develop an inner and an outer layer. At this stage, doctors call this hollow sphere a blastocyst. The inner layer expands and presses against the tough outer layer until it gives way and breaks up. This happens around the sixth day after fertilization. Once the cells of the inner layer are exposed, they secrete an enzyme that erodes part of the lining of the uterus, allowing it to implant. When the blastocyst implants, it is then known as an embryo.

The lining of the uterus

By now the pregnancy hormone progesterone will have stimulated the growth of lots of new blood vessels in the lining of the uterus, ready to nourish the embryo. The outer layer of the embryo carries on breaking down cells in the lining of the uterus, allowing it to burrow further in. It also stimulates new blood vessels to grow, creating the beginnings of the placenta. Ectopic pregnancies (see pp.44–5), where the embryo implants somewhere other than the uterus (this is usually in the fallopian tube) normally occur at around this time.

Around 13 days after fertilization has taken place, a yolk sac is visible attached to the embryo. This will act as a rudimentary circulation system for the embryo until its own circulatory system is up and running. Different types of cells

---

The first week

You may not even know you're pregnant, but amazing things are happening in that first week.

Step by step

- Fertilization begins when a sperm penetrates the egg.
- Fertilization takes about 24 hours.
- The fertilized egg (or zygote) begins to divide into 16 cells.
- It leaves the fallopian tube and enters the uterus.
- Three to four days after fertilization, it starts to burrow into the blood-rich lining of your uterus.
- At around day eight, the placenta starts to grow.

Parents**Talk...**

"I had my suspicions I was pregnant before I did a test, even though we'd only been trying for a few weeks. It sounds like a real cliché, but the second I saw the line on the test, I just knew that my life was never going to be the same again. And it was an enormous change, but one I've never regretted."
Sinead, 27, mom to two-month-old Lily

"We'd only been trying for two months when I got my big fat positive. I was actually shaking when I saw the blue line. Sam was away on business so I had to keep it a secret for four days. I didn't want to let him know by phone so I went to meet him at the airport. I sat him down in a coffee shop to tell him."
Jen, 26, mom to Charlie

are starting to develop in the embryo and these will go on to form the various parts of your baby's body. A stalk is also forming between the developing placenta and the embryo. This will later become part of the umbilical cord.

Next, a thin line of cells, known as the "primitive streak," start to organize themselves down the center of the embryo. From now on this primitive streak will develop symmetrically on either side of this central line. By the time you would normally be expecting your period, the embryo is just 0.4 millimeters (mm) in length—barely visible to the human eye. Its head end is wider than the tail end and its cells are now organized into three layers that will later develop into baby's organs and tissues. The neural tube—from which the brain, backbone, and spinal cord and nerves will sprout—develops in the top layer. The heart and the circulatory system begin to appear in the middle layer. The third layer starts to create the lungs, intestines, and beginnings of the urinary system. Strange as it may seem, your doctor will calculate your baby's gestational age (and your due date) from the first day of your last period. This is because it's often difficult to know exactly when your egg was fertilized. So, although it's only about two weeks since you conceived, you are now considered to be four weeks pregnant. In the following days, the embryo's heart, no bigger than a poppy seed, will begin to beat and pump blood.

Gradually the beat will become stronger and more regular. Major organs, will begin to grow, the neural tube that connects the brain and spinal cord will close, upper and lower limb buds will begin to sprout, and your baby's facial features will start to form.

Conception and implantation

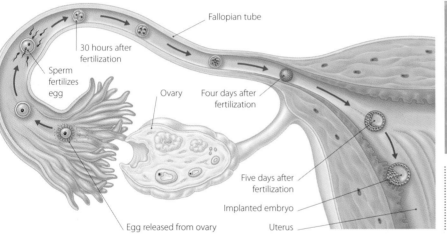

Fallopian tube

30 hours after fertilization

Sperm fertilizes egg

Ovary

Four days after fertilization

Five days after fertilization

Implanted embryo

Egg released from ovary

Uterus

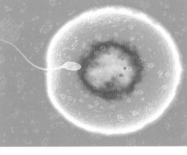

Sperm fertilizing egg This egg has left the ovary and entered the fallopian tube where it is being fertilized. The egg starts dividing (see below) and travels to the uterus where it implants itself in the uterine wall.

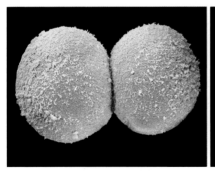

About 30 hours after fertilization, this egg is at the two-cell stage and has not yet implanted in the uterus.

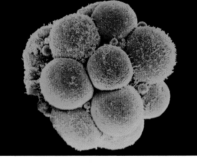

Four days after fertilization, the 16-cell blastocyst is dividing rapidly. It now looks a bit like a blackberry.

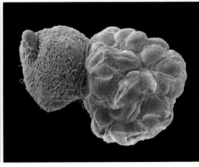

Five or six days after fertilization, the dividing cells break out of the tough outer shell that surrounds the fertilized egg.

Am I pregnant?

If you're extremely tuned in to your body's rhythms, you may suspect that you're pregnant soon after conception. But most women won't experience any early pregnancy symptoms until the fertilized egg attaches itself to the wall of the uterus, several days afterward.

Signs you may be pregnant

For most women, the first sign of pregnancy is a missed period. But there are other telltale signs.

It's a cliché, but food cravings really can be a sign of pregnancy. Don't rely on them, but if you've got other signs of pregnancy, start counting the days from your last period.

You may notice changes in your breasts. They can become tender to the touch, similar to the way they feel before your period, only more so. The skin around your nipples may also get darker.

If you're lucky, nausea and vomiting won't hit you until a few weeks after conception. But as early as a couple of days following conception, you may begin feeling nauseated. And not just in the morning, either—pregnancy-related nausea can be a problem morning, noon, or night. You may also notice that your sense of taste changes.

Fatigue is another sign of early pregnancy. High levels of the hormone progesterone can make you feel as if you ran a marathon when all you've done is worked a day at the office. And you may find that you're running to the bathroom a lot—this is caused by rising levels of the pregnancy hormone hCG (see p.74).

About six to eight days after ovulation, you may have implantation bleeding—some pinkish, brownish discharge from your vagina—and possibly some cramping. This is caused by the egg burrowing into the lining of the uterus. You might also have spotting around the time you expect your period.

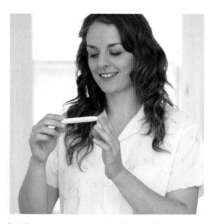

A home pregnancy test is usually accurate once you have missed a period.

All you need now is a positive pregnancy test (see opposite). If you've waited until at least the first day of a missed period and a blue line appears in the test window, congratulations—you're in the family way!

ParentsTalk...

"The first sign I had that I was pregnant was the nausea and sickness, and it struck any time, day or night. I was constantly exhausted too—I could have happily fallen asleep at my desk at work during the first few weeks."
Vidja, 28, first-time mom

"My breasts were so sore—it was the first thing I noticed. They were tender to the touch, and much bigger too."
Helena, 23, mom to year-old Alex

"Before I took my test, I felt really bloated and needed to go to the bathroom a lot. I had cramping too,

and I wasn't sure if it was period pains or early pregnancy symptoms."
Anne, 28, mom to six-month-old twins

"My first symptoms were light spotting and cramping. Then, when my period didn't arrive, I took a test."
Jo, 31, mom to seven-month-old Barney

Home pregnancy tests

A standard home pregnancy test detects the hormone hCG in your urine. This hormone is first secreted about six days after fertilization, when the egg implants in the uterus. Levels of hCG build up rapidly, but if you have a negative result when you first test, it's possible that your hCG levels are still too low to be detected. You may want to wait a few days and then repeat the pregnancy test again.

Some pregnancy tests are more sensitive than others and so are usually more expensive. Concentrations of hCG are given in milliInternational Units (mIU). A test with a sensitivity of 20 IU/L is more sensitive than one that has a sensitivity of 50 IU/L.

You can test at any time of day, and as early as the first day of your missed period with most tests. Avoid drinking too much just before testing since this could dilute the hCG in your urine. Over-the-counter medicines, such as acetaminophen, shouldn't affect the result: fertility drugs containing hCG may.

Directions vary with different brands, so read them carefully. Some ask you to urinate in a cup and then place a sample into a testing well using a dropper. Or you may need to urinate directly onto a stick. Some change the urine sample's color, others show pink or blue lines, reveal a red plus or minus sign, or indicate "pregnant" or "not pregnant" in a window.

If you follow the directions to the letter, home pregnancy tests are 97 percent accurate. But mistakes do happen, which is why some kits come with two tests. If the test comes back negative but you still suspect you're pregnant, wait a few days, read the directions carefully, and try again. False positives (when the test says you're pregnant but you're not) are rare.

Your expected date of delivery (EDD)

Find the first day of your last period on the shaded bar. Beneath it you'll see your expected date of delivery or EDD—also called your due date. Your EDD is arrived at by counting on nine calendar months and seven days (40 weeks) from the first day of your last normal period. If your menstrual cycle is shorter or longer than 28 days, your expected date of delivery may be earlier or later. An expected date of delivery based on a dating scan (see p.136) is more accurate than one that is based on your last period.

January	1	2	3	4	5	6	7	8	9	10	11	12	13	14	15	16	17	18	19	20	21	22	23	24	25	26	27	28	29	30	31
Oct/Nov	8	9	10	11	12	13	14	15	16	17	18	19	20	21	22	23	24	25	26	27	28	29	30	31	1	2	3	4	5	6	7
February	1	2	3	4	5	6	7	8	9	10	11	12	13	14	15	16	17	18	19	20	21	22	23	24	25	26	27	28			
Nov/Dec	8	9	10	11	12	13	14	15	16	17	18	19	20	21	22	23	24	25	26	27	28	29	30	1	2	3	4	5			
March	1	2	3	4	5	6	7	8	9	10	11	12	13	14	15	16	17	18	19	20	21	22	23	24	25	26	27	28	29	30	31
Dec/Jan	6	7	8	9	10	11	12	13	14	15	16	17	18	19	20	21	22	23	24	25	26	27	28	29	30	31	1	2	3	4	5
April	1	2	3	4	5	6	7	8	9	10	11	12	13	14	15	16	17	18	19	20	21	22	23	24	25	26	27	28	29	30	
Jan/Feb	6	7	8	9	10	11	12	13	14	15	16	17	18	19	20	21	22	23	24	25	26	27	28	29	30	31	1	2	3	4	
May	1	2	3	4	5	6	7	8	9	10	11	12	13	14	15	16	17	18	19	20	21	22	23	24	25	26	27	28	29	30	31
Feb/Mar	5	6	7	8	9	10	11	12	13	14	15	16	17	18	19	20	21	22	23	24	25	26	27	28	1	2	3	4	5	6	7
June	1	2	3	4	5	6	7	8	9	10	11	12	13	14	15	16	17	18	19	20	21	22	23	24	25	26	27	28	29	30	
Mar/Apr	8	9	10	11	12	13	14	15	16	17	18	19	20	21	22	23	24	25	26	27	28	29	30	31	1	2	3	4	5	6	
July	1	2	3	4	5	6	7	8	9	10	11	12	13	14	15	16	17	18	19	20	21	22	23	24	25	26	27	28	29	30	31
Apr/May	7	8	9	10	11	12	13	14	15	16	17	18	19	20	21	22	23	24	25	26	27	28	29	30	1	2	3	4	5	6	7
August	1	2	3	4	5	6	7	8	9	10	11	12	13	14	15	16	17	18	19	20	21	22	23	24	25	26	27	28	29	30	31
May/June	8	9	10	11	12	13	14	15	16	17	18	19	20	21	22	23	24	25	26	27	28	29	30	31	1	2	3	4	5	6	7
September	1	2	3	4	5	6	7	8	9	10	11	12	13	14	15	16	17	18	19	20	21	22	23	24	25	26	27	28	29	30	
June/July	8	9	10	11	12	13	14	15	16	17	18	19	20	21	22	23	24	25	26	27	28	29	30	1	2	3	4	5	6	7	
October	1	2	3	4	5	6	7	8	9	10	11	12	13	14	15	16	17	18	19	20	21	22	23	24	25	26	27	28	29	30	31
July/Aug	8	9	10	11	12	13	14	15	16	17	18	19	20	21	22	23	24	25	26	27	28	29	30	31	1	2	3	4	5	6	7
November	1	2	3	4	5	6	7	8	9	10	11	12	13	14	15	16	17	18	19	20	21	22	23	24	25	26	27	28	29	30	
Aug/Sept	8	9	10	11	12	13	14	15	16	17	18	19	20	21	22	23	24	25	26	27	28	29	30	31	1	2	3	4	5	6	
December	1	2	3	4	5	6	7	8	9	10	11	12	13	14	15	16	17	18	19	20	21	22	23	24	25	26	27	28	29	30	31
Sept/Oct	7	8	9	10	11	12	13	14	15	16	17	18	19	20	21	22	23	24	25	26	27	28	29	30	1	2	3	4	5	6	7

Pregnancy following IVF

Discovering you have a baby on the way is a hugely emotional moment for any couple. But for couples who have been through IVF, joy at finally being pregnant can be mixed with anxiety about the next nine months. For now, just look after yourself and take each day as it comes.

ParentsTalk...

"I know that everything is okay with my pregnancy now but I'm so overly protective. I'm worried that being on my feet all day could hurt my baby. I keep telling myself that it's our one and only baby so it's probably normal to be this crazy."
Emma, 28, pregnant after IVF

"I have to go back in at 32 weeks to discuss my birth plan. I know I want a natural active birth since I'd like something in this pregnancy to be natural."
Leah, 31, pregnant after IVF

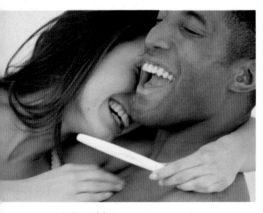

A positive pregnancy test is even more welcome if you've been trying to get pregnant for a while, but it can cause concern, too.

Pregnant at last

A positive pregnancy test after IVF can seem like a miracle. But for many couples, the joy of conceiving can be quickly replaced with more worry. Am I really pregnant? Is my baby OK? You'll probably feel anxious about every twinge or change in symptoms. For you and your partner, nine months will probably feel like a very long time.

Reassurance

The first scan will help to reassure you. You should have an ultrasound between six and 11 weeks to confirm that the embryo has implanted. From seven weeks onward a heartbeat will be visible but it may be detected as early as six weeks. As tiny as your embryo is, seeing it for the first time on a sonogram with its heart beating, will probably do more than anything to put your mind at rest.

At your first appointment, your doctor will explain to you when you will have your prenatal appointments. For some women who have had IVF, care will be just the same as if they had conceived naturally, though many doctors treat all IVF assisted conceptions as high risk. It can feel very strange to have quite long periods between appointments after the busy schedule you had during your IVF cycle.

Remember, you can always call your doctor between appointments if you have any concerns or questions at all.

If you had any complications in a previous pregnancy, or if you have any preexisting health problems (see pp.22–3), you will be monitored more closely during your pregnancy, and if your IVF has resulted in a twins pregnancy, you will also see your doctor more frequently.

Taking care of yourself is important in any pregnancy and you may feel that you want to be particularly careful. Make sure you follow a healthy diet with plenty of fresh fruit and vegetables. Experts are divided about safe levels of caffeine and alcohol in pregnancy, so you may feel you want to err on the side of caution and cut them out entirely.

Most importantly, try to relax and make the most of your pregnancy. You've probably battled hard to get here.

Fact: Nearly 500,000 babies conceived through IVF were born in the US between 1985 and 2006, according to the American Society for Reproductive Medicine. The average cost of a cycle is $12,400.

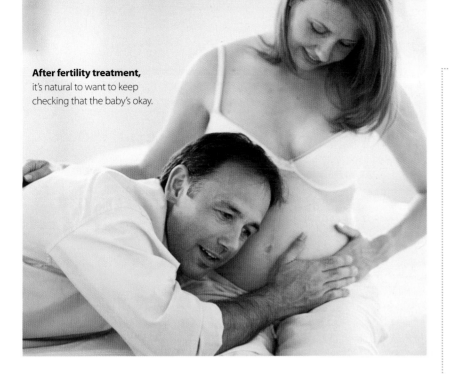

After fertility treatment, it's natural to want to keep checking that the baby's okay.

Dad's **Diary**

Dads get anxious too

"We tried to get pregnant for five years before we did with our third round of IVF. The relief when we got our positive test results was immense. You can't begin to imagine. Men's feelings are often forgotten when it comes to fertility treatment, which is understandable when I think about some of the invasive treatments that Libby had to go through—not to mention the hormonal and emotional effects of it. I often felt guilty that I didn't have to endure much more than the occasional blood test and sperm sample. It was difficult for us both. The thought that I might never be a parent was as upsetting for me as it was for Libby."

The risks

One of the first things you will probably worry about when you find out that you are pregnant following IVF is the risk of miscarriage. Miscarriage is no more common after IVF than after a natural conception, but it's also no lower. Sadly, about 15 percent of known pregnancies end in miscarriage, usually in the first 13 weeks of pregnancy (see pp.42–3).

Multiple pregnancy

If you've had more than one embryo placed in your uterus, you'll have a higher than usual chance of having twins or triplets. Around one in four couples will have twins after successful IVF, compared with approximately one in 80 of the general population. Though many couples consider this a blessing, multiple pregnancies do increase your risk of miscarriage and other complications such as premature labor, preeclampsia, and pregnancy-induced high blood pressure.

IVF also puts you at increased risk of having an ectopic pregnancy, where an embryo implants in your fallopian tube or your abdominal cavity. This is more likely to happen if you've had problems affecting your fallopian tubes previously. Your first ultrasound will confirm that your embryo has implanted in your uterus and not in your fallopian tube. If you haven't yet had an ultrasound and you have any vaginal bleeding or stomach pain, call your doctor.

Unfortunately, the fertility drugs used to stimulate egg production themselves can have severe side effects. You will need to be closely monitored while you are taking them to ensure you do not develop ovarian hyperstimulation syndrome (OHSS). This is potentially a dangerous condition, which can go on for weeks into early pregnancy. It can mean that you will have to stay in the hospital while your overly stimulated ovaries settle down.

 Active mom

Waiting those first few weeks can be difficult after IVF, especially if you're used to a carefree life.

"We've waited so long for this pregnancy; I really want our beanie to stick. I've been having a few cramps and some vaginal discharge, but it's white—no blood or anything so that makes me feel better. I'm just terrified that the clear stuff will change and I'll see blood. The doctor says there's nothing to worry about but I can't help it. I've tried to get a scan but my doctor says there's no point until six weeks. I even tried to go at another facility but they said the same thing. What's reassuring me is that I've got swollen and sore boobs, some nausea, and headaches. I know those are all good signs, but I won't feel better until I go for that six-week scan and see a heart beating on the screen."

Is it twins (or more)?

If you're expecting twins, you're certain to have lots of questions and probably some worries, too. We'll answer your concerns on everything about a multiple pregnancy, from conception and prenatal care, to how your pregnancy will differ from a singleton pregnancy.

How twin/multiple births occur

About one in 32 births are twin births these days. Nonidentical, or fraternal, twins start off from two different eggs that are fertilized by two different sperm. Identical twins are more rare. They start off as one fertilized egg, which then splits into two.

Influencing factors

There are various factors that can increase your chances of having a multiple birth. Your age is important. If you're in your 30s or older you have a greater chance of having twins or more. As you age, you naturally produce more ovulation-stimulating hormones, which may trigger your ovaries to release several eggs at once instead of just one.

Heredity is another important factor. Nonidentical twins tend to run in families, usually—but not always—on the mother's side. If twins run in your mother's family, you're more likely to have a set yourself. They also occur more often in African ethnic groups.

Identical twins, which are the result of a single fertilized egg splitting, don't tend to run in families.

Size matters, too. A US study revealed that there was a significant increase in nonidentical twin births to mothers who had a BMI of 30 or above, or to those who were in the top 25th percentile for height.

Nowadays, most women who give birth to multiples have undergone some type of fertility treatment, although one treatment— IUI (intrauterine

---

How twins are conceived

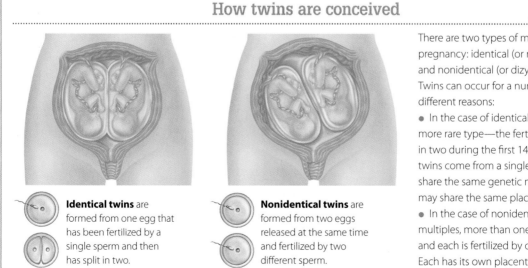

Identical twins are formed from one egg that has been fertilized by a single sperm and then has split in two.

Nonidentical twins are formed from two eggs released at the same time and fertilized by two different sperm.

There are two types of multiple pregnancy: identical (or monozygotic) and nonidentical (or dizygotic). Twins can occur for a number of different reasons:

● In the case of identical twins—the more rare type—the fertilized egg splits in two during the first 14 days. Since the twins come from a single egg, they each share the same genetic make up and may share the same placenta.

● In the case of nonidentical twins or multiples, more than one egg is released and each is fertilized by different sperm. Each has its own placenta.

insemination), where sperm are injected into a woman's uterus—doesn't increase the risk of a multiple pregnancy unless you're also taking fertility drugs.

If you're taking a fertility drug, prepare for the possibility of twins. The drugs stimulate your ovaries, increasing the odds that you'll release several eggs at the same time. Up to 13 percent of women taking the fertility drug clomiphene have a multiple pregnancy.

Newer fertility techniques, such as ICSI (intracytoplasmic sperm injection)

and GIFT (gamete intrafallopian transfer), also increase the chances of a multiple pregnancy. Like IVF, these can involve more than one embryo being put into a woman's uterus or fallopian tubes.

The rate of identical twins also increases after IVF for reasons that we don't yet fully understand, but the vast majority of IVF twins are nonidentical.

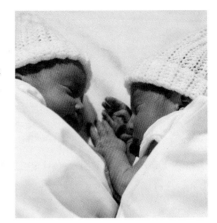

Twins may provide extra work and you'll need more rest before they arrive, but they'll also give you extra joy and excitement.

What's different about a multiple pregnancy

Early on in pregnancy you may suspect you are having twins if you have gained a lot of weight, your uterus is big for your due date or you are suffering a lot from nausea and vomiting. As your babies grow, you will probably become tired easily and need extra rest. And you will carry more weight than women who are pregnant with one baby, so you might get annoyed with feeling so big.

Digestive problems

Nausea and vomiting can be more of a problem if you are expecting twins because you have higher levels of the pregnancy hormone hCG (see p.74), which triggers nausea and vomiting. In the early stages, higher levels of the hormone progesterone can make you feel short of breath. You might also be more likely to have constipation or suffer from gas and bloating.

Later in pregnancy

Later in your pregnancy there is more of a strain on your muscles because you are carrying additional weight, so back pain might be a problem. Anemia is more common with twins and it can

make you feel very tired. Make sure that you eat iron-rich foods and take iron supplements if they are recommended.

The danger signs to look out for are the same as in any pregnancy. You do need to be alert to any unusual or worrying symptoms, though, because the risk of some complications, such as premature labor and preeclampsia, is higher when you are expecting twins.

Trust your instincts and, if you're not sure about a symptom, or just don't feel right, call your doctor.

Get as much rest as you can, ask people for help at home, and remember to enjoy the little things in life. You will need lots of energy both during your pregnancy and after your babies are born, so it's a good idea to get into the habit of taking care of yourself now.

Parents**Ask...**

I'm expecting twins. Will I have extra prenatal care?

You'll be offered extra scans to see how your babies are positioned, how well they are growing, or whether any complications are developing. Regular blood pressure and urine tests are important too.

How much weight will I gain?

You're likely to gain more weight than mothers of one baby. As in any pregnancy, try to eat a healthy, balanced diet.

What are the risks?

Premature birth (before 37 weeks) occurs in about half of twin pregnancies. Call your

doctor if you think you are in labor or go straight to the hospital. Preeclampsia is also more common with twins. This potentially dangerous complication is usually detected by blood pressure and urine tests, but symptoms include severe headaches, vision problems, and sudden swelling of your feet, ankles, face, and hands.

Will my labor be induced?

Some doctors argue that it's safer to plan for your twins' birth at about 37 to 38 weeks of pregnancy, either by induction or by planned cesarean. But this is not as common these days. Discuss your options with your doctor.

Miscarriage

Sadly miscarriage is all too common, affecting about 15 to 20 percent of pregnancies. But that doesn't make it any easier to bear if it happens to you. Here's how to reduce your risk of pregnancy loss and how to spot the signs if the worst does happen.

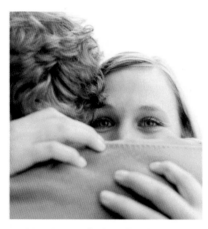

Miscarriage can be heartbreaking but you can take action to prevent it from happening to you and can learn to recognize the signs.

ParentsTalk...

"We held out until 10 weeks to tell friends and family our thrilling news, but a week later I miscarried. We were heartbroken—and what was worse was that we'd allowed ourselves and our friends and family to get excited about it."
Julia, 30, pregnant for a second time

"It takes time to get back on your feet after a miscarriage. I went back to work after a week, then had to take a month off to recover properly."
Louise, 28

What is a miscarriage?

Miscarriage is the loss of a baby in the first 24 weeks of pregnancy. Sadly, it's common; about 15 to 20 percent of known pregnancies end in miscarriage. About 98 percent of women who miscarry do so in the first 13 weeks.

The risk factors

Research suggests that you are more likely to miscarry if you smoke, drink more than four cups of coffee a day, or drink a lot of alcohol. You also have a higher risk of miscarriage if you:

- Have had more than one miscarriage, though this is not a significant risk.
- Have fibroids (noncancerous growths of the uterus).
- Have an abnormally shaped uterus.
- Have lupus.
- Have diabetes, kidney disease, or thyroid disease (if these conditions are well managed by you and your doctors, the risk of miscarriage is much lower).
- Have an infection in early pregnancy, such as rubella, listeria, or chlamydia.

Age also plays a role. Older women are more likely to conceive babies with chromosomal abnormalities, and these pregnancies are more likely to be lost.

Why miscarriages happen

Doctors still don't know why miscarriages happen. Probably at least half of all miscarriages in the first

If you think you're miscarrying

If you think you may be miscarrying, call your doctor or hospital.
Do not hesitate to contact your doctor or the hospital immediately if:

- The bleeding is very heavy.
- You begin to feel feverish and generally unwell.
- You have severe, one-sided abdominal pain—this may be a sign that you have an ectopic pregnancy.

To help with the strong period-type cramping pains, rest, take analgesics and use a hot water bottle to help ease the discomfort.

If the bleeding is not that heavy, or if there is no pain, then you do not need to rush to the hospital, but it is a good idea to contact your doctor anyway. She may want to see you at her office the next day, to examine you to check that you are physically all right.

trimester are the result of chromosomal abnormalities. Miscarriages that occur after 20 weeks may be the result of an infection, an abnormality of the uterus or placenta, or a cervix that is not strong enough to keep the uterus tightly closed.

The signs

The most obvious signs of miscarriage are periodlike pains, cramping, and bleeding (which may include blood clots). Some miscarriages are only discovered by chance during a routine prenatal visit, when the doctor cannot find the baby's heartbeat.

Sometimes you may have some spotting—losing very small amounts of blood from your vagina. Spotting in early pregnancy is common and usually nothing to worry about. Often, it's simply "breakthrough" bleeding when your period would have been due, caused by the hormones that control your menstrual cycle; or "implantation" bleeding—when the fertilized egg implants in the wall of the uterus.

With any spotting, bleeding, or severe pain, you should call your doctor. It could be a sign that you are going to miscarry.

Reducing the risk

By far the best way to reduce your risk of miscarriage is to quit smoking before you become pregnant (see p.118). This may be the hardest thing you've ever had to do, but it will be worth it.

Caffeine and alcohol

Even if you are already pregnant, it is still extremely worthwhile quitting smoking, and cutting down on caffeine and alcohol, both of which are possible additional factors in miscarriage. The March of Dimes recommends that pregnant women should have no more than 200 milligrams (mg) of caffeine (about one 12-ounce cup of coffee) a day since caffeine consumption is linked to miscarriage as well as to low-birthweight babies.

There is also research that links even low levels of caffeine intake to miscarriage, so if you are really concerned, you may want to cut out caffeine entirely, just to be on the safe side. Although the research isn't absolutely clear, it also seems possible that drinking more than one to two units of alcohol once or twice a week may increase your risk of miscarriage.

If you've had a miscarriage before, your doctor or midwife might suggest that you try to rest as much as possible during the first couple of months of your pregnancy. You might also be advised to avoid sex until your pregnancy is well established. If you think this is going to cause problems with your partner, ask your doctor to talk to the two of you together so that he can understand why it's necessary.

If you know you have a weak cervix because that caused a previous miscarriage, you may be able to have a stitch put around it to keep it closed until your baby is ready to be born. This is called a Shirodkar suture or cerclage.

Sadly, there is not much that can be done to prevent a miscarriage once it is underway. Dealing with it is very hard, but it may be some comfort to know that most women do manage to get pregnant again, and go on to have a normal, full-term pregnancy.

200 mg is the maximum amount of caffeine that pregnant women should have a day, according to the March of Dimes. That's one cup of coffee, two cups of tea, or five glasses of caffeinated soda. This follows research linking caffeine consumption to miscarriage and low- birthweight babies.

Active mom

If you love your sports, be extra careful when you're exercising to protect your baby.

"I've led a really active life ever since I was a child. I love the great outdoors and often go on activity vacations. When I found out I was pregnant, though, I knew I'd have to make some changes for the safety of my baby.

I've had to give up the horseback riding; it's been a long time since I fell off a horse, but I don't want to take the risk because I know that it could cause a miscarriage. Plus, I know that my center of gravity will change as my baby grows, which will increase the risk of a fall.

But because I've always exercised regularly, my doctor says it's safe for me to continue with my more pregnancy-friendly pursuits. I love going on really long walks, and I've started to swim more often. I'm thinking of joining a yoga class for pregnant women too.

Most importantly, though, I listen to my body and I stop exercising if I feel too tired or too out of breath."

Ectopic pregnancy

Ectopic pregnancy affects roughly one in 50 pregnancies in the United States. Sadly, it always ends in pregnancy loss, but most women who are affected will later go on to have healthy pregnancies. Here's how to spot the signs early.

Signs of ectopic pregnancy

Most affected women experience symptoms of an ectopic pregnancy about two weeks after missing a period. Signs to watch out for include:

The first signs

● Unusual vaginal bleeding. The blood is often different from your normal period—the blood may look red or brown like the color of dried blood, and may be continuous or intermittent, heavy, or light.

● One-sided pain in the lower abdomen that is severe and persistent.

When the fallopian tube ruptures

If an early diagnosis is not made, the tube may rupture and you may have the following symptoms:

● Sudden, severe pain gradually spreading out across the abdomen.

● Sweating; feeling light-headed or faint; diarrhea or blood in your stools.

● Collapse or shock as a result of severe internal bleeding.

● Shoulder tip pain, which is also a sign of internal bleeding.

If you have any of these symptoms, see your doctor immediately or go straight to the hospital.

What's going on?

An ectopic pregnancy is one that develops outside the uterus. It happens in roughly 2 percent of all pregnancies in the United States.

Almost all ectopic pregnancies implant in one of the fallopian tubes. As the pregnancy grows, it causes pain and bleeding and, if it's not recognized in time that you have an ectopic pregnancy, the fallopian tube can rupture, causing internal bleeding. An ectopic pregnancy is a life-threatening emergency. In rare cases it can be fatal. Sadly, the pregnancy itself never survives as it always has to be completely removed.

Symptoms often start about two weeks after a missed period. The most common reason for an ectopic pregnancy is when the fallopian tube has been damaged. This causes a blockage or narrowing, which prevents the egg from reaching the uterus. Instead, it implants in the wall of the tube.

Risk factors

You are more likely to have an ectopic pregnancy if:

● You have tubal endometriosis, which increases the risk of scarring and adhesions in the tubes.

● You have had any abdominal surgery.

● You have had pelvic inflammatory disease (PID)—this can cause scarring to the fallopian tubes (there are signs of PID in about half of all ectopic pregnancies that occur).

● You are pregnant following IVF.

● You have an intrauterine system (IUS—also sometimes called a coil or IUCD) or if you are taking the mini-pill.

● You smoke.

● You have had a previous ectopic pregnancy (your risk increases from one in 100 to one in 10).

● You are an older mom.

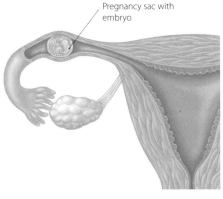

Pregnancy sac with embryo

In most ectopic pregnancies the blastocyst (see p.34) implants in the fallopian tube. Once diagnosed, the pregnancy must be removed.

Symptoms

It can be difficult to recognize if you are having an ectopic pregnancy, since it may begin with the sort of signs you associate with your period starting or a threatened miscarriage, such as cramping and slight bleeding. Early symptoms include unusual vaginal bleeding (it may be the color of dried blood). You may also have severe, persistent one-sided pain in the lower part of your abdomen. Shoulder tip pain, which can be felt where the shoulder meets the top of the arm, is another sign. This can happen if there is internal bleeding which will irritate other internal body organs, such as the diaphragm. If the ectopic pregnancy isn't diagnosed early enough and the fallopian tube ruptures, you may feel sudden, severe pain gradually spreading out across your abdomen. You may also start sweating and feeling faint, and you may have signs of shock, such as a weak, racing pulse; pale, clammy skin; and dizziness or fainting. You may also have diarrhea or blood in your stools. Pain in your shoulder, particularly when you lie down, is a red flag for a ruptured ectopic pregnancy.

How it is treated

You may need serial blood tests to measure the levels of the hCG hormone (see p.74) in your blood. If the levels of hCG are lower than they would be in a normal pregnancy, it can be a sign of ectopic pregnancy.

Further tests

You may have a vaginal ultrasound examination, since the pregnancy may not show up using an abdominal scan. If this does not confirm what is happening, you will probably be given a laparoscopic examination. This is where a narrow viewing instrument is put into your abdomen.

If an ectopic pregnancy is discovered, the surgeon can sometimes use laparoscopy (keyhole surgery) to remove the pregnancy, leaving the tube intact if at all possible. If the tube has ruptured, doctors usually recommend full abdominal surgery, because it's the quickest way to stop blood loss.

Whether the tube and pregnancy are removed entirely, or the pregnancy is removed and the tube repaired, depends on how damaged the tube is, the health of your other fallopian tube, and your desire for future pregnancy.

In a few cases where the tube has been saved, the pregnancy continues to grow and needs treatment with the drug methotrexate, which terminates pregnancy. If the pregnancy is clearly ectopic and the embryo is relatively small, you may be given the drug methotrexate. This is injected into a muscle and reaches the embryo through your bloodstream. It ends the pregnancy by stopping the cells of the placenta from growing. Over time, the tiny embryo is reabsorbed into your body.

If you're too far along for methotrexate or laparoscopic surgery, you'll need major abdominal surgery. You'll be given general anesthesia and an ob-gyn will open your abdomen and surgically remove the embryo. (As with laparoscopic surgery, your tube may be preserved or may need to be removed, depending on the situation.) After the operation, you'll need about six weeks to recuperate.

ParentsAsk...

Will an ectopic pregnancy affect my future fertility?

The answer to this is yes, possibly. If your fallopian tubes are undamaged after an ectopic pregnancy, then your chances of conceiving again remain the same as before. If one of the tubes ruptured or was badly damaged, your chances of conceiving again are reduced, particularly if your other tube has already been compromised by PID or endometriosis.

Some 65 percent of women will conceive again within 18 months of an ectopic pregnancy, but if both your fallopian tubes were damaged or ruptured, you may need to think about IVF treatment. Women who've had a laparoscopy should normally wait three to four months before trying to conceive again. If you have had abdominal surgery, it's best to wait for six months to allow scarring to heal.

Organized mom

If you've had an ectopic pregnancy there are places you can go for help and support.

"My ectopic pregnancy was really heartbreaking. I wanted to try for another pregnancy but was terrified it would happen all over again. My doctor was great. He put me in touch with the Ectopic Pregnancy Foundation. Knowing the facts helped me come to terms with what had happened—and plan for the future. Talking online to other women who'd had a similar experience was invaluable —they gave me so much support. It's easier to cope when you know you're not alone, and that others have gone on to have healthy pregnancies."

Getting ready for pregnancy

Staying safe and healthy

Your pregnancy diary

Birth and beyond

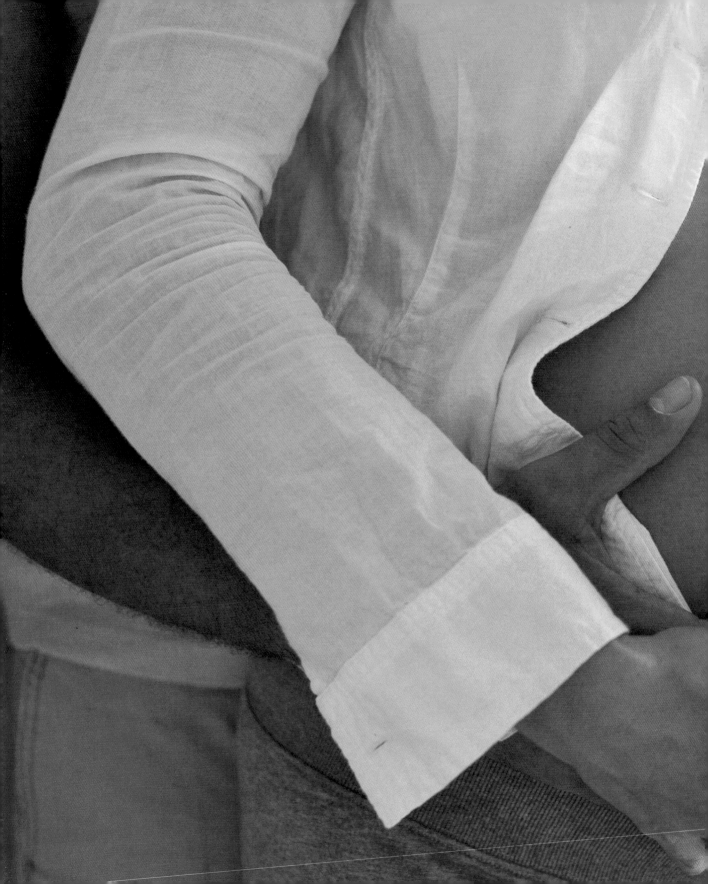

Staying safe and healthy

Healthy eating for you and baby

Now that you're a mom-to-be, it's important to make sure that you and your developing baby are getting all the nutrients you need. That means eating a healthy, balanced diet that's rich in vitamins and minerals. You'll also need to avoid certain foods that could be harmful.

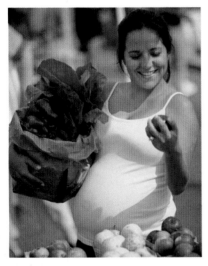

During pregnancy, eating your recommended seven daily portions of fruit and vegetables is even more important.

What should I be eating?

Although you're pregnant, don't think that you have to eat for two. The average woman needs only about 300 extra calories a day, fewer during the first trimester.

Recommended diet

According to the Food Guide Pyramid, to keep you and your baby well nourished, you should aim to eat:

● Two to four servings of fruit and three to five servings of vegetables a day—fresh produce is best for fiber and important nutrients.

● Six to 11 servings of bread, cereal, rice, and pasta—choose whole-grain versions if possible. Getting plenty of fiber helps prevent constipation.

● Two to three servings of foods rich in protein, such as lean meat or chicken, and fish in moderation (see p.53), plus iron-rich eggs, beans, and lentils.

● Two to three servings of calcium-rich dairy foods, such as milk, cheese, and yogurt. Indulge sparingly in fats, oils, and candy.

As far as snacks are concerned, try eating a banana rather than chocolate, or frozen-fruit sorbet instead of whole-milk ice cream. And if you desire the occasional treat, don't feel guilty—just enjoy every bite!

ParentsAsk...

Do I need a supplement?

Most women—especially those in the throes of morning sickness—can benefit from taking a prenatal vitamin and mineral supplement to make sure they get important nutrients during pregnancy.

What should it contain?

A good supplement will contain more folic acid, iron, and calcium—vital for your baby's development—than a general multivitamin supplement. It will also contain the plant-derived form of vitamin A (betacarotene). The animal form, retinol, can be harmful to unborn babies in large doses.

Should I take probiotics?

Two studies found that probiotics taken during pregnancy may help to prevent atopic eczema from developing in babies. More research is needed, but if you have a family history of allergies you could ask your doctor for advice.

 Active mom

If you're a more than usually active pregnant mom, you should eat when you're hungry.

"Despite all those stories about 'eating for two', it turns out that you don't need many extra calories for the first six months of pregnancy. But since I'm very athletic, my doctor said I should eat when I'm hungry and that plenty of fruit and vegetables and lots of water would help keep my energy up."

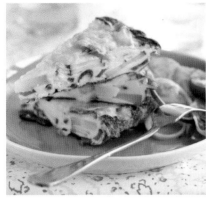

Iron-rich eggs are a healthy choice during pregnancy, but make sure omelets and frittatas are all well cooked.

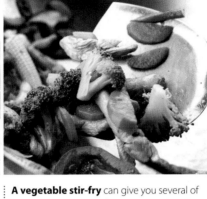

A vegetable stir-fry can give you several of your "seven a day." Stir-fries are a healthier, less fatty choice than deep-fried foods.

When choosing a dessert, keep sugar to a minimum since it's full of "empty" calories with no nutritional value. Honey's a better choice.

Appetite fluctuations

You may find your appetite fluctuates as your pregnancy progresses:

- In the first few weeks your appetite may drop dramatically and you may not want real meals, especially if you are suffering from nausea or sickness.
- During the middle part of your pregnancy your appetite may be the same as before you were pregnant or slightly increased.
- Toward the end of your pregnancy your appetite will probably increase, but if you suffer from heartburn or a full feeling after eating you may find it helpful to have small frequent meals instead of three meals a day.

Healthy weight gain

Weight gain varies from woman to woman and depends on many different factors. Women whose pre-pregnancy weight was in the healthy range for their height should gain between 25 and 35 pounds, gaining one to five pounds in the first trimester and about one pound per week after that Most women gain the least weight during the first trimester, then steadily increase, gaining most weight during the third trimester when their baby is growing the most.

Although you may be tempted, dieting during pregnancy isn't good for you or your baby. Diets can leave you low on iron, folic acid, and other vitamins and minerals. Remember, weight gain is one of the most positive signs that you are having a healthy pregnancy.

Small frequent meals

Even if you're not hungry, chances are your baby is, so you should try to eat every four hours. And if nausea and vomiting, food aversions, heartburn, or indigestion make eating a chore, eating five or six small meals, rather than the usual three larger ones, may be easier on your body.

Folic acid

The B vitamin folic acid is particularly important during pregnancy. Lack of it has been linked with neural tube birth defects, such as spina bifida. The US Public Health Service, the Centers for Disease Control, and other experts recommend that women should take 400 micrograms (mcg) of folic acid in a supplement from the time they start trying to get pregnant until the 12th week of pregnancy. You also need to have a good intake of the naturally

occurring form of folic acid—folates—from the food you eat. Leafy green vegetables, such as cabbage, broccoli, and greens, are all good sources. Other sources include black-eyed beans and bran flakes.

Tips for safe eating out

There is no reason why you can't eat safely in a restaurant. Here are a few pointers as to what to choose:

Starters Avoid raw fish and go for cooked dishes, such as crab cakes or shrimp. Pâtés and soft cheeses are best avoided.

Main courses Steak tartare, sushi, and other raw meat are risky. Opt for meat or fish that is cooked thoroughly.

Desserts Soufflés, mousses, and chilled chocolate puddings may contain raw eggs. Tiramisu often contains raw egg white as does homemade ice cream. Crème brulée and caramel custard are fine, because the eggs have been cooked.

Getting ready for pregnancy

Staying safe and healthy

Your pregnancy diary

Birth and beyond

Pregnant and vegetarian

With careful planning, a vegetarian diet during pregnancy can provide all the healthy nutrients you need.

Iron and calcium

Your body requires a little more protein during pregnancy, and this is easily provided by following a healthy, varied

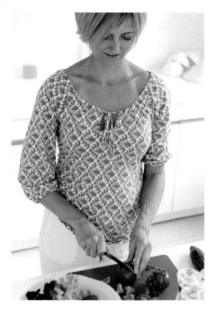

vegetarian diet. However, vegetarians should be extra careful to ensure that they have an adequate intake of iron and calcium. Both are very important during pregnancy (see p.121).

Vegetarian moms-to-be should be particularly careful to include plenty of iron in their diet since vegetable sources of iron are not as well absorbed as iron that is found in meat. Good sources include peas, beans, green vegetables, dried fruit, and fortified breakfast cereals.

Try to have some food or drink containing vitamin C, such as a glass of fruit juice, with any iron-rich meals since this helps your body absorb the iron. Avoid drinking tea with iron-rich foods since this contains tannin, which reduces absorption. If your iron levels become low, your doctor may advise you to take iron supplements.

The best sources of calcium are dairy foods, such as milk, cheese, and yogurt. Aim to have three servings per day.

The vitamin C in salads helps your body absorb all-important iron from other foods.

Vitamin D is essential for calcium absorption and can be obtained from sunlight, margarine, and dairy products. You may want to consider taking a vitamin D supplement.

There are some nondairy sources of dietary calcium, such as dark green vegetables, sesame seeds, and some fortified soy products. Generally, calcium is not as well absorbed from these foods so, if you do not eat dairy foods, it's a good idea to take a calcium supplement.

During pregnancy you'll need about an extra 300 calories a day to support your rapidly growing baby—less during your first trimester. You can bump up your calorie intake by eating more cereals, peas, beans, nuts, seeds, dairy products (unless you're a vegan), and starchy vegetables, such as potatoes.

You can get the 71 grams of protein you need each day during pregnancy by having three cups of milk or soy milk, one cup of tofu, four cups of brown rice, and a cup of yogurt. And don't neglect omega 3 fatty acids, found in fish, flax seeds, and walnuts.

Parents**Ask...**

Can I diet when I'm pregnant?
Dieting to lose weight during pregnancy isn't advised, but you should follow a healthy low-fat, low-sugar diet. It might help to see a registered dietitian with experience of working with pregnant women to find out how to eat well.

How many calories do I need?
Your daily calorie requirement depends on how active you are, but most pregnant women need 1,800 to 2,100 calories per day. In pregnancy you only need an extra 300 calories a day, less in the first trimester.

Can vitamin B6 help relieve my morning sickness?
Vitamin B6 helps some women, but no one really knows why. It helps the body metabolize certain amino acids (proteins), which may reduce nausea. You can get it from food sources such as bananas, brown rice, lean meats, poultry, fish, avocados, whole grains, corn, and nuts, as well as from a supplement. You need about 1.9 mg a day when pregnant; most prenatal vitamins contain at least 100 percent of the recommended amount. Talk to your doctor if you're not sure you're getting enough.

Single mom

There are plenty of ways to save money on your shopping bill and make good food go further.

"I earn a good salary but I still need to watch what I spend. I find it helps to make a shopping list and stick to it. I eat a mainly vegetarian diet since it's cheaper, but I treat myself to some good, lean meat a couple of times a week. I also tend to go for the supermarket's own brand. I really can't taste any difference."

Pregnant and plus-sized

Your weight may not have any affect at all on your pregnancy or your baby's birth, but being overweight or obese could put you at higher risk of certain pregnancy complications. Some of the most common of these are:

- gestational diabetes
- gestational hypertension (high blood pressure)
- preeclampsia
- premature labor
- a large baby (macrosomia)

When it's time to give birth, having a high body mass index can mean you are more likely to have:

- an assisted birth (by forceps or vacuum)
- a cesarean section
- shoulder dystocia (where the baby's shoulders get caught on the mother's pubic bone during birth)

Preventing problems

Most of these health conditions and situations are manageable though, and some are preventable. Ideally, you should lose weight before you get pregnant since research has shown an association between dieting during the first three months of pregnancy and babies born with neural tube defects, regardless of the mother's size. But if you are pregnant, there's still plenty you can do to help yourself and your baby.

Exercise

Regular exercise is one of the most effective ways to manage your weight, particularly when combined with a healthy diet.

As long as you get the go-ahead from your doctor, you can engage in mild to moderate exercise. Stick to low-impact activities like walking or swimming, stay well hydrated, and talk to your doctor about the length of exercise sessions.

Talk to your doctor about your risk factors. Do you have a history of high blood pressure or of diabetes? Is there a family history of larger babies? You can work with your doctor to give yourself the best chance of having a healthy baby.

Healthy eating for working moms

However busy your job, you can make time to eat well at work by following some simple steps.

- Keep some healthy nibbles and drinks in your desk drawer to satisfy hunger pangs throughout the day: try fruit, crackers, organic no-added-sugar cereal bars, seeds, and nuts. Bread rolls, cartons of fruit juice, mineral water, and sticks of cucumber or carrot are also great working day snacks.
- If you can, take your lunch into work so you can be sure you're eating a balanced meal. Transform your usual sandwich into something more interesting by using different breads every day, and fresh fillings such as watercress, arugula, and grated carrot. Or try a salad—pasta and couscous give you a prolonged release of energy. Add vegetables and salad ingredients for added nutrients. For a hot meal, try soup, made fresh or ready made, with a whole-wheat roll. Baked potatoes are great fillers, too—eat with salads or baked beans.

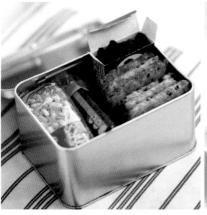
Keep a box filled with healthy snacks in the drawer of your desk for those moments when you have an attack of the munchies.

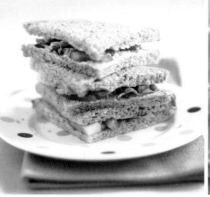
Making your own healthy sandwiches to take to work ensures you'll always eat a balanced meal at lunchtime.

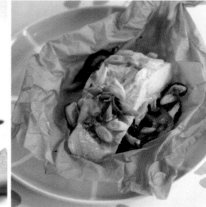
A salmon parcel is a quick, easy, and healthy meal to make for dinner when you get home after a long day at work.

Getting ready for pregnancy

Staying safe and healthy

Your pregnancy diary

Birth and beyond

What's safe to eat?

It sometimes feels as though the list of foods you can't eat when you're pregnant grows longer every day. Try not to worry too much. Just remember that the risks to you and your baby are low and you can avoid them entirely by taking a few sensible steps.

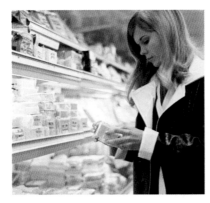

Cheese is an important source of calcium when you're pregnant, but you should be careful which you choose.

Laid-back mom

It may never occur to you before you get pregnant that some foods can be bad for your baby.

"Finding out what I could and couldn't eat when I was pregnant was a revelation. Now I make sure any meat I eat is thoroughly cooked—no more rare steaks for me! Or soft-boiled eggs. And I try not to eat too much oily fish, though I never ate more than a couple of portions a week. Cheese is a tricky one—I've cut out all the moldy cheeses. But I don't worry too much. As long as you're careful, food-related infections are quite rare."

Why what you eat may be bad for your baby

Confused about which cheeses are safe in pregnancy? Or whether you can drink alcohol? Here's all you need to know to keep you and your baby safe from harm.

Alcohol

Heavy drinking, particularly binge drinking (five or more units of alcohol at one time), during pregnancy can seriously affect your developing baby. The risks of drinking much less, however, aren't clear cut. Even so, all public health officials in the United States recommend that pregnant women, as well as women who are trying to conceive, play it safe by steering clear of alcohol entirely.

Caffeine

If you have too much caffeine in your diet your risk of miscarriage goes up and your baby could have a lower birth weight. Researchers recommend no more than 200 milligrams (mg) a day— about one cup of coffee.

Diet sodas

Diet sodas are generally okay in moderation, as long as you're mindful of the caffeine. You might want to be wary of the sweeteners in them, however.

Artificial sweeteners

Artificial sweeteners such as aspartame (NutraSweet) and Sucralose (Splenda) are considered safe; you may want to avoid saccharin, which was linked to birth defects in rats when consumed in very high amounts.

Raw or undercooked meat

Raw, rare, cured, and undercooked meat or poultry of any kind is best avoided. It may contain salmonella bacteria, which can cause severe food poisoning, or the toxoplasmosis parasite, which can be harmful to your unborn baby.

Raw or undercooked eggs

Eating soft-boiled or raw eggs is not recommended because of the risk that the eggs may carry salmonella bacteria. To stay safe, boil a medium-sized egg for at least seven minutes, fry eggs on both sides, and poach eggs until they are completely set.

Cheese and dairy products

Cheese is an important source of protein and calcium for pregnant women but the following kinds, made from unpasteurized milk, need to be avoided:

- Soft, mold-ripened cheeses, such as Brie or Camembert.
- Blue-veined cheeses, such as Danish Blue, Stilton, Roquefort, Gorgonzola.
- Soft, unpasteurized cheeses, such as Chabichou and queso blanco fresco.

These cheeses provide a perfect environment for harmful bacteria, such as listeria, to grow. However, thorough cooking should kill any listeria, so it's safe to eat these cheeses in well-cooked food. All hard cheeses, including cheddar, Gruyère, and Parmesan, are safe to eat. Yogurt, buttermilk, cottage cheese, ricotta, cream cheese, and processed cheese (such as American) are also safe.

Fish

Seafood is sometimes contaminated with environmental pollutants so it's recommended that pregnant women avoid eating too much oily fish, since it tends to contain more pollutants than white fish. You should eat some, though, so that you and your baby can benefit from the omega-3 fatty acids and other vitamins and nutrients it contains. Just enjoy it in moderation and choose from wild salmon, trout, flounder, sole, tilapia, catfish, whitefish, and sardines.

You should avoid eating shark, king mackerel, swordfish, and tilefish entirely because of their high levels of mercury, which could harm your baby's developing nervous system. You also need to limit the tuna you eat to no more than six ounces of light tuna; it's best to avoid albacore (or "white") tuna and tuna steaks, since they can have three times as much mercury as light tuna.

Deli meats

It's not safe to eat precooked meats such as deli meats, hot dogs, and pâté when you're pregnant unless they're heated until steaming hot. These foods can cause listeriosis.

Shellfish

Most shellfish are safe to eat, provided they have been thoroughly cooked. Raw shellfish are a common cause of food poisoning so avoid them completely while you are pregnant.

Prepared salads

Make sure to wash these again before use. There is a chance that they may carry the toxoplasmosis parasite or listeria bacteria. Be wary when eating salad from a deli counter—if you don't feel that it has been prepared in a hygienic manner, then don't eat it. Look out for staff with an obvious cold.

Parents**Ask...**

Is it safe to eat sushi when you're pregnant?

Sushi that uses cooked fish, such as steamed crab and cooked eel, is generally fine but raw sushi can be unsafe. There is a small risk of getting a parasitic infection from raw fish. While the risk is small, contracting a food-borne illness could cause serious complications for you or your baby. There's also the risk of toxins: Bluefish, mackerel, mahi-mahi, and tuna can carry a histamine toxin that may cause flushing, dizziness, and burning of the mouth and throat.

Herbal teas

Most herbal tea bags bought from supermarkets and which contain common ingredients, such as lemon, are thought to be safe for use in pregnancy, though excessive amounts of any teas could cause health problems for you or your baby. Anise, catnip, chamomile, ephedra (also call ma huang), lemongrass, mugwort, raspberry leaf, rosemary, sage, and stinging nettle leaf, among others, are all best avoided.

Foods to avoid when you are pregnant

Figuring out what you can and can't eat when pregnant is confusing to start with. Just follow these simple rules.
- **Cheese** Steer clear of blue-veined cheeses, Brie, and Camembert and avoid unpasteurized soft cheeses, too.
- **Eggs** Avoid raw or undercooked eggs. Salad dressings sold in supermarkets, such as mayonnaise, are safe. Beware of "homemade" products, such as chocolate mousse: these may contain raw egg.

- **Deli meats and pâté** Avoid all pâté, whether made from meat, fish, or vegetables, and deli meats.
- **Meat and meat products** Make sure meat is cooked thoroughly. Cured meat products, such as salami, also carry a risk and are best avoided.
- **Seafood** Oily fish in particular is good for you and your baby since it gives you all the benefits of omega-3 fatty acids, but you should limit your intake to a

maximum of two portions a week to lower the risk from pollutants and steer clear of raw fish altogether.

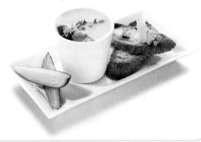

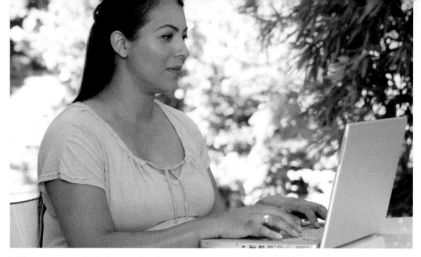

If you are worried about a food scare, you can search for reliable information online.

Food hygiene in pregnancy

During pregnancy, it is especially important to avoid the germs responsible for food poisoning:

● **Personal hygiene** Washing your hands before and during food preparation (especially if you are handling raw meat or poultry) prevents the spread of bacteria.
● **Keep foods at the right temperature** Take bought chilled and frozen foods home quickly and put them straight into the fridge (below 41º F/5º C) or freezer (below 0.5 ºF/−18º C).
● **Store food safely** Store raw and cooked foods separately in the fridge. Put raw meat on the bottom shelf, where it can't drip onto cooked food.
● **Cook foods thoroughly** Cook until food—especially meat and poultry—is piping hot with steam coming off it.
● **Beware of cross contamination** Clean work surfaces with soapy, hot water before preparing food, and after contact with raw meat or poultry.
● **Eating out** Look out for dirty public areas, staff with dirty hands or an obvious runny nose, or raw foods displayed next to ready-to-eat foods.

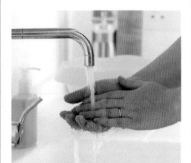

Always wash your hands before and after you prepare food to reduce your risk of getting food poisoning.

Food scares: how to tell the good from the bad

The papers are full of scare stories and lots of them are about food. Remember the "hotdogs give you cancer" story? Stories like this are worrying, but you should take many of them with a grain of salt. Next time you see a worrying headline, you should ask yourself the following questions:

● **Is the advice backed up by a trustworthy organization?**
The US Food and Drug Administration, for example, issues new guidance from time to time. Visit the relevant website or look for links from reliable news websites to ascertain the facts.

● **Is the report based on a true account of the facts?**
Sometimes the media picks on one aspect of a much larger topic. Editors often publish an unbalanced view of an issue that hasn't really been proven yet.

● **What is the source of the story?**
From time to time, companies issue press releases that support the use of their products. These may not give a truly balanced picture of a certain issue. Also, experts sometimes have an investment in the findings of a research study. If the findings are shown in a certain light, it could help sell a drug or product he or she has just patented.

● **Is the story really based on conclusive evidence?**
Experts around the world often report their research findings in special journals and at conferences. Sometimes the media reports the findings of very small research studies when, in fact, evidence from much larger studies is needed before the issue can be accepted as fact.

● **Is it really new?**
Sometimes the same old issues are paraded out again and again. For example, the media may report an inquiry into an issue. There isn't any new evidence yet, but the same panic-inducing headlines are released without adding anything new.

If you have asked yourself all these questions and you are still not sure what to do, don't be afraid to ask for some advice. Perhaps a visit to your doctor may help.

ParentsTalk...

"I'm never entirely sure if I'm eating something that health experts might suddenly decide is bad during pregnancy. I was sticking to the 300 mg of caffeine a day rule (three cups of coffee) during my pregnancy—but when I was 32 weeks the rules changed to 200 mg a day. I panicked, thinking I'd just spent the first 32 weeks of my baby's life impairing his growth. But I was assured by the experts' advice that no harm would have come to my baby. So why did the rules change?

Maybe it's that the guidelines are often overly cautious to compensate for those moms who like things in excess!"
Bel, mom to two-month-old Adam

"We have a history of food allergies in our family and I decided to cut out peanuts entirely when I was pregnant—even though the advice says it's probably okay to eat them. They're difficult to avoid though—they seem to crop up as an ingredient in more foods than you might think."
Jennifer, 30, mom to Max and Cameron

"Having followed the advice to the letter with my first son, only to discover he has a peanut allergy, I decided to continue eating them when I was pregnant with my second baby and he is fine. I don't know whether eating the peanuts helped or not, but the advice is so vague it's difficult to know what to do sometimes."
Madeleine, 37

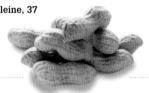

If there are allergies in the family

Some experts believe that avoiding allergens, such as peanuts, during pregnancy may reduce your child's risk of allergies. However, there's no evidence to back this up.

Precautions during pregnancy

An allergic reaction is when the body overresponds to some substance causing breathing problems, wheezing, rashes, and other, sometimes dangerous, symptoms. Allergic conditions include eczema, asthma, and hayfever, plus allergic responses to certain foods. Nonfood substances, such as pollen, dust mites, and bee or wasp stings, can also trigger allergies.

Before an allergy can develop, a child first has to be sensitized by contact with a trace of an allergen, such as peanut. Some believe that this may occur during pregnancy, when a tiny amount of the allergen crosses the placenta. However, there's no definite evidence yet.

A review of studies of high-risk pregnant women who avoided common allergens, such as eggs and cow's milk, during pregnancy found that this was unlikely to reduce the risk of allergies in children. On the other hand, exclusive breast-feeding for the first six months of your baby's life does help to lower her risk of allergies.

It's fine to eat peanuts while you're pregnant, if you aren't yourself allergic to peanuts. There is no evidence to suggest that eating or not eating peanuts while you are pregnant will affect your baby's chances of developing a peanut allergy.

Despite this advice, you may still feel reluctant to eat peanuts, and that's understandable. Talk to your doctor if you have a family history of allergies and are worried about the effect eating

peanuts will have on your baby. It's also worth remembering that, as long as you're eating a healthy balanced diet during your pregnancy, excluding peanuts from your diet will not do you or your baby any harm.

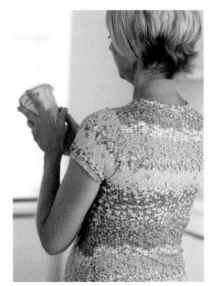

If you have food allergies in your family, you'll probably want to check food labels.

Fitness during pregnancy

Staying active has lots of benefits, both during your pregnancy and when it comes to giving birth. Whether you were a regular gym bunny before you got pregnant, or more of a couch potato, we've got tips on how to exercise safely with a baby-belly.

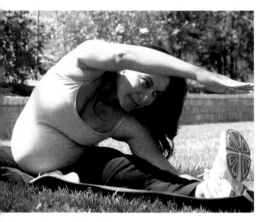

Stretching tones muscles and gives you flexibility, both of which will help you to cope better with pregnancy and childbirth.

Staying active

Why exercise in pregnancy? One reason is that exercise strengthens your cardiovascular system, so you don't tire as easily. Staying active will also:

● **Help prepare you for the rigors of childbirth** Giving birth requires stamina. The better shape you're in, the stronger you'll be to enable you to deal with childbirth.

● **Reduce stress and lift your spirits** Exercise can boost your levels of serotonin, a brain chemical linked to mood, which puts you in better spirits.

When you're feeling a little blue, try putting on your favorite CD and kicking up your heels in the living room, or sign up for a low-impact dance class (make sure you let your teacher know that you are pregnant).

● **Reduce pregnancy discomfort** Exercise stretches and strengthens your muscles, which will help your body to better deal with the various aches and pains of pregnancy.

● **Fend off the pregnancy blues** By the sixth or seventh month, pregnancy can become downright tedious. Finding a new healthy activity appropriate for pregnant women may be the answer.

● **Help you sleep better** When you are carrying all that extra weight, finding a comfortable position to sleep in at night can be a real challenge. Exercise will help to lull you into a deeper, more restful slumber.

● **Improve your self-image** Although you know it's for a good cause, watching the scale creep its way up to numbers you've never seen before can be disheartening. Staying active can make you feel less frumpy.

● **Help you get your body back faster after birth** For many of us, this alone is reason enough to embark on a pregnancy exercise regimen.

Tips for a safe workout

To keep you and your baby safe while you're exercising:

● Always check with your doctor before you start a new exercise plan.

● Wear loose-fitting, breathable clothing and supportive shoes, and make sure your maternity bra is doing its job.

● Warm up before exercising to avoid straining your ligaments.

● Keep moving—standing motionless can cause blood to pool in your legs, making you dizzy.

● Drink lots of water before, during, and after exercising—to make sure you don't become dehydrated.

● Don't do deep knee bends, lunges, or full sit-ups in case of ligament strain.

● Avoid overdoing it—slow down if you can't comfortably carry on a conversation.

● If you feel uncomfortable or are in pain, stop immediately. You're working your body, not punishing it.

● Avoid exercising while flat on your back after the first trimester—besides being uncomfortable, this position can affect the blood flow to your uterus.

● Get up from the floor slowly—getting up quickly can make you dizzy.

● Cool down to give your heart a chance to return gradually to its normal rate.

Swimming is a great exercise during pregnancy. You get a cardiovascular workout while the water supports your body weight.

Active mom

If you've always exercised, it should be safe to continue your pre-pregnancy exercise routine.

"I've always been heavily into athletics and weight training, so I was so happy to learn that healthy, well-conditioned women who exercised before pregnancy can continue throughout pregnancy without it affecting their baby's health or development. And what was even better, I read that weight-bearing exercise throughout pregnancy can reduce the length of your labor and decrease birth complications. What's not to like about that? So I plan to keep up my exercise routine and I'm looking forward to a shorter labor! It must be better than the marathon I ran last year."

What exercise is safe when you're pregnant?

The following exercises are fairly safe for expectant mothers, although some of them may not work for you during the last few months of your pregnancy. To be safe, consult your doctor before embarking on any of these activities.

• **Walking** One of the best cardiovascular exercises for pregnant women, walking keeps you fit without jarring your knees and ankles. It is a safe exercise to do throughout the nine months of pregnancy and can easily be built into your day-to-day schedule.

• **Jogging/running** Going for a jog is the quickest and most efficient way to work your heart and your body. You can tailor it to your schedule—running 15 minutes one day when that's all you can fit in, and 30 when you have more time.

• **Yoga and stretches** Yoga and stretching can help maintain muscle tone and keep you flexible with little, if any, impact on your joints. Be careful not

to overdo it though. You will be more supple as a result of the effects of the hormone relaxin (see p.75), so don't hold the stretches for too long or try to develop your flexibility too much.

• **Swimming** This is ideal because it exercises both large muscle groups (arms and legs), provides good cardiovascular benefits, and allows you to feel blissfully weightless.

• **Water aerobics classes** Exercising while standing in water is gentle on your joints and can help lessen swelling in the legs, which is a common symptom in late pregnancy.

• **Pilates** Pilates can be useful in pregnancy because it targets the abdomen and pelvic floor muscles and these muscles can weaken during pregnancy. Many Pilates exercises are performed in a "hands and knees" position. This helps to take a lot of stress off your back and pelvis, and, toward the

end of your pregnancy, can help to position your baby ready for delivery.

• **Low-impact aerobics** One good thing about joining an aerobics class is that it gives you a consistent time slot when you know you'll do some exercise. If you sign up for a class specifically designed for pregnant women, you'll get to enjoy the camaraderie of others just like you, and can feel reassured that it's safe for you and your baby.

• **Weight training** If weight training is already part of your exercise routine, there's no reason to stop although you will need to avoid using heavy weights and assuming certain positions.

• **Dance** Dancing will certainly get your heart pumping, but steer clear of dance movements that call for you to leap, jump, or twirl, and avoid sudden changes of direction. If you decide to sign up for a class, tell your instructor that you are pregnant.

Relaxation during pregnancy

Pregnancy brings its own stresses, including worries about whether or not your baby is okay, how the birth will go, and how your relationship with your partner will change once your baby is born. Discover below why it's important to relax, plus some tips for a chilled-out pregnancy.

Why relaxation is important

Feeling stressed and nervous is not unusual in pregnancy. The occasional periods of stress we all experience from time to time do not harm your baby but some experts believe that prolonged, severe stress in early pregnancy can increase your chances of complications, such as preeclampsia and premature birth. Research has also shown a link to hyperactivity in preschool children when the mother had long-term anxiety and stress during pregnancy, so seek help and support if you have a problem.

Talk to your doctor about how you are feeling. Often, your doctor will have advice on methods of relaxation. Doctors can rule out the possibility that an illness or a problem with the baby is causing your problems or can arrange for you to see a counselor if you need to talk through your worries.

Joining a support group in your area might help, too. Ask your doctor about local support groups, and check for prenatal yoga classes at gyms, health clubs, and the YMCA.

Getting the sleep you crave

Pregnancy often brings with it a multitude of sleep disturbances. To help make your nights more serene, make your bedroom inviting and relaxing, keep it cool and reduce light and noise as much as possible.

When you get home from work, try to have a leisurely evening meal and do something quiet, such as reading a book or relaxing in a nice warm bath. If you have a "to do" list, complete what you can by dinnertime then leave the rest of your list for the next day so that you have time to unwind before heading for bed. And avoid exercising in the evenings, because exercise too close to bedtime can cut down on deep sleep. If you are troubled by nausea or trips to the bathroom at night, see pp.162–3 for some advice on how to avoid these pregnancy problems.

Finally, if you really can't sleep, listen to soothing music or read a magazine until you're drowsy enough to go back to bed. Or you may want to try some self-help—guided imagery, deep breathing, or muscle relaxation.

Stress survival tips

It is best to do all you can to avoid long periods of stress when you are pregnant. These tips show you how.
- Make time to rest.
- Try deep breathing—it really helps.
- Find a friendly ear to talk through your concerns.
- Relax with a massage or reflexology.
- Get information about the birth.
- Share your relationship worries with friends with young babies.
- Start or finish work earlier to avoid rush hour, or try and work from home a couple of days a week.
- Get your finances in control to avoid worrying about them (see p.21).
- Eat foods that increase your levels of the anti-stress hormone serotonin, such as a glass of warm milk.
- Treat yourself to the occasional trip to the movies or weekend break.

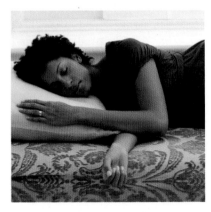

If you have trouble sleeping at night take daytime naps—even if you can only manage it on weekends.

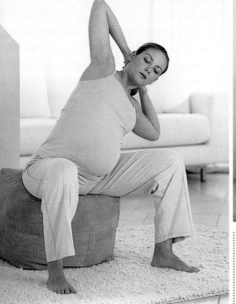

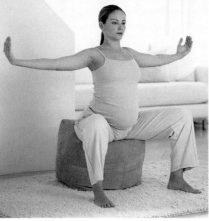

Sideways stretch *(left)* Place your hands behind your head. Inhale and stretch to the left, keeping your back straight and your elbows back. Repeat on the other side.
Back stretch *(above left)* Inhale, sit upright, and extend your arms to the sides. Exhale and

turn your hands upward in a receiving gesture. Hold for a few minutes.
Groin stretch *(above)* Sit in front of a chair and bring the soles of your feet together. Lean back onto the seat. Place cushions under your back for support if needed.

Yoga—ideal for relaxation

Yoga combined with a cardiovascular exercise such as walking can be an ideal way to maintain fitness when you're pregnant. When you stretch or do yoga, you're toning your muscles and limbering up with little, if any, impact on your joints—good news for pregnant women. Check for a special pregnancy yoga class near you or let your yoga instructor know that you are pregnant.

Yoga is also great for breathing and relaxation, which can help you adjust to the physical demands of labor, birth, and motherhood. One of the first things you learn in a yoga class is how to breathe fully. Yoga breathing techniques require you to take in air slowly through your nostrils, filling your lungs entirely, and then exhaling completely until your abdomen compresses.

Learning how to do yoga breathing primes you for labor and birth, because it trains you to stay calm when you most need it. When you're afraid—during labor, for example—the body produces adrenaline and shuts down the

production of oxytocin, a hormone that makes labor progress. Yoga training will help you fight the urge to tighten up when you feel the pain, and will show you how to breathe, instead.

As with any other exercise in pregnancy, you must always be careful. Avoid any movements that involve lying flat on your back after the first trimester, since this decreases blood flow to the uterus. Also avoid movements that overstretch the abdominal muscles. The pregnancy hormone relaxin, which allows the uterus to expand, also acts on other connective tissue, so you might tear or strain a muscle. If you find you have pain in your back, hips, or pelvis, you should modify your postures.

Try to find a special pregnancy yoga class. If you choose to go to a general class, tell the teacher that you are pregnant and ask if she is trained to teach pregnant women. To find an prenatal yoga class near you, ask your doctor if there's one in your area, or check with nearby gyms or the YMCA.

Green mom

Massage and aromatherapy are great for helping you relax when you are expecting.

"I love having a massage even if it's just one from my boyfriend at the end of a long day. I'm definitely going to make time for a few while I'm pregnant. I'm sure my baby will appreciate it too.

In fact, for my birthday my mom gave me a gift certificate for a treatment at a spa that offers special massages just for women who are pregnant. I'm really looking forward to that. And if they do aromatherapy massage there, I might book one of those as well. I've heard that some of the oils aren't suitable during pregnancy (see p.95), so you need to go to someone who's qualified and knows which oils are okay."

Safety at home

When you're newly pregnant it's natural to be wary of the cleaning products and toiletries you normally use without a second thought. Is it safe to clean the oven now? Can you still use aromatherapy oils? Here's how to keep you and your baby safe around the house.

How safe is my home?

While we usually see them as places of safety, it can feel as though your home is full of potential hazards once you're pregnant. Here are some dos and don'ts:

Cleaning products

In general these are safe. Just make sure you have good ventilation and wear gloves. Avoid cleaning the oven, though, as it's hard to get good ventilation in such a tight space. If any fumes make you feel nauseated, choose products that are environmentally friendlier, such as vinegar and bicarbonate of soda.

Paint

Painting exposes you to many chemicals, but it's difficult to know the exact risks. It's safest to let someone else do any painting, but if you do decide to do it yourself:
- Limit the time you spend doing it.
- Use low VOC or no VOC paint.
- Keep the windows open and don't sleep in a newly painted room.
- Wear gloves, long pants, and a long-sleeved shirt to protect your skin.
- Don't eat or drink where you work so you won't take in any chemicals.

Aerosols and air fresheners

Recent research found that preschool children whose mothers used aerosols and air fresheners most frequently during pregnancy were more likely to wheeze persistently in early childhood. While the researchers don't recommend tossing out the aerosols and air fresheners just yet, they do recommend:
- Wearing gloves when using indoor aerosol products.
- Reducing your aerosol use.
- Opening windows whenever you are using aerosols.

ParentsAsk...

Is it safe to use cat litter?
Cat feces can carry the toxoplasmosis parasite, which may harm your developing baby, so experts recommend you avoid emptying the cat litter tray. If you have to do it, wear rubber gloves and wash hands and gloves afterward.

Are aromatherapy oils safe?
These may be natural, but there are some you shouldn't use while pregnant. Rather than using them at home, you may want to go to a professional aromatherapist so that you're sure the

oils used are safe (see p.95). Ask around for a personal recommendation for a registered practitioner with experience in working with pregnant women.

Are electric blankets safe?
Probably, although some studies show that raising a pregnant woman's body temperature to 101° F (38.3° C) or higher for an extended period can increase the risk for miscarriage or neural tube defects. But it's very unlikely that a heated blanket would elevate your body temperature high enough to endanger your baby.

Green mom

Safety in pregnancy is an added reason to use "green" household cleaning products.

"I've always played it safe when it comes to cleaning products, but now that I'm pregnant I make sure I stick to old-fashioned things—white vinegar for cleaning glass and unblocking showerheads and sinks, lemon juice instead of degreasers and bleach, and bicarbonate of soda for everything from removing stains on the carpet to cleaning the toilet seat."

Can I take that medicine?

If you have, or develop, any of the following conditions during pregnancy, check out whether the over-the-counter or prescribed medicines used to treat them are safe for you and your baby. If you have a question about the safety of any medication during pregnancy, ask your doctor or visit the Organization of Teratology Information.

● **Aches and pains** You'd be lucky to get through pregnancy without at least a headache but you're limited in your choice of pain relief. Aspirin should be avoided, as it has a blood-thinning effect, and ibuprofen isn't recommended since it may affect your unborn baby and prolong labor. Acetaminophen is considered safe as long as you stick to the recommended dosage and only use it occasionally.

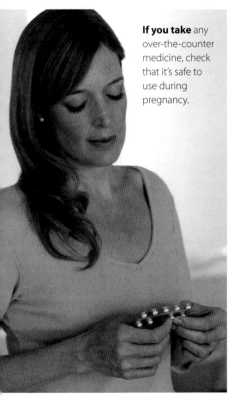

If you take any over-the-counter medicine, check that it's safe to use during pregnancy.

● **Acne** Benzoyl peroxide and salicylic acid are the main ingredients in over-the-counter acne treatments and these are safe to use in pregnancy. However, if you're taking oral treatments for acne you must be sure that you check with your doctor that these are okay during pregnancy.

● **Asthma** Not only is using asthma inhalers safe during pregnancy, it's recommended to keep your asthma under control. Uncontrolled asthma can result in too little oxygen getting to your baby, increasing the risk for low birthweight and other problems.

● **Colds** Avoid medicines that contain alcohol. Also avoid the decongestants pseudoephedrine and phenylephrine, which can affect blood flow to the placenta. Good cold relief options include guaifinesin, dextromethorphan, cough drops, and Vicks VapoRub.

● **Constipation** Laxatives and stool softeners are low-risk, along with psyllium, polycarbophil, and methylcellulose.

● **Coughs** Speak to your pharmacist before taking a cough medicine, since they tend to contain several different ingredients, some of which aren't recommended in pregnancy.

● **Cystitis** Your doctor can prescribe antibiotics that are safe to use during your pregnancy.

● **Diarrhea** Loperamide and kaolin-and-pectin remedies such as Imodium and Kaopectate are okay to use.

● **Eczema** Emollients are safe to use, as is hydrocortisone cream to calm an occasional flare-up. But if you get a skin infection, your obstetrician will need to prescribe a safe antibiotic.

● **First aid** Hydrocortisone and polysporin are generally safe.

● **Flu** Check with your pharmacist before taking any over-the-counter flu medications. Some might not be suitable. Pregnant women should be vaccinated for swine flu since they are at greater risk of developing a severe case. Be diligent about washing your hands thoroughly before eating, after sneezing, and after going to the bathroom. If you think you may have the flu, call your doctor—don't just show up at her office as you then run the risk of exposing other patients to the infection.

● **Hayfever and allergies** Speak to your doctor to find out which antihistamine is best to take during pregnancy, since some may raise your blood pressure. Chlorpheniramine, loratadine, and diphenhydramine, along with ephedrine and pseudoephredine, are usually okay to use.

● **Heartburn and indigestion** Try simple remedies first such as drinking a glass of milk or peppermint tea. If this doesn't help, antacids for heartburn and simethicone for gas pain are safe to use.

● **Insomnia** Sleep aids containing diphenhydramine and doxylamine succinate are low-risk.

● **Yeast infections and other fungal infections** Check labels carefully. Safe antifungal agents include clotrimazole, miconazole, terbinafine, tiocanazole, butenafine, and undecylenic acid.

Fact: An uncontrolled asthma attack is more dangerous to your baby than the risks of taking asthma medication during pregnancy. Uncontrolled asthma can result in your baby getting too little oxygen.

Getting ready for pregnancy

Staying safe and healthy

Your pregnancy diary

Birth and beyond

Safety at work

For most pregnant women, there's no reason why you shouldn't continue working for as long as you are able. But you need to make sure that the kind of work you do, and your working conditions, won't put your own or your baby's health at risk.

How safe is my workplace?

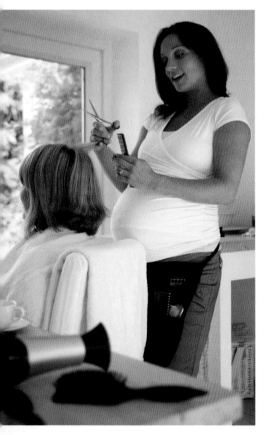

If your pregnancy is uncomplicated or low risk, and you work in a safe environment, you can work until close to your due date if you wish. However, if your job is strenuous or exposes you to toxic substances, you may need to request reassignment.

Potential hazards

Some studies have shown that women who work physically strenuous jobs during pregnancy—including heavy lifting and standing for long periods—are more likely to deliver prematurely, have lower-birth-weight babies, and develop high blood pressure during pregnancy. Discuss any concerns about your job with your doctor.

If you do have a strenuous job, you'll have to decide how you can best accommodate your pregnancy, perhaps by switching to a less physically taxing job or exchanging tasks with a co-worker. Take occasional sick or vacation days if needed to relieve fatigue.

Legally, you can work as long as you want and can choose when to start maternity leave. But if you have a high-risk pregnancy or develop complications, your doctor may order you to stop working early.

If you do develop complications, talk things over with your doctor. You may

Some occupations pose a special risk to you and your unborn baby. Make sure your employer carries out a risk assessment.

be advised to stop if you've previously given birth to more than one premature baby, have either diabetes or high blood pressure, have a history of miscarriage, or are expecting twins.

Toward the end of your pregnancy, you may get tired very quickly, so take it as easy as possible. If you can afford to start your maternity leave a week or two before your due date, you might consider using the time to rest, prepare, and indulge yourself. Remember: This may be the last quality time you have for yourself for a while.

Single mom

If you need to work as long as possible for financial reasons, ensure that you're safe at work.

"Being a single mom and needing to earn, I'm planning to work for as long as I can—right up until the week my baby's due if possible! I'll have to change my duties at work, though. I often help out in the warehouse and sometimes end up having to lift things. Luckily, my boss has made arrangements for me to remain on desk duties until my maternity leave."

If you work in a field where you come into contact with known reproductive hazards such as lead, mercury, organic solvents, certain biologic agents, and radiation, you'll need a reassignment—preferably even before you conceive. These teratogens can cause miscarriage, preterm delivery, structural birth defects, and abnormal fetal and infant development. You're likely to come into contact with these hazards while working in places such as computer chip factories, dry-cleaning plants, rubber factories, operating rooms, darkrooms, tollbooths, and printing presses, to name a few.

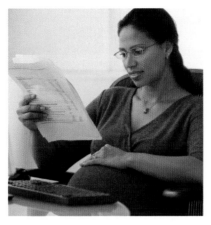

Make sure your workplace is comfortable and that you can take regular breaks. And accept any help your co-workers offer.

Staying comfortable at work

Coping with nausea and vomiting at work can be difficult. If you are prone to vomiting, keep wipes and mouthwash in your desk drawer. If no one knows your news yet, you could come up with a few convincing lines about "food poisoning."

Practical tips

During the first and third trimesters, you may have other symptoms like fatigue and absent-mindedness. It might help you to talk to a colleague who has been through this too and can support you. If there's a working parents' group in your workplace, join it to get some support.

Your pregnancy, though visible, can still be private. You may welcome the interest from colleagues and enjoy the opportunity to talk about your growing baby. On the other hand, you may prefer to keep your pregnancy personal and not to discuss it at work.

To make sure you stay comfortable throughout your working day:
- Put your feet up. Keep a box or stool under your desk.
- Wear comfortable shoes. You might try maternity or support hose, too.
- Dress comfortably.
- Seek the support of fellow mothers.
- Take breaks. Stand up and stretch if you've been sitting; sit down and raise your feet if you've been standing.
- Drink a lot. Keep a tall water glass at your desk, and refill it often. (This will also give you a chance to take a break.)
- Evaluate your office space. Working at a computer won't harm your developing baby, but pregnant women are more susceptible to carpal tunnel syndrome (numb, achy fingers), so try to make your workplace as comfortable as possible.
- Rest, rest, rest. Don't overly exert yourself at home or at work.
- Eat properly. Keep a supply of healthy snacks in your drawer (see p.51).
- Reduce stress. If you can't eliminate stress at work, find ways to manage it, such as deep-breathing exercises, stretching, or simply taking a short walk.
- Accept help. If your colleagues offer to help, make the most of it!

Your rights at work

Some employers are very accommodating when it comes to their employees' pregnancies, but others are far less compassionate. No one can discriminate against you because you're pregnant—employers have to comply with the Pregnancy Discrimination Act.

If you can't do the things you used to do—for example, standing for long periods of time or doing heavy lifting—your employer has to treat you just as he would any other employee with a temporary disability. If you ask for a less strenuous assignment, you can't be refused.

Still, your boss isn't required to make it easier for you to do your work. She doesn't have to give you extra breaks or change your work schedule, for example. If you feel your employer is being especially hard on you, it's up to you to decide whether to continue working at the job, based on what's best for your family and your growing baby. You might want to talk to your human resources department.

ParentsAsk...

Is it safe to use a computer?

It's impossible to prove that using a computer in pregnancy is 100 percent safe, but research has so far failed to find any evidence of harm. So you can be pretty confident that it's safe to use a computer while you are pregnant. However, when you do, make sure you take care of your general health and comfort. Take regular breaks and adjust your chair and monitor so your forearms are roughly horizontal, your back is well supported, and your feet are flat on the floor or a footrest.

Getting ready for pregnancy

Staying safe and healthy

Your pregnancy diary

Birth and beyond

Rights and benefits at work

As a working mom-to-be, you're entitled to certain rights and benefits during pregnancy and beyond. Don't leave it to chance, though. Make sure you keep up-to-date on what rights you're entitled to. You also need to know about the money you might be able to claim.

What are my rights?

It's always nerve-racking telling the boss you're pregnant. But it's worth doing it sooner rather than later. Once you've told your employer, it is against the law for them to dismiss you, treat you unfairly, or lay you off for any reason connected with pregnancy, childbirth, or maternity leave. It doesn't matter how long you have worked for them or how many hours you work.

Before taking maternity leave

Federal law requires you to notify your employer at least 30 days before you plan to begin your maternity leave. Most women prefer to wait until after the first trimester, when the risk of miscarriage is lower, to tell their employers they're pregnant—but you can let your boss know whenever you're comfortable doing so.

Maternity leave

Maternity leave, now often called parental or family leave, allows mothers and fathers time off from work for the birth or adoption of a child. Paid maternity leave is unusual in the United States. Most likely, you'll use a combination of short-term disability (STD), sick leave, vacation, personal days, and unpaid family leave.

The Family and Medical Leave Act (FMLA) entitles most workers to up to 12 weeks of job-protected medical leave for birth or adoption, but it doesn't cover those who work for smaller companies and guarantees only unpaid leave. A few states have enacted paid family leave.

Not all allow women to take short-term disability leave to cover pregnancy, birth, and postpartum recovery.

Short-term disability (STD)

Short-term disability is meant to cover your salary—or some of it—when you can't do your job due to illness, injury, or childbirth. Many large employers and unions offer it, as do several states. Six weeks is the standard amount of time for pregnancy. Some plans allow more if you've had complications or a cesarean. Many also cover bedrest before birth.

State STD benefits typically cover half to two-thirds of your salary. The cover for pregnancy usually lasts four to six weeks but can last up to 12 weeks.

The portion of your salary you get from your employer's coverage is taxable, but no income taxes will be taken out of your checks, so you'll owe the money in April. Money from a state disability program is generally not subject to federal or state income taxes. If you pay for disability insurance yourself, the benefits are also tax-free.

Extending leave

If you've accrued vacation, personal, or sick days, you may want to use them to extend your leave. You may also be

Working mom

If you're working full-time, it's important to figure out when to tell your employer you're pregnant.

"To be absolutely sure that I gave my employer enough notice, I let both human resources and my manager know about my pregnancy by the 15th week before the week that my baby was due. I was nervous about it, but then was thrilled to discover that I could choose exactly when to start my maternity leave. In the end, I decided to let it go as late as possible. That way, I knew I'd be able to enjoy some extra time at home with my baby after the birth."

eligible for unpaid disability leave. If you're unable to return to work when your STD coverage runs out, certain states allow you to take some unpaid pregnancy disability leave. Your employer is required to hold your job for you until you're able to return (or the leave runs out). Your employer may require that you use up your sick days before taking unpaid disability leave.

Unpaid leave

Ask your company's human resources department about the FMLA, which requires many companies to allow men and women 12 weeks of unpaid leave after the birth or adoption of a child. At the end of your leave, your employer must allow you to return to your job or a similar job with the same salary, benefits and working conditions.

Even if you're not eligible under the FMLA, you may still be eligible for leave under your state's provisions (usually more generous than the FMLA), or under your company's family leave policy.

Your employer may require that all the paid leave that you take counts toward the 12 weeks required by the FMLA. But some states and employers allow you to take the full 12 weeks as well as whatever paid leave you take.

You can use your unpaid leave in any way you want during your pregnancy or during the year after your child is born. You can take it all at once or, as long as your employer agrees, you can spread it out over your child's first year and reduce your normal weekly or daily work schedule.

Benefits

With the FMLA, your company must keep you on its health insurance plan while you're on leave but it may or may not contribute to your premium. If you tell your company that you don't plan to return to work, or if your job is eliminated while you're gone, your employer may stop paying your premiums and may even require you to pay back the money spent to maintain your health insurance while you were on leave.

The FMLA doesn't require employers to allow you to accrue benefits or time toward seniority when you're out on leave. The clock may stop on things like vacation accrual and the amount of time you can say you've been with the company in order to qualify for things like raises based on seniority, additional vacation days, participation in your company's 401k plan or vesting of your company's matching investment, or vesting of stock options.

Finally, you won't be able to contribute to your 401k or flexible spending account while you're on leave.

Filing a complaint

If your employer balks at providing benefits that you're certain you are entitled to, gently let your employer know more about these laws. If reason doesn't work and you believe you're entitled to leave, contact your regional office of the Labor Department's Wage and Hour Division to file a complaint. A phone call from the Labor Department to your employer can usually resolve most problems.

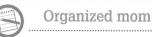

Organized mom

You need to be organized to be sure you claim all your pregnancy rights and benefits.

"I didn't know what rights or benefits my company had in place so I checked with my human resources department before I even started trying to get pregnant. I wanted to be sure everything was in place and had all my ducks in a row before I conceived.

It turns out that I have good benefits but I'll have to tack on some unused vacation time if I want to spend more than three months at home."

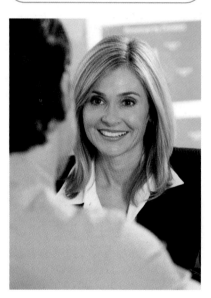

Telling your boss you're pregnant may be a bit nerve-racking, but is essential to ensure you get all the maternity benefits available.

Getting ready for pregnancy

Staying safe and healthy

Your pregnancy diary

Birth and beyond

"Your company **must continue to keep you** on its **health insurance plan** while you're on leave, but it may or may not **contribute to your premium**."

Environmental hazards

Everyday things can suddenly have you worrying about safety when you are pregnant. We round up some of your most common safety worries so that you can feel clear about what does pose a risk to you and your baby, and what doesn't.

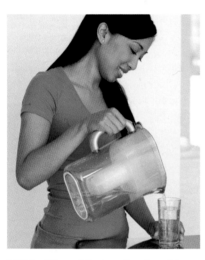

Water filters claim to reduce harmful contaminants such as chlorine and lead in tap water.

Playing safe

You can't live in a sterile bubble during your pregnancy, so start thinking about how to protect your developing baby and minimize the risks of exposure to chemicals and radiation. Talk with your doctor and review exposure information provided by the Organization of Teratology Information Specialists.

Lead and mercury

Various chemicals in our environment can cause birth defects. These are known as "teratogens" and include lead and mercury. How poisonous or harmful a teratogen is depends on different factors, including the amount you're exposed to and when in the pregnancy you are exposed.

You may be exposed to lead if your work or hobbies include ceramics, jewelry making, printmaking, stained glass, electronics, or glassblowing. Lead exposure can also happen during home redecorating if old paint is removed.

The most common way for people to be exposed to mercury is by eating contaminated fish. The highest levels of mercury are found in large fish at the top of the food chain, such as swordfish, shark, and marlin.

Insect repellents

Mosquito repellents often use diethyl-3-methyl benzamide (DEET), but little information is available on any harmful effects in pregnancy. A 2001 study conducted in Thailand showed no adverse effects to mother or baby when moderate amounts were used in the second and third trimesters. But because DEET is considered toxic in high doses, it's still recommended that pregnant women either avoid such repellents or use only small amounts.

As a natural alternative try using an oil that contains citronella, since this is considered safe for pregnant women.

ParentsAsk...

Is it safe to use cell phones?

The short answer to this question is that cell phones probably are safe to use in pregnancy. Research suggests that there is no risk to health from cell phones in the short term, but no one is certain of their long-term effects yet.

Cells emit low levels of "non-ionizing" electromagnetic radiation as do televisions, computers, and microwave ovens. Experts agree that this radiation is unlikely to harm a developing baby. However, if you want to err on the side of caution, you can reduce your exposure from your cell phone by keeping your calls short or by sending a text or using a landline instead.

Is it safe to walk through airport screening machines?

The metal detectors in airports use a low-frequency electromagnetic field to look for metal objects. This exposure is considered safe for everyone, including pregnant women. The same holds true for the wands that are sometimes passed over individual passengers.

X-rays

Most diagnostic X-rays (dental X-rays, for example) do not expose your baby to high enough levels of radiation to cause a problem. While fetal exposure over 10 rads (a rad is the unit of measurement for absorbed radiation) may increase the risk of learning disabilities and eye abnormalities, it's rare for a diagnostic X-ray to exceed 5 rads.

Experts still recommend that women postpone getting unnecessary X-rays until after giving birth. However, if your doctor feels X-rays are needed for your particular medical situation, it may ease your mind to know that the amount of radiation your baby receives will most likely be well within the safe range. On the day of the test, make sure the radiographer knows you are pregnant so she can shield you properly.

If your work involves you being around radiation, you should talk to your supervisor about ways to reduce or eliminate your exposure. You may want to discuss the possibility of wearing a special kind of film badge that monitors the amount of radiation you receive. If you're concerned that your employer isn't addressing safety issues, you should contact your local office of the Occupational Health and Safety Administration, the government agency responsible for safety in the workplace.

Dry-cleaning chemicals

Worries about dry-cleaning chemicals often stem from research that suggested dry-cleaning machine operators had a higher rate of miscarriage than other women. The risk did not apply to other dry-cleaning workers or to women who had their clothes dry cleaned.

The risk occurs because the organic solvents used in dry cleaning can pass through the placenta. Perchloroethylene (perc), a commonly used dry-cleaning fluid, has also been associated with male fertility problems.

Tetrachloroethylene is another solvent sometimes used in commercial dry cleaning. Several studies have found an association between inhalation of tetrachloroethylene and an increased risk of miscarriage and infertility.

If you're pregnant, you'd be wise to minimize your exposure to organic solvents at work. Ask your employer to change your job for the duration or carry out a risk assessment at your workplace.

Laid-back mom

Feeling anxious when pregnant is natural, but it helps to find a way to deal with your worries.

"You know what they say about a trouble shared being a trouble halved? Well, my mom reminded me of that when I was worrying about whether or not our baby was going to be healthy after I had a small show. I'm not usually a worrier, but I couldn't help thinking something was horribly wrong or that I was about to have a miscarriage. So I talked about my concerns to Ian and it turns out he was worrying about the same thing.

Once we'd talked about it together, we agreed that the best thing was to go and see our doctor to try to arrange a scan, just to be sure. I know they say that a scan can't detect every possible problem, but they arranged for us to have one within a few days. I must say, just seeing that fuzzy outline of our growing baby on the screen made us feel a whole lot better!"

ParentsTalk...

"We both decided to cut down on smoking before we started trying to get pregnant. It was really tough at first. But as soon as we found out I was pregnant, it gave us both a very good reason to stop entirely."
Julia, 34, mom to seven-month-old Zoe

"In the early weeks, I have to admit to having the occasional sneaky cigarette when my wife wasn't looking. She'd smell the smoke on me, though. In the end I realized that it wasn't fair to her when she was doing so well at quitting."
Leon, 29, dad to four-month-old Zac

"Quitting smoking was a whole lot easier for me—I found even the smell of it made me feel sick in first three months anyway. And once I'd banned smoking in the house, it was easier for Ben to give up too!"
Hannah, 28, pregnant for the second time

"I knew the risk to the baby of smoking during pregnancy—and we didn't want our baby to be exposed to smoke once he was born, either. There's no better incentive."
Kallie, 29, mom to two-month-old Dan

"Quitting smoking when there's a baby on the way is simply a no-brainer. Giving up was much easier with each other's support."
Frances, 27, mom to month-old Sam

Getting ready for pregnancy

Staying safe and healthy

Your pregnancy diary

Birth and beyond

The body beautiful

After the first trimester, lots of women start to "bloom" and enjoy glowing skin, thick shiny hair, and strong nails. Others aren't so lucky and find themselves struggling with unmanageable hair and blotchy skin. Here are the changes to expect as the weeks pass.

Your skin, hair, and nails

Your appearance changes when you are pregnant, often for the better. However, you may also have to adjust your beauty regimen as you cope with minor problems related to your skin, hair, nails, and teeth.

Your new skin

Glowing skin is one of the great beauty bonuses of being pregnant. However, other, perfectly normal, skin changes may not do as much for your looks. The good news is that they generally clear up soon after your baby is born. Here's an idea of what to expect.

Stretch marks

Thin reddish or brownish (depending on your skin color) lines of stretch marks usually appear on the abdomen, breasts, and thighs. They affect at least half of pregnant women and may appear as you put on more weight and cause the skin to stretch. Higher levels of hormones also disrupt your skin's protein balance, making it thinner.

After pregnancy, the pigmentation in the stretch marks gradually fades, and the streaks become lighter than the surrounding skin. This takes time.

Some lucky women have more elastic skin than others, meaning they won't get stretch marks, but for most of us they are simply a fact of pregnancy. Try to minimize them by avoiding putting on weight too quickly, rubbing oil or cream rich in vitamin E over your abdomen to keep it supple, and eating a healthy diet that is rich in vitamins E and C, and in zinc and silica, to help keep your skin healthy.

After your baby is born, topical medications such as tretinoin (Retin-A) and glycolic acid may help to reduce the

Mellow mom or high-maintenance mom?

Are you a mellow mom or high-maintenance (HM) mom when it comes to beauty treatments? Read on to find out.

On hair
Mellow: put off visiting the hair salon for fear of scaring him with your wild mane.
HM: enjoy a weekly trim and blowdry at an upscale salon, reading *Vogue* while your highlights are touched up.

On pregnancy pampering
Mellow: feel grateful to have 10 minutes of peace in the bathroom with a gossip magazine and a splash of bubble bath.
HM: make it a priority to relax and enjoy regular facials and soothing massages at the spa.

On skin care
Mellow: ditch any pretence of having a cleansing, toning, and moisturizing routine in favor of an extra 10 minutes in your cosy bed.
HM: love your pregnancy glow and buy a new collection of cleansers and lotions to make the most of it—along with plenty of new cosmetics.

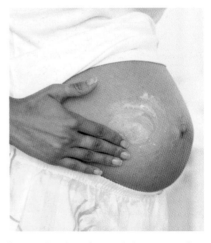

Keep the skin of your abdomen supple and reduce stretch marks by rubbing with a cream or oil that is rich in vitamin E.

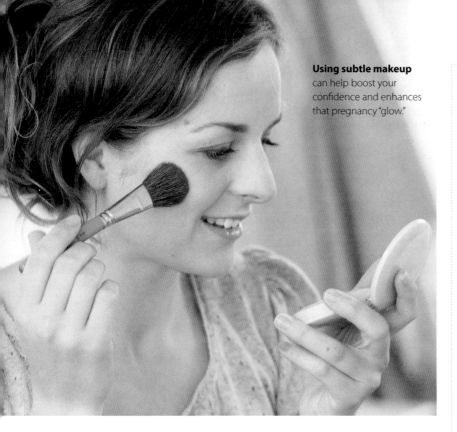

Using subtle makeup can help boost your confidence and enhances that pregnancy "glow."

ParentsTalk...

"With my second pregnancy, the hair on one side of my head, just above my ear, became curly! After having my second baby, I had my hair cut shorter, hoping that would calm it. But that just made it worse and curly all over! I've finally found a stylist that can make it straight, so I'm off to buy some hair straighteners!"
Claire, 35, mom to Mabel and Joelly

"I had problems with my hair. Imagine already having thick hair—and it just getting thicker and thicker! It was also really dry and I looked awful. I kept getting it cut but it didn't make any difference. Not long after having my baby my hair returned to normal and I got it thinned."
Amy, 29, mom to six-month-old Laura

"My hair with my first baby was great! My sister-in-law decided she'd update my look halfway through my pregnancy, and gave me a great crop, a la Posh Spice (short and spiky). But as my belly grew bigger, I looked like a weeble, with a tiny pea-head on top!"
Mel, 34, mom to Lucy and Freddie

appearance of stretch marks. Retin-A is not safe to use during pregnancy and is best avoided while breast-feeding.

Chloasma

Also known as the "mask of pregnancy," chloasma describes the appearance of brown patches of pigment on the neck, cheeks, and forehead. Darker-skinned women have lighter patches. They are caused by the increased production of melanin, the tanning hormone, which protects the skin against ultraviolet light.

Exposure to sunlight will darken the patches, making them more obvious, so protect your skin with a high-factor sunscreen (SPF 30 or more) and a hat when you go out (see pp.96–7). If you are worried that the patches look unsightly, try using a tinted foundation to blend them with your skin. They will begin to fade within three months of your baby's birth.

Linea nigra

The linea nigra is a dark, vertical line, up to a half inch wide, that may appear down the middle of your stomach, often crossing the navel. It tends to appear around the second trimester and is caused by changes in the skin pigment where your abdominal muscles stretch and separate slightly to accommodate your baby as it grows.

The line may darken in sunlight, so you should use a high-factor sunscreen (SPF 30 or more) or avoid the sun completely, especially during the hottest part of the day.

The line should fade within a few weeks of your baby's birth, although it may need a gentle rub to remove any dry skin. Sometimes it can take up to a year to disappear; occasionally it may never fade completely. Other areas with pigmentation—such as your nipples, moles, and freckles—may darken too, but these should also fade.

Glowing skin

The "bloom" or "glow" that's said to accompany pregnancy is not just a myth. Your skin retains more moisture, which plumps it up, smoothing out any fine lines and wrinkles. The pinkish glow that makes you look radiant is due to increased amounts of blood in your body. This may make you feel slightly flushed sometimes.

Another downside is that you may look a little bit puffy from water retention and, unfortunately, any red patches that you already have on your face may become more visible. The solution is not to cut down on drinking water to counteract the fluid retention—your body needs fluids—but simply to rest as much as you can. Any red patches will calm down once you've given birth, but meanwhile if you want to hide them, you could try using a tinted moisturizing foundation.

ParentsTalk...

"I use a commercially available oil for stretch marks and soak in a baby oil bath every night."
Emma, 25, mom-to-be

"I didn't use anything more special than an ordinary baby oil. Listen to your body and take note of areas of skin that are getting a bit tight, then moisturize those parts— several times in a day if you can manage it. Making sure that the skin is elastic will help."
Phoebe, 29, mom to month-old Jake

"I've heard and read that drinking plenty of water is good for preventing stretch marks. I certainly plan to give it a try."
Jenny, 26, mom-to-be

"My stretch marks didn't show until the end of my pregnancy. I used cocoa butter on my hips and belly twice a day, which may have helped, but personally I wouldn't worry about them too much. They fade eventually."
Safa, mom to nine-month old Josh

Spider veins

Small, thin veins that lie close to the surface of the skin may become more noticeable in pregnancy. They tend to run in families and, sadly, don't usually go away after the birth. They can be just faint red lines or else develop as a circle kind of like a spider's web, hence the name spider veins. The good news is they aren't harmful, and are reasonably easy to cover with makeup.

Laser treatment can successfully remove spider veins in the legs—but you shouldn't have this done when you're pregnant. Some complementary therapists say that eating a diet rich in vitamin C will help strengthen capillaries, and that taking extra vitamin E might help, too. However, no studies support either of these suggestions, but it's well worth having a good diet that gives you plenty of these vitamins.

Acne in pregnancy

Pregnancy can sometimes trigger acne. This can come as a shock, as many of us will not have experienced acne since our teenage years. Higher levels of certain hormones can encourage the production of sebum—the oil that keeps our skin supple—and too much sebum causes pores to become blocked, resulting in oily skin and pimples.

To ward off problems, you should cleanse your facial skin regularly with a gentle cleanser and use an oil-free moisturizer. If you prefer to avoid using skin products, keep your skin fresh and clean by patting it dry rather than rubbing, so that you minimize the irritation to the acne.

Don't use acne creams or treatments unless your obstetrician advises you to do so—some of them cannot be used when you are pregnant. A few weeks after your baby is born, your skin should return to its pre-pregnancy condition.

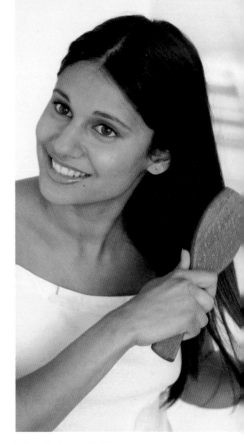

Your hair may look better than ever now that you're pregnant. Pregnancy hormones help to reduce the rate of hair loss.

Ask your doctor before using any over-the-counter lotions or gels to treat your acne. It's particularly important to avoid the oral prescription drug Accutane (isotretinoin), which can cause serious birth defects. You must also avoid tetracycline, doxycycline, and minocycline, which can cause teeth and bone abnormalities in the fetus.

Your hair

During the second trimester, you might notice that your hair looks full and healthy. This isn't because you're growing more but because, thanks to the pregnancy hormones, you're just losing less.

Some women worry about using hair dyes in pregnancy. The chemicals in both permanent and semi-permanent hair dyes have been around a long time.

Getting ready for pregnancy

Staying safe and healthy

Your pregnancy diary

Birth and beyond

No research shows they harm unborn babies, so coloring your hair during pregnancy is probably safe. If you apply the dyes safely (using gloves in a well-ventilated room, and not leaving solutions on for long periods of time), you don't absorb much of the chemicals into your system. However, you may want to wait until after the first trimester, just to be on the safe side.

Another option is highlighting, painting, or frosting your hair. You absorb hair coloring agents into your system through your skin (scalp), not through your hair shaft. So any process that puts less of the chemical in contact with your scalp reduces your exposure to the compounds in dyes.

Vegetable hair dyes are another alternative to chemical dyes when you are pregnant. However, many actually contain the same synthetic chemical compounds found in permanent and semi-permanent dyes. Pure henna, a semi-permanent vegetable dye in various colors, is the exception.

This dye is considered to be very safe. If you like to use an eyelash or eyebrow tint, have a patch test for sensitivity, even if you've had the treatment before without a problem.

Once your due date is approaching, it's a nice idea to book a consultation and cut with a good stylist. You'll be starring in lots of photos alongside your baby over the next few weeks, and there won't be time to have your hair done once she's born. Your stylist can help you find a lower-maintenance style that will see you right through those first few weeks of living with your baby.

Your nails

Around the fourth month, your nails may start to grow faster than usual. This is due to the effects of pregnancy hormones. Your fingernails may become softer or more brittle than usual, and you may notice tiny grooves along the base of the nail. Don't worry; they should return to normal within a few months after giving birth.

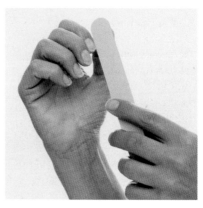

Pregnancy hormones can make your fingernails more brittle, so always file them gently to prevent them from breaking.

Handy makeup camouflage tips

Pregnant women are beautiful, but their skin can also become blotchy, prone to acne, and dry or oily. You don't have to grin and bear it, though, thanks to the wonders of makeup.

● Adjust your skin-care regimen. Add more moisture to combat dryness or change to oil-free products if your skin is feeling oily.

● Apply corrective concealer with a brush to cover hyperpigmentation. Then lightly spread foundation or tinted moisturizer over your whole face.

● When you're lacking a healthy glow apply a pretty shade of blush or a light touch of bronzer over your face.

● If your eyelashes appear a little sparse, invest in a good pair of eyelash curlers. Finish by applying lots of lengthening and thickening mascara.

● Apply a shimmery highlighter over your cheek- and brow-bones for an extra sparkle.

● Keep your beauty routine simple—you'll need it for when you don't have so much time to beautify!

Your dental health

Gum problems are a common concern in pregnancy. You may find that your gums bleed when you brush or floss them. This is because the hormone progesterone softens your gums and your increased blood supply makes them more likely to react to the bacteria in the plaque that forms on your teeth.

Take good care of your teeth in pregnancy, partly to avoid bleeding gums (gingivitis) developing into a more serious condition called periodontitis. One study has shown that infection can progress from your gums into your teeth and jaw bones, and may possibly cause premature labor in some mothers.

Brush your teeth thoroughly but gently. If you brush them too vigorously you can damage your fragile gums. Make sure you brush your teeth at least twice a day. You should try to brush after every meal, preferably within 20 minutes of eating or drinking anything. Use a brush with soft bristles or, better still, an electric or battery-operated toothbrush. Use fluoride toothpaste, and floss at least once a day. Eat a well balanced diet and avoid carbonated or sugary drinks.

If you haven't seen your dentist recently, schedule a visit for a thorough cleaning and checkup. And be sure to let her know that you're pregnant.

Pregnancy weight gain

Piling on the pounds during pregnancy is difficult for the body-conscious among us, but it's a sign that your pregnancy is progressing well. Too much weight gain, though, isn't good either for you or your baby, so try not to indulge too often in comforting sugary snacks.

Don't pile on the pounds

First and foremost, it is important to accept that you are going to put on weight during pregnancy! You are meant to because your body is growing and changing to give your baby the best possible start in life.

The amount of weight you should gain will depend on how heavy you were before you became pregnant. Or, more accurately, on what your body mass index (BMI) was.

Your doctor can help you calculate your BMI. If you would like to have a try at doing it yourself, here's how it's done:
1. Divide your weight in pounds by your height in inches squared.
2. Then multiply by 703. If you're 5'5" and weigh 150 pounds, your BMI would be 150 divided by 4225, multiplied by 703, for a BMI of 24.96.

Here's how your BMI is classified:
BMI less than 18.5—Underweight
BMI 18.5 to 25—Ideal
BMI 25 to 30—Overweight
BMI 30 to 40—Obese
BMI greater than 40—Severely obese

The Institute of Medicine recommends that women aim for weight gain related to their BMI before they became pregnant:
● If your pre-pregnancy weight was in the healthy range for your height (a BMI of 18.5 to 24.9), you should gain between 25 and 35 pounds, gaining 1 to 5 pounds in the first trimester and about 1 pound per week for the rest of your pregnancy for the optimal growth of your baby.

What makes up your pregnancy weight gain

Your weight at the end of pregnancy compared to what it was before you became pregnant is considerable. Here's where the extra weight comes from:
● At birth, your baby will weigh approximately 7¼ pounds.
● During pregnancy, the muscle layer of your uterus grows dramatically and weighs an extra 2 pounds.
● The placenta (afterbirth), which keeps your baby nourished, weighs around 1¼ pounds.
● Your blood volume increases and weighs an extra 2¾ pounds.
● Your breasts are busy creating milk-producing tissue and, at birth, will weigh an extra ¾ pound.
● You have extra fluid in your body, and amniotic fluid around the baby, weighing 5¾ pounds.
● Plus, you will lay down some fat during your pregnancy to provide you with extra energy for breast-feeding. This comes to about 5½ pounds.

These are only average figures. The actual amount of weight you should gain will depend on how heavy you were before you became pregnant. Your age, race, and height will also influence how your body will change over the next nine months.

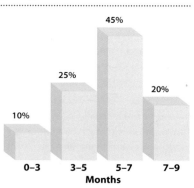

This chart shows at what stage of your pregnancy you will put on weight, and what percentage of your total pregnancy weight gain should occur when.

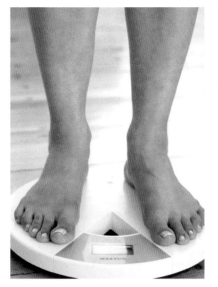

Accept that you will gain weight during pregnancy, but eat a healthy, well-balanced diet to protect yourself and your baby.

ParentsTalk...

"I think the reason I was getting so depressed was because so much of my sense of identity was in my self image. I really had to pull myself together and realize that the first of my many sacrifices as a parent had to be my figure for a few months. It's worth it for a baby. I'm now trying to just stay healthy rather than slim by going swimming twice a week to keep my fitness level up."
Kate, 25, mom to two-month-old Bea

"One thing that drives me crazy is when you see someone that you haven't seen for a while and the first thing they say is, 'Wow, you're huge.' Like I hadn't noticed! I feel like saying, 'I do have another person growing inside of me you know. What's your excuse?'"
Emma, first-time mom-to-be

"I knew I was overeating early in my pregnancy so I started walking, swimming, and basically doing whatever I could to keep active. I've come to accept the weight gain and now I simply plan to get back to my normal weight within a year after the birth. I am sure I can do it!"
Polly, mom to four-month-old Daisy

• If you were underweight for your height at conception (a BMI below 18.5), you should gain 28 to 40 pounds.
• If you were overweight for your height (a BMI of 25 to 29.9), you should gain 15 to 25 pounds. If you were obese (a BMI of 30 or higher), you should gain between 11 and 20 pounds.
• If you're having twins, you should gain 37 to 54 pounds if you started at a healthy weight, 31 to 50 pounds if you were overweight, and 25 to 42 pounds if you were obese.

Limiting your weight gain
Women with a high pre-pregnancy BMI should try to limit their weight gain. Putting on a lot of weight could increase your risk of getting high blood pressure (see pp.229–30), gestational diabetes (see p.229), and having a big baby.

Don't try to diet, though. Research shows that, for a pregnant woman who is overweight—or who has put on a lot of weight in the first half of pregnancy—a low-calorie diet does not reduce your chances of developing high blood pressure or preeclampsia.

Instead, get some advice from your doctor about how to eat a sensible, nourishing diet. It's far better to stick to a normal, well-balanced diet (see pp.120–21, 148–9 and 182–3) and just cut out things such as cookies, candy, and ice cream, which are loaded with calories and are low on nutritional value. Just eat sensibly, keeping in mind that a pregnant woman needs approximately 2,500 calories a day.

If you are underweight, you risk having a small baby who may have lots of problems. If you are already pregnant, speak to your doctor and ask for advice on the best diet for you and your baby.

In 2002, the American Association for Cancer Research reported a study showing that women who put on a lot of weight during pregnancy and don't lose it again afterward are at increased risk of developing breast cancer after menopause. Experts recommend that women should pay attention to their lifestyle during pregnancy and especially to getting regular exercise. They also recommend women try to lose any excess "baby weight" after having their baby and before menopause.

Losing the weight
Much of that weight will be gone pretty soon after you give birth. Mothers usually lose half of their pregnancy weight gain by six weeks after delivery.

For the rest, remember that it took nine months to put on the weight, and it can take just as long or longer for it to come off. A healthy diet combined with regular exercise is the best way to shed the pounds—and keep them off.

Don't start cutting back on calories right away, though. Being the mother of a newborn requires lots of energy—and that means giving your body all the nutrition it needs. If you're patient and give your body a chance to do its work, you may be surprised at how much weight you lose naturally, especially if you're breast-feeding.

Getting ready for pregnancy

Staying safe and healthy

Your pregnancy diary

Birth and beyond

Hormones in pregnancy

Hormones play a vital role in maintaining your pregnancy and kickstarting labor. From telling your body that pregnancy has begun, to relaxing ligaments so that your baby can pass through the birth canal, here's how your body's chemical messengers do their amazing job.

What do the hormones do?

Hormones are substances formed in our body and carried in the blood to other parts of the body to make them perform specific tasks. They are vital in pregnancy, creating a variety of physical and mental effects. We blame everything from mood swings to swollen ankles and varicose veins on "hormones," but which hormones are responsible and what do they do?

Human chorionic gonadotropin (hCG)

Your body makes large amounts of the hormone hCG in early pregnancy (see p.36). This hormone plays a key part in your baby's development, makes your periods stop, and maintains the high levels of progesterone that are needed for a healthy pregnancy.

It is also thought that hCG is the hormone that is responsible for nausea and vomiting.

Fact: Around 8 out of 10 women feel sick in pregnancy, and about half actually vomit. The cause is unknown, but it's thought to be connected to the hormone hCG. Other hormones, such as estrogen and thyroxine, are also thought to be responsible.

Human placental lactogen (hPL)

Made by the placenta, this hormone may help to prepare your breasts for breast-feeding. The hormone hPL also ensures your body uses less glucose, which leaves more for your baby. This hormone can block the action of insulin in your body. Your pancreas usually creates more insulin to compensate, but occasionally it doesn't, which can result in gestational diabetes (see p.229).

Estrogen

Your estrogen levels increase tenfold during pregnancy. Among other effects, estrogen ensures that the uterus can receive and maintain a fertilized egg. High levels mean that some women find their skin improves during pregnancy. Estrogen makes your breasts swell and makes your vagina extra sensitive. It also makes your blood clot more easily. Obstetric cholestasis (see pp.230–31) is a rare condition related to a liver problem. It's believed to be associated with high levels of estrogen.

Progesterone

When you become pregnant your ovaries produce more progesterone, which helps keep the lining of your

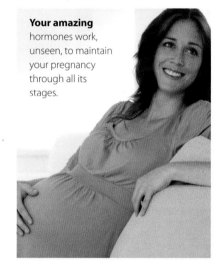

Your amazing hormones work, unseen, to maintain your pregnancy through all its stages.

uterus thick for implantation of the fertilized egg. Later, the placenta produces progesterone, which causes your blood vessels to relax or soften. This can make your gums swell and become inflamed, which leads to frequent, easy bleeding, especially when you floss or brush.

Progesterone also swells your nasal passages, can lead to varicose veins, and may raise your core body temperature, so you feel hot. It can also affect your gut, causing bloating, indigestion, heartburn, and constipation.

Both progesterone and estrogen are thought to be partly responsible for pregnancy mood swings, but general stress and fatigue, coupled with the fact that you're going through a major life change also play a large part.

Relaxin

During pregnancy you produce a hormone called relaxin, which softens your ligaments, allowing the joints in your pelvis to open so your baby can be born. Sometimes, however, relaxin can cause problems where the joints open up too far, and become unstable, causing back and pelvic pain. Higher levels of relaxin in your body can also make you more prone to injury, which is why it's not a good idea to start a strict exercise regimen when you're pregnant.

Melanocyte stimulating hormone (MSH)

This hormone, together with estrogen and progesterone, is responsible for some skin changes during pregnancy. For example, it produces the linea nigra, a dark, vertical line down the middle of your stomach (see p.69). The line usually appears around the second trimester where your abdominal muscles stretch and separate a little, to make room for your growing baby. The line fades within a few weeks of your baby's birth.

MSH may also affect pigmented areas, such as freckles, nipples, and moles, which may darken. You may also get chloasma, the "mask of pregnancy" (see p.69). This is brown patches of pigmentation that appear on your forehead, cheeks, and neck. All these conditions usually fade a few months after your baby is born.

Oxytocin and endorphins

Oxytocin and endorphin levels rise in pregnancy. These hormones help us to feel happy, and help us deal with stress and pain. They rise sharply during labor—preparing you for birth. Oxytocin triggers contractions and stimulates the flow of breast milk.

Hormonal changes

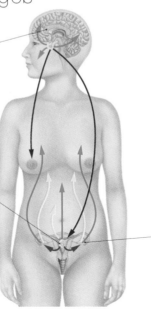

Pituitary gland produces oxytocin, endorphins, and MSH, and helps to prepare the breasts for breast-feeding

Placenta produces hCG, hPL, and relaxin

Hormones affect the whole body, but specific hormones are secreted during pregnancy—from the moment of conception through to birth—to act on specific parts of the body.

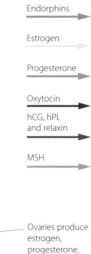

Endorphins →

Estrogen →

Progesterone →

Oxytocin →

hCG, hPL and relaxin →

MSH →

Ovaries produce estrogen, progesterone, and relaxin

Getting ready for pregnancy

Staying safe and healthy

Your pregnancy diary

Birth and beyond

Staying positive

You've taken the pregnancy test and shared the good news with everyone. They all say, "Congratulations! You must be so happy." Yes, you are glad you're expecting, but you're downright unhappy sometimes. Don't worry—these ups and downs are a very normal part of pregnancy.

Emotions and mood swings

Are you fine one minute and in tears the next? Welcome to the club—it's quite common to have major fluctuations in your emotions during pregnancy.

Progesterone and estrogen, the hormones that regulate the reproductive cycle (see pp.28–9), are thought to be partly responsible, but much of your moodiness is simply because pregnancy is a time of tremendous change. You may be overjoyed at the thought of having a baby one day, then just as quickly begin wondering what on earth it is that you've got yourself into.

Even when a baby is very much wanted, many ecstatic mothers-to-be find that concerns about the future momentarily cloud their happiness. You may be worried about how your relationship will be affected, the health of the baby you're carrying, and how you'll handle future financial challenges. Some of the minor problems of pregnancy, such as heartburn, fatigue, and frequent urination, can also be a burden.

You may also find that your dreams seem more bizarre than usual, filled with images of sex, talking animals, and huge, towering buildings, for example. This is completely normal. These dreams may provide a way for your subconscious to deal with any fears and insecurities you may have about pregnancy and motherhood. Or they may just be sleep disturbances caused by indigestion, hormones, or aches and pains.

For a few women, pregnancy mood swings can turn into depression. You're more vulnerable if there are aspects of your life that aren't going well. For instance, you are more likely to suffer from depression if you aren't getting along well with your partner, or you don't have a partner living with you. If you feel you may have depression, speak to your obstetrician.

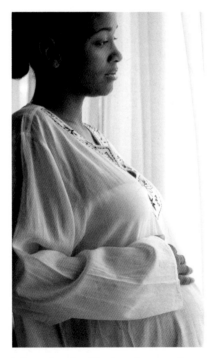

Pregnancy is a life-changing experience so it's perfectly normal for you to feel up some days and down on others.

Single mom

Being a mom on your own is a real challenge, so you need to find ways to stay upbeat.

"There are days when I wonder what the hell I'm doing and others when I'm so happy that I'm pregnant. Maybe I would be like this even if I wasn't on my own but I'm sure it's making the worry worse. I try to keep busy and I've started writing my worries down. It helps to stop me from going over the same thoughts again and again. Then when I've written it down I put it away and get on with something else.

My main worry is that my little girl will grow up not having a daddy. My doctor offered to write a note getting me out of work for a week, but I think that would make me feel even more isolated than I feel already."

Managing your mood swings

Mood swings tend to be most pronounced in the first 12 weeks of pregnancy. However, they should gradually diminish as you figure things out and as your body adapts to the hormonal onslaught.

If you're down in the dumps, do something that makes you feel good. Take a nap, go for a walk, or see a movie with a friend. Talk your feelings through with your partner, friends, and family or, if you prefer, with your obstetrician. Talk therapy is one of the best antidotes. Don't be hard on yourself. Pregnancy is a life-changing event. It's bound to make anyone—even a mom who's wanted a baby for years—feel overwhelmed and anxious sometimes.

Talking to a good friend about your anxieties can help you deal with them.

If you feel like your mood swings are more than run-of-the-mill, it may be a good idea for you to see a counselor or therapist. About 10 percent of expectant women battle mild to moderate depression throughout their pregnancies. If you often or consistently feel blue, you may fall into this category.

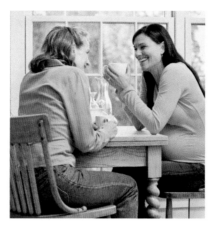

Getting ready for pregnancy

Staying safe and healthy

Your pregnancy diary

Birth and beyond

Dad's **Diary**

More than baby blues
"My wife had postpartum depression after our first son was born. Sarah had enjoyed her pregnancy—and was so excited about becoming a mom. But after we brought Harry home, she got anxious and irritable. She'd cry over the slightest problem. We'd read about the baby blues and thought that, with some rest and time, she'd be soon be back to normal. But things only got worse. It took a while to convince her that she needed help. I don't think she would have gone if I hadn't offered to go with her. The doctor prescribed some medicine and I took a couple of weeks off to help take care of Harry, do housework, and just generally be there for her. That helped her—and it helped me feel like I could actually do something to support her."

Need professional help?

Pregnancy is usually a positive time, but not for every woman. About one in 10 women suffers from bouts of depression during pregnancy.

There isn't a simple set of symptoms which add up to depression; it varies from person to person. Some people have a low mood all the time, others feel irritable and tearful, or feel useless and want to withdraw from life. Possible triggers for depression include:
- stressful life events
- low income
- problems with the pregnancy
- complications that you've had in a previous pregnancy
- infertility or previous pregnancy loss
- abuse—past or present
- having a family or personal history of depression

To ward off prenatal depression, or to manage it once you have it:
- **Take it easy** Read a book, have breakfast in bed, or meet up with a friend. Don't feel guilty: taking care of yourself is an essential part of taking care of your baby.
- **Get active** Exercise can help lift your mood and is a recognized therapy for mild and moderate depression.
- **Talk it out** Keep the lines of communication between you and your partner free and clear.
- **Consider therapy or counseling** If you have tried everything you can for two weeks to try to snap yourself out of a low spell, but nothing seems to work, seeing a therapist or a counselor may help. You should talk to your doctor about this.

Knowing when you need help

These are just some of the symptoms that you may have if you're suffering from depression:
- inability to concentrate
- anxiety
- extreme irritability
- sleep problems
- extreme or unending fatigue
- a desire to eat all the time or not wanting to eat at all
- a sense that nothing feels enjoyable or fun any more
- difficulty making decisions
- persistent sadness

If you're feeling suicidal, or disoriented, unable to handle your daily responsibilities, or if you're having panic attacks, talk to your doctor immediately.

First-time parents

If this is your first baby, no doubt you're incredibly excited, but also a little nervous. Try to relax and enjoy your pregnancy. Your obstetrician is there to support you throughout and you can learn all you need to know about giving birth at your local childbirth classes.

Your childbirth classes

For first-time parents, pregnancy, and the arrival of your baby, is a giant step into the unknown. Childbirth classes can be a great help to you. They come in a variety of forms, but all have the same aim—to help prepare you and your partner for labor, birth, and early parenthood. Most hospitals offer classes, or you can take one through an independent organization. (When attending classes other than those run by your hospital, check that the teacher is properly trained.) If an online class better suits your schedule or your budget, you can try the one offered at

BabyCenter. Childbirth classes not only help you focus on your pregnancy and forthcoming labor and birth, they're also a great place to meet other parents-to-be. After everyone's births, you'll have a network of friends in place whose babies are the same age as yours.

Your doctor can tell you about classes in your area. They can vary considerably—for example, they may be between three and six sessions of different lengths in the afternoon or evening, or the course might take place over a weekend. They can get very booked up so ask about them early on.

The classes should include some of the following:

● Information about the process of labor and childbirth.
● Signs of labor.
● What-to-expect details of medical procedures and interventions.
● Advice on relaxation techniques.
● The opportunity to learn about and experiment with different birth positions.
● A guide to pain relief choices and techniques for coping with pain.
● The chance to learn and try out massage skills and breathing techniques.
● Time to ask questions and to rehearse the variety of decisions you may have to make during labor.
● Some indication of the changes you might experience after the birth and in early parenthood, including the basics of taking care of a newborn.

Classes may include a tour around the labor unit of your hospital. This gives you the chance to get familiar with the layout and to find out how things are done there.

Whatever class you decide to attend, the idea is that both you and your partner will acquire the skills and confidence you need to make birth and the early days with your baby a really positive experience.

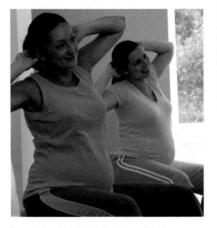

Your local childbirth class will help prepare you for the next few months, and it's a great place to meet other moms-to-be.

ParentsAsk...

How will we ever manage on a single income?
When crunch time comes and that second income vanishes, parents often find it financially easier than they had expected. If you add up the cost of your working wardrobe, commuting, lunches, coffees, and more, you'll be amazed at how much you can save. And remember, too, that if you do decide to go back to work after you've had your baby, child care will probably eat up a large part of your salary.

Getting ready for pregnancy

Staying safe and healthy

Your pregnancy diary

Birth and beyond

The challenge of stopping work

Whichever way you do it, babies are expensive. If one of you decides to stay at home you lose one salary or, if you both work and you're not lucky enough to have family or friends caring for your baby, you have to pay for child care.

But money isn't the only factor when making your decision. In general, society encourages mothers to return to work—all your friends may go back and you may feel pressure to do the same. Yet running a family home and taking care of children is much harder work than many other jobs so working may be an attractive option. Around half of all mothers have returned to work by the time their child reaches the age of one.

Decisions about whether to return to work are often made by looking back on our own childhood. It may be that we don't want to give up as much as our mothers gave up for us, or maybe our mother held down a responsible job and wasn't around that much for us.

Flexibility is an issue, too. Some jobs are flexible, while others are more difficult to adapt to family life. If you work in an office, for example, and your company has a rigid approach to overtime and early morning meetings, there's a risk that you will be resented by colleagues if you have to leave at 5 pm to pick up your children every day.

For some women there's the need to know that they are financially independent and can continue climbing the career ladder. Staying at work can also provide insurance for the future. Although life may be more difficult short term, the long-term prospects are better.

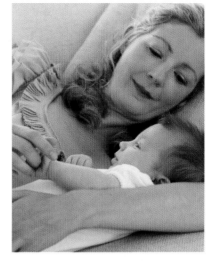

Staying at home with your baby is not always easier than the job you were doing before, so try not to feel pressured to return to work if you don't want to.

The role of dads

During those early weeks, it can be hard for dads to work out how to get involved. Here are our top tips for being the best possible dad from the word go:

- **Educate yourself** Read all you can on pregnancy and babies. It isn't rocket science, but you've got homework to do.
- **Practice, practice, practice** Learn how to do it just like mom. So get in there and change that dirty diaper, give your baby a bath, and do your best to comfort him when he's fussy.
- **Take the time** Once you're back at work, make spending time with your baby a regular part of your evening and weekend routine.
- **Step in** It's vital for your baby, and for your partner's sanity, that you take over some of the chores.

- **Stand your ground** If your partner criticizes your attempts at helping—which she will, without realizing it—gently remind her that you can handle it, as long as she gives you the chance.
- **Be a breast-feeding partner** If your partner is breast-feeding, bring your baby to her for feedings and, once breast-feeding is well established, you could give the occasional bottle of expressed milk. Your partner will be eternally grateful and you'll get some baby-bonding time.
- **Get physical** Fathers interact differently with their baby to mothers: dads' high-energy physical play is the perfect counterpoint to moms' gentler, nurturing care. So don't hesitate to offer a game of airplane, horsey, or other time-tested dad-and-baby pastimes.

Dad's **Diary**

Coming to terms with fatherhood

"In the final months of my wife's pregnancy, people would corner me in the elevator at work and say things like, 'So, are you enjoying your last days?', as if I had terminal cancer. A lot of people fear parenthood as the death knell of their creative ambitions.

I started compiling a mental list of activities that I'd never done and now would never get around to doing. Joining the foreign legion, joyriding, going on tour with my favorite band, climbing Mt. Everest! I quickly realized that all these things actually sounded horrible, and I found the idea of dividing my spare time between 'Goodnight Moon' and a box of Lego quite appealing. All those dreams—that best-selling novel! That winning goal in the World Cup final!—time to let go!"

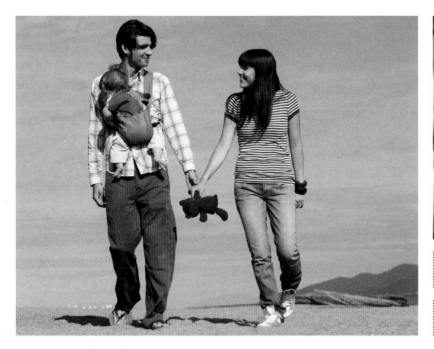

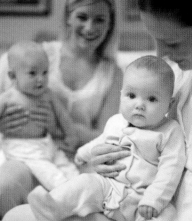

Meeting other moms (above) who have babies the same age as yours can be a social lifesaver during that first year.

Making time for each other (left) and involving dad in the care of your baby can help solidify your new family.

Is there life after baby?

Yes! But it won't be the same as the life you have now. You and your baby will be on a round-the-clock cycle of feeding, diaper changing, and comforting and there just won't be a moment for anything else. A typical newborn sleeps for between 16 and 20 hours in a 24 hour period, but that will be in bits and pieces throughout the day and it will never feel like enough time to get anything done. As time goes on, and your baby begins to settle into a routine, you should be able to carve a little space for yourself in his days. Until then, it's really important to give yourself time to adjust and don't expect too much of yourself. If you have fed your baby, changed his diaper, and cuddled him you will have done enough. So what if you aren't even dressed!

The feeling that your time is not your own is one of the hardest things to get used to when you're a new parent but

there are lots of other adjustments to be made, too. You and your partner will have to get used to each other as parents and that can be a difficult process. He may feel jealous of the attention you give to your baby and if you've given up work, even if only temporarily, you may feel jealous of his life outside the home. On the plus side, you will see a whole new side of each other as you grow together as a family.

You may think that having a baby means the end of your social life but that need not necessarily be the case. However, if going out used to mean going for a drink after work you'll find you need to make some new daytime friends. Moms with babies the same age as yours will be a lifeline during your baby's first year and there are lots of classes and activities you will be able to take your baby to. Far from having no

social life you may find that you're busier than ever—even if big nights out are a thing of the past. If you're planning to go back to work when your maternity leave finishes you may find you feel differently after your baby is born. You may want to work part-time or you may decide that you want to embark on a new career entirely. So there is undoubtedly life after having a baby, but perhaps the best approach is to keep an open mind as to what that life will be.

51% of women who give birth to their first child return to work within four months, according to the US Census. As of 2002, 55 percent of all mothers were working six months after giving birth, increasing to 64 percent by a year.

Avoiding isolation

During those early days with your newborn you can feel quite isolated. Just getting out of the house can be hard enough; the thought of being social and making new friends can seem impossible. Don't worry, there are lots of ways of meeting new "mom friends." And the great thing about meeting other new moms is that they know just how you feel.

The first obvious port of call is your doctor and the maternity department of the hospital where you delivered. The hospital may offer breast-feeding or support groups for new parents where you can talk, ask questions, and enjoy some company. If your hospital doesn't offer those services, your doctor can help you find local support groups.

Another good source of new friends are mother-and-baby groups. To find one in your area, looks for ads in newspapers and parenting publications, and check with your local hospital, child-care cooperatives, universities, libraries, churches, synagogues, and other community organizations. Also, go online to find resources in your area.

Look out for baby-signing classes, baby music groups, and mother-and-baby swimming classes, as well. Some movie theaters now have special mother-and-baby showings of the latest film releases, and many libraries have story times for babies and toddlers.

An easy way to meet local moms is to simply go outside: Pack your baby in her stroller and head to a park, to a children's museum, or around the neighborhood. A warm greeting could be the start to rich friendships, for you and your baby.

Getting some help

It can be hard to get the help you need during those first few weeks with a new baby. You feel like you're suddenly trying to juggle 100 things at once, while being the most exhausted you have ever been. The best guests will ask you what they can do to help. You shouldn't be afraid to tell them.

The truth is that your guests are there to see your baby. Take advantage of this and let them bill and coo over your little one while you use the time to take that relaxing bath you've been craving or take a nap. When guests phone to say they're on their way, don't dash around making coffee and cleaning up. They'll be only too glad to help out with those things when they arrive.

If you know that guests will be arriving in the next few days, phone them and ask them to stop off at the supermarket on their way over to pick up any groceries that you need. It may feel bold asking, but it will be a lifesaver until you feel able to face the stimulation of the supermarket yourself.

Even better, put out the word that you would really appreciate a few home-cooked meals. When you're a new mom (or any mom for that matter!), there's nothing better than tucking into a delicious meal that someone else has gone to the trouble of cooking.

If mom is coming to visit, ask her to bring some essential groceries with her.

Working mom

It's perfectly normal to worry about how having a baby might affect your career.

"I'm still unsure if I'll go back to work after my baby's born. I know I'll definitely take at least six months maternity leave, but I haven't decided whether I'll go back to work part-time, full-time—or at all.

The idea of us living on just one income is something I'm struggling to get my head around, although I'm sure there are ways to save money. If I stay home I won't do my coffee-shop run every day to begin with, and we could spend less on vacations.

But it's more than just the money. I've worked very hard to get where I am today and I worry that, if I don't go back to work, it'll take me years to get my next promotion. My company has a fairly child-friendly policy, and I've got the option to go back part-time, but I feel you have to be seen to be totally committed to the job.

I guess I'll have to wait until after the baby is born and see how I feel then."

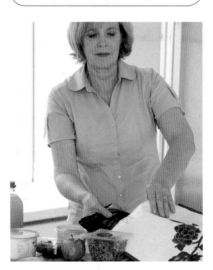

Coping with a sibling

Those first weeks with a newborn are always hectic, but even more so if you already have a toddler. Make your new baby's entrance into the world easier by preparing your toddler in advance for her arrival. With luck this will help to keep sibling rivalry at bay.

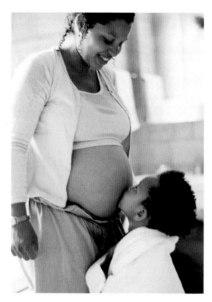

Encourage any interest your toddler shows in your developing baby. It can help him deal with any jealousy he will feel.

Be prepared

Once you've told your toddler he's going to have a sibling, let him decide how much he wants to talk about it or be involved in the preparations.

He may be curious about what the baby is doing in there: "Is she moving around?" Let him feel the baby kicking once her movements are strong enough. Also consider taking him to an ultrasound scan so he can see the baby. It will help to make it more real for him.

Keep your talk about the new baby light and positive. If you want to explain your fatigue, for example, you could say, "Growing a baby is hard work. I sometimes felt tired when you were growing inside, too." Toddlers like to hear about themselves and learning

about any similarities will help him to feel closer to the baby. You can also tell your toddler stories about what he was like when he was a baby. Explain how excited you were when he was born so he understands that he was once the baby who got the special attention.

As you get more focused on the impending labor, your toddler may become clingy, develop new fears, and even regress slightly. This is all perfectly

Top tips for coping with more than one

- Prepare as much as possible—for example, cook and freeze meals while you're still pregnant so you've a supply of nutritious food to see you all through the early post-birth days.
- Lower your expectations—it doesn't matter if the dusting doesn't get done, if there are crumbs on the floor, or you wear un-ironed clothes.
- Help your toddler feel included—let him play with the baby's things and unwrap presents that arrive for her.
- Regularly reassure your toddler that you love him and that having the new baby hasn't changed your feelings toward him.

Parents**Ask...**

How should I break the news to our toddler?

When you're ready to tell him about the pregnancy, keep the language positive and simple. For example, "There's a baby growing inside Mommy. You are going to have a little sister or brother next year." Perhaps start reading him stories about babies or siblings or talk about his friends and their little siblings.

Can I leave my toddler alone in a room with my new baby?

It's probably sensible to stay nearby in the early weeks in case your baby is the subject of any misplaced attention. If you have to move out of the room where the children are for more than a few moments, encourage your toddler to come and help you, or distract him from the baby by offering him some activity.

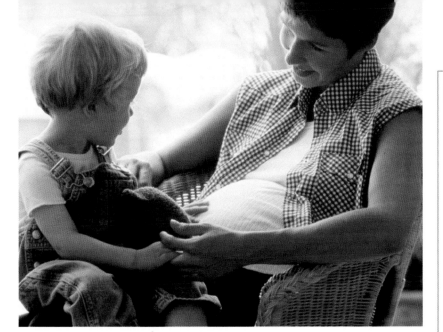
Children like to hear stories about when they were smaller. Telling him how you felt when he was in your belly helps to make him feel closer to your unborn baby.

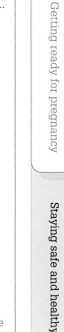

normal. Lots of love and affection will help him to regain his confidence, so try to spend as much time as you can with him during these last few weeks before your new baby is born.

Dealing with jealousy

It can be especially hard for a toddler who thinks he's the center of the universe to welcome a new baby into his home. Desperate to win your attention, he may react by misbehaving, regressing, or even by giving his new sibling a few less-than-subtle pinches, prods, or smacks.

Rather than scolding him, acknowledge his feelings by saying something like, "I know you wish I wouldn't spend so much time with the baby, but she needs her diaper changed right now. As soon as I've finished we'll read a story together." Set aside time each day to do something just with him, even if it's only a few minutes drawing or playing. If he is aggressive toward the new baby, intervene right away. Tell him plainly that his behavior is not acceptable and that it's never okay to hurt the baby. It may help you both to give him a time out until he is calmer.

> ### Organized mom
> ....
> *Even the most organized moms need some help when they're expecting a second baby.*
>
> "We thought we could manage by ourselves when we were having Tom, but when crunch time came, we realized we'd need some help. Mom had said she'd watch Emma when I went into labor, and fortunately she lives nearby, so as soon as I got a few twinges I called her to warn her. We were determined that we should tell Emma about her new brother, so although Mom was busting to break the news, we made sure she didn't. When I gave the word, she brought Emma to see us in the hospital. I like to think Tom was a nice surprise!
>
> My best friend Jo was great, too. She made some meals and put them in the freezer while I was in the hospital and she did a quick tidy up before I got home. That's what friends are for."

Blended families

While marriage breakdown is a sad fact of life for many people, one in two divorced parents goes on to remarry or re-partner. When new partners have a baby together it can be difficult for existing children. They often see it as a signal that their parents will never get back together, and might be jealous of the new baby. To make the arrival of a new baby easier:

● You and your partner should tell your children about the new baby together—it's not a good idea to let them find out from anyone else.
● Once everyone knows, spend plenty of time with your children and stepchildren, reassure them that you still love them and that will never change.
● Decide with your partner how to describe the relationship between existing children and the new baby—will they be half-siblings or just siblings?
● Once baby arrives, give your other children opportunities to help take care of him and to choose gifts, names, and clothes. Don't force them if they're reluctant—they may need more time.
● In the early days, set aside some one-on-one time each day to spend with your children.

Sex in pregnancy

Nausea and fatigue can put a dampener on your love life during the first trimester of pregnancy. But once you are feeling up to it, there's no reason why you and your partner shouldn't enjoy a normal sex life, even when your growing belly starts to get in the way.

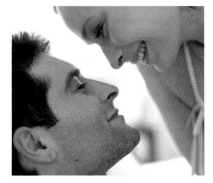

It's perfectly safe to have sex when you're pregnant, but your libido—and his—may fluctuate wildly with every stage.

Parents**Talk...**

"I must say I found my wife's pregnant body really sexy. And knowing that we'd made a baby really brought us closer together. I think we had our best sex ever."
Tom, 31, dad to six-month-old Ethan

"I was totally turned off by sex for the first three or four months of my pregnancy. Besides the fact that I felt sick most of the time, I just wasn't interested anymore. Things really improved during the second trimester, though—much to my boyfriend's relief!"
Nadia, 20, pregnant for the first time

Where's my libido gone?

During pregnancy, sex is even better for some women, not as good for others. Increased blood flow to the pelvic area can cause engorgement of the genitals and heighten the sensation. But the same engorgement gives other women an uncomfortable feeling of fullness after intercourse ends. Sometimes, women find sex painful during pregnancy.

Also, some women feel abdominal cramps during or after intercourse because orgasm can set off a wave of contractions. This may be particularly noticeable in the third trimester. It can be off-putting but give it a few minutes and the tightening of your uterus will ease; just like it does when you have Braxton Hicks contractions.

The big changes in your body are bound to change your sex life. Some women, finally free from worries about conception and contraception, feel sexier than ever. But others are just too tired or nauseated to make love, especially in the first trimester. Some women find that their libido is at a high in the second trimester but, there is always a wide variety in how women feel and how sexually active couples are.

All these feelings and experiences are perfectly normal—every woman is different, and it's just as normal to experience either more or less desire at the various stages of pregnancy.

It's not uncommon for men to feel just as sexually attracted to their partner in the first two trimesters but then to feel less interested in sex in the third trimester. But don't worry: this doesn't mean necessarily that he doesn't find you attractive anymore. Your partner's desire may be dampened by fear that sex can hurt the baby. Or he may be worried about you and your unborn baby's health, feel apprehensive about the burdens of parenthood, or even feel self-conscious about making love in the presence of your unborn child.

Is it safe?

Sex is perfectly safe during a normal pregnancy, and you can keep on making love right up until your water breaks if you feel like it. If you're feeling sexy and well enough, having sex during pregnancy may be good for your relationship now and after your baby has arrived. But check with your doctor first if you're having any problems, such as a low-lying placenta (placenta previa) or bleeding, or if you have a history of cervical weakness. There are situations when sex isn't a good idea (see opposite).

Lovemaking in later pregnancy

Desire sometimes wanes in the third trimester as birth, labor, and your belly loom large, or you may simply feel unattractive or worried as to whether your partner is satisfied sexually. Yet it is possible to have an active sex life throughout pregnancy.

As your pregnancy progresses, you may find that the missionary position (man on top) is no longer comfortable. You'll need to be inventive. Below are some time-tested positions and tips for making love late in pregnancy:

● **Lie sideways** Lying partly sideways allows your partner to keep most of his weight off your uterus.

● **Use the bed as a prop** Your belly isn't an obstacle if you lie on your back at the side or foot of the bed with your knees bent, and your bottom and feet perched at the edge of the mattress. Your partner can either kneel or stand in front of you.

● **Lie side-by-side in the spoon position** This allows for only shallow penetration. Deep thrusts can become uncomfortable as the months pass.

● **Get on top of your partner** This puts no weight on your abdomen and allows you to control penetration.

● **Enter from a sitting position** This position is another one that keeps the weight off your uterus. Try sitting on your partner's lap as he sits on a (sturdy!) chair.

Have faith—where there's a will, there's a way. With some experimenting, you and your partner are sure to find a technique that works for you.

When not to have sex during pregnancy

There are some important circumstances in which you may be advised not to have intercourse. These include if you have experienced:

● bleeding
● abdominal pains or cramps
● broken water
● a history of cervical weakness
● a low-lying placenta after 20 weeks (placenta previa)

You may also be advised to avoid sex if your partner has genital herpes. If you catch this for the first time when pregnant, there's a risk it could affect your developing baby.

Parents**Ask...**

Will sex harm the baby?

Perhaps the most common reason couples cut back on sex during pregnancy is a fear that they'll hurt the baby. If you're concerned about that, you can stop worrying right now. Your baby is safely cushioned in an amniotic fluid-filled sac and, unless you're having very rough sex, you have almost no chance of injuring anyone. There are some important circumstances, however, when you may be advised not to have sex (see above).

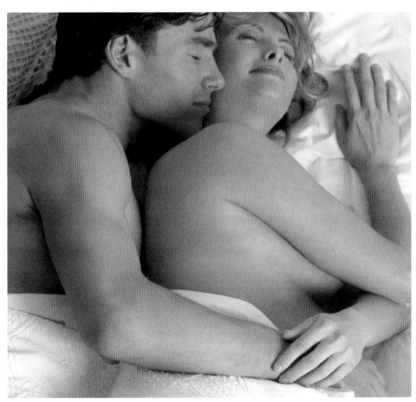

Although your belly may get in the way when you try making love later in pregnancy, there's no reason why you shouldn't experiment to find a more comfortable position. And don't worry—making love cannot hurt your baby; he's cushioned in his amniotic sac.

Getting ready for pregnancy

Staying safe and healthy

Your pregnancy diary

Birth and beyond

Style, fashion, and comfort

Being pregnant doesn't mean you can't look fabulous. In fact, having a belly can give extra impact to your outfits—you'll find that you can try different styles to complement your new shape. Here's how to get that special va-va-voom.

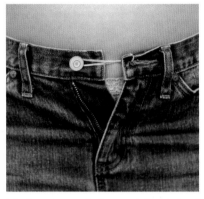

A short-term solution to a tight waistband is to loop a rubber band through the buttonhole then loop it around the button.

Stylish at each stage

For the first three months or so, you'll probably be able to wear your usual clothes. You may have to leave the top button undone on your skirts and pants, but you can hide that by leaving your shirts untucked. When your waistband gets too tight, loop a rubber band through the buttonhole and then wrap it around the button. This will provide a crucial extra bit of breathing room.

If your bust grows quickly, opt for loose tops or wear suit jackets open over a T-shirt or shirt to disguise it. You'll also almost certainly need to invest in a few good maternity bras (see pp.92–3).

Pashminas and wraps are great pregnancy accessories. They drape over your belly and distract attention, so you can go sleeveless or wear something low cut, safe in the knowledge that you can cover up. You can find simple, dressy wraps in the accessories area of most department stores.

Mixing and matching

Once you enter the Awkward Zone—that time in your pregnancy when you're a bit big for your normal clothes, but not big enough for real maternity wear—it can be quite frustrating. You will usually find you can get around this problem with:

- A few pairs of pants and skirts with elastic or drawstring waistbands in a size larger than you usually wear. You could ask your larger friends—discreetly!—if they have anything they could lend you for a week or so.
- Low-rise trousers that will sit nicely below your belly.
- A wrap dress that accentuates your curves and accommodates your belly in its various stages of growth.
- Sweaters, cardigans, loose shirts, and pretty, floaty tops.

Long tops work especially well at this awkward stage, gracefully hiding your growing belly without drawing attention to it. If you haven't shared your news with your work colleagues yet, dressing in this way might buy you a little more time.

After the word on your pregnancy is out, you might as well make life easier by dressing the part. Now it's time to hit the stores. You could try buying five items of clothing in similar fabrics and complementary shades: pants, a skirt, a jacket, a dress, and a top. If you shop carefully, these can form the basis of your wardrobe over the next few months and you can even mix and match them with a few non-maternity items to mix it up a bit.

Accessorizing

Beads, bangles, bags, ribbons, scarves, shoes—the possibilities are endless. The most basic maternity wardrobe can be brightened up with accessories. Think belts that sit below your belly, colorful beads to cheer up a plain black dress, an armful of trendy bracelets.

You can dress an outfit up or down, and the best thing about accessories is that you'll still be able to wear them after the baby is born, unlike those enormous pants that suddenly remind you of a military parachute. And it doesn't matter how big you get, you'll never outgrow that must-have handbag.

Perfect footwear

The ligaments that control your lower back are softened during pregnancy, so they are more at risk of being stretched and damaged. The problem with high heels is that they alter your posture and put a strain on this already

weakened area. This could contribute to lower back pain, which can be severe.

Flat or low-heeled shoes are therefore a better bet. They will ensure that you are comfortable and will minimize the strain on your back. To compromise, you could spend part of the day in heels and keep a pair of low-heeled shoes in your bag to change into when you get tired.

Shop around for elegant, flatter-heeled shoes that can be worn with lots of outfits. Ballet-style leather pumps look great with skirts, pants, or jeans, but snuggly suede boots are equally versatile. Retro-style sneakers often look nicer than their sporty cousins and are perfect for walks or weekends away.

All in all, it's best to save your high heels for special occasions, especially since your feet can get wider in pregnancy so, if you have a much-loved pair of Manolos, they may stretch and not fit you afterward. The horror!

Top tips for comfortable clothes

Your changing body shape requires some wardrobe changes. These tips cover the essentials for comfort.

● Good underwear is a must. See our advice on choosing maternity bras on p.93. You may be able to keep wearing regular bras, though, but go for fittings throughout your pregnancy to make sure you're wearing the right size.
● Maternity underpants are brilliant because they stretch as your belly grows. Low-slung hipster pants, or even briefs that can fit under your belly, are other good options.
● When buying maternity jeans, go by the size you were before you became pregnant. These jeans come in many different styles and fits—choose from those that fit over your belly, on it, or under it.

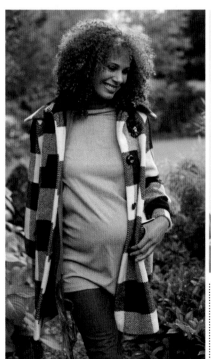

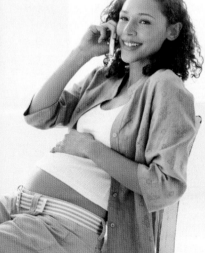

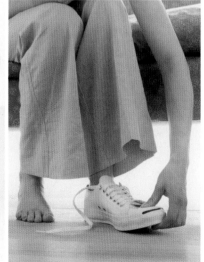

Low-rise trousers (above) work well, sitting either on top of your belly or below it. **Wearing a long cardigan or coat (left)** and leaving it open—weather permitting!—can save you from buying a new coat or jacket. And it looks super-stylish, too.

As your center of gravity changes and the ligaments in your abdominal area stretch, you'll find that high heels can give you a backache. Your feet can get wider, too. Invest in a couple of pairs of flat or low-heeled shoes or sneakers.

Getting ready for pregnancy

Staying safe and healthy

Your pregnancy diary

Birth and beyond

Maternity wear

Tops are a snap when you're pregnant, but, as your belly grows, pants and skirts are a bit more of a challenge. Investing in a couple of pairs of maternity pants, and perhaps a nice maternity suit, will help you look great at home, at work, and when you're out for the evening.

What to look for in pants

You won't find many women's wardrobes that don't have a pair or three of jeans in them, so why should it be any different when you're pregnant? A well-fitting pair of maternity jeans makes an invaluable addition to your wardrobe. Below are a few tips to remember before you buy them:

● Fit varies from style to style and from brand to brand so make sure that you try before you buy.

● Buy your normal size jeans, but make sure they are maternity jeans: don't be tempted just to go for a bigger size jean.

● Don't put style over comfort: go for what you will be happy wearing for at least 12 hours a day.

● There are plenty of styles to choose from, not just leg styles (bootcut, straight leg, or boyfit, for example) but also the way the style sits over or under your belly.

● Some styles may fit better at different stages of pregnancy, so think about getting two different styles.

● Go for reasonably priced pairs rather than expensive ones. That way you won't feel too guilty if you get only six months' wear out of them.

At work, you may be able to get away with swapping a jacket for a softer cardigan or tunic top, but good work pants are essential. When shopping for work pants:

● There is no need to spend a fortune on maternity pants. Remember, you will only be wearing them for around six months, although if you have more than one child you may be able to wear them for subsequent pregnancies.

● Choose two different colors of pants to make your pregnancy work wardrobe more versatile.

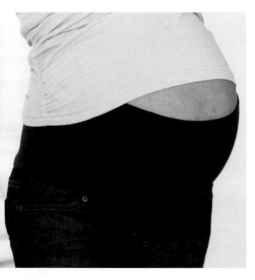

Buying a pair of real maternity jeans is best. You won't find a larger size of your normal jeans nearly as comfortable.

You'll have to get yourself a few maternity clothes, but you don't need to spend a fortune.

"After weeks and weeks of declaring that I will never spend money on maternity clothes that I'll only wear for a month, I finally had to give in.

All my tops started to roll up so I could feel a breeze on my belly. I sorted through my closet and had to put most of my clothes in a suitcase because nothing fits. Even my baggy tops don't fit over my boobs. A few weeks ago I was able to wear my pants and not close the button, but now the zipper won't even close so I've been forced into buying some new clothes.

Having said that, I still don't want to spend a fortune on maternity clothes. Fortunately, there are lots of reasonably priced—and fashionable—lines available now, and I've even managed to borrow a few items from some of my friends who've had babies recently.

Besides, as everyone and their uncle keeps telling me, I'll probably have to continue to wear my maternity clothes for some time after the baby's born, so at least I'll get my money's worth."

Maternity clothes on a budget

You deserve to look and feel good during your pregnancy. It's not always easy, though, especially when clothes and finances are getting tight. Before you dismiss the idea of clothes entirely and head for the nearest tent shop, below are some top tips for looking great on a budget while you're pregnant:

● **Buy basics** Investing in a few "key" items of maternity wear that can be mixed and matched will take you a long way. Try two pairs of well-cut pants, a pair of yoga pants, a plain skirt or dress, a cardigan or jacket, a plain sweater that can be worn over most outfits, two casual tops, and a nicer top for special occasions.

● **Throw a clothes-swapping party** Ban all men from your house and invite over all your pregnant friends, plus those friends who are already moms. The latter should have some maternity clothes that they feel more than happy to part with, and might actually want to borrow some of your clothes in exchange. The swap does not need to

be permanent, and you could turn it into a fun evening by sharing stories and even playing silly games.

● **Borrow your partner's clothes** If you're just relaxing at home, raid your partner's closet. His shirts and sweaters may well be big enough, and you can save your own clothes for when people will actually see you. The elastic waist on men's boxer shorts and pajama bottoms makes them comfortable to wear in bed—and if you can distract

your partner's attention long enough, his bathrobe might come in handy too.

● **Get online** If you're a fan of internet shopping, the web is a real treasure trove. Some sites offer exchange services for women who no longer want their maternity clothes, while others sell discontinued lines and ex-catalogue clothing for a fraction of their original prices. If you're a fan of auctions, go online for a vast selection of maternity wear at very reasonable prices.

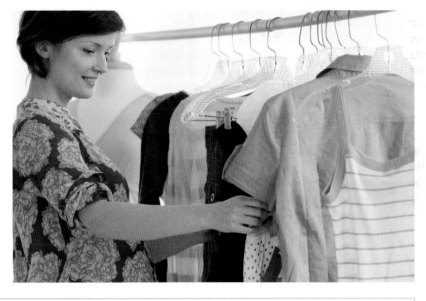

Secondhand stores are a good source of clothes when you're pregnant. Recycling is good for your budget and the planet.

Getting ready for pregnancy

Staying safe and healthy

Your pregnancy diary

Birth and beyond

Mellow mom or high-maintenance mom?

Mellow moms put fashion aside for nine months, while high-maintenance (HM) moms delight in a reason to shop.

On jeans
Mellow: squeeze into your trusty old jeans for as long as possible, even though the top button's popped off.
HM: dash to a lavish maternity store for custom top-of-the range jeans.

On maternity shopping
Mellow: track down bargains, borrow from friends, and wear your partner's shirts.
HM: buy a whole new wardrobe and enlist a team of personal shoppers.

On shoes
Mellow: squeeze your swollen ankles into some rather large and clumpy flats.
HM: make some sacrifices for impending

motherhood— like reducing the heels on your Jimmy Choos by half an inch.

On underwear
Mellow: abandon thongs for the next nine months for fear of losing them somewhere they shouldn't be(!)
HM: spend a fortune on new, expensive lingerie that flatters your belly and makes you feel sexy.

Special occasion wear

Being pregnant doesn't mean you can't look gorgeous. Whether you're after the perfect Little(ish) Black Dress, or something floor length and fabulous, it really is possible for moms-to-be to look fab on a night out.

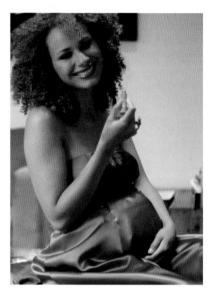

Try a stunning empire waist dress for a big night out. If you don't want to splurge for a single occasion, you could rent.

Evening wear

For evening wear, keep it simple with pants or a skirt and a pretty top. Not only will you look great but you can mix the separates with the rest of your maternity wardrobe to give you maximum use from them. Also, a pretty top can be a great way to show off that extra cleavage you have!

A wrap dress can adapt to all the different stages of your pregnancy just by loosening the ties. Wrap dresses can be quite figure hugging, so be prepared to show off your belly. You can try using different accessories to make your outfit really special.

A classic empire waist dress has been a wardrobe staple for fashionistas for years. Dresses like this that pull in under your bustline then flare out can really flatter your pregnancy figure. For best effect, look out for one cut on the bias (across the grain of the fabric).

If you don't like the idea of buying an outfit you are unlikely to get wear out of, look into renting a dress. This could be a more economical way of looking fabulous on a special occasion.

Wedding day

If you are getting married, it's time to really go for it. Your wedding day is one of the most important days of your life and being pregnant doesn't mean you can't still look the part. Look for dresses that have been specifically designed for pregnant women since they are more likely to be flattering for your belly. You can find beautifully simple ones if you are going for a low-key affair, or classic floor-length gowns for something a little bit more dressy. There are also pregnancy wedding dresses for rent if you prefer.

Parents**Talk...**

"There are no stores in my town that stock extra-large maternity clothes. I can't keep buying the next size up. Even worse, I just got back from my vacation to find that nothing fits, other than the shorts I took with me. They're not exactly work wear! Help!"
Louise, 27, first-time mom-to-be

"You should try eBay if you don't want to spend loads of money on new clothes. They always have lots of maternity stuff for sale to suit all shapes and sizes."
Jodi, 27, mom to William and Anna

"I'm a larger lady and was mostly able to get away with my normal clothes. I did need something new to wear for a wedding at the end of my pregnancy though. I went to a chain store specializing in big sizes, and bought a lovely skirt and top. I was so pleased."
Vicky, 26, mom to 11-month-old Alexander

"About halfway through my pregnancy, I couldn't fit into any of my normal clothes and couldn't find a single item to buy. The only option left seemed to be an old smock dress that I found stashed at the back of my wardrobe! What would 'fashionistas' say?"
Rachel, 31, mom to 18-month-old Hugh

"Luckily, I discovered the plus-size maternity lines at a couple of chain stores. Finding them saved me from the fashion police! I feel almost human again."
Jackie, 30, first-time mom-to-be

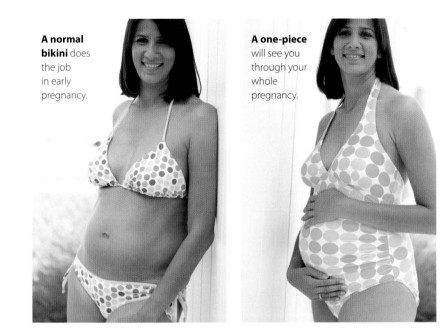

A normal bikini does the job in early pregnancy.

A one-piece will see you through your whole pregnancy.

Active mom

You want sports clothes while you're pregnant? Some ordinary sports clothes adapt well.

"I was disappointed to find that there's not much choice in the stores for sporty pregnant moms, except for basic stuff like yoga pants and cami tops. So it was a relief to discover that low-slung tracksuit bottoms sat happily under my belly. And they were super comfortable in the last weeks of my pregnancy. Sports T-shirts with built-in shelf bras helped stop my breasts from taking on a life of their own, too."

Maternity swimwear

Swimming is a great way to stay in shape and healthy during pregnancy, so it's definitely worth taking the plunge. If you're planning a last romantic trip before baby arrives, naturally you'll want to look gorgeous on the beach. Normal swimsuits aren't stretchy enough to see you much past your first trimester, so invest in a maternity swimsuit early on. Below is a list of what's available:
- **The one-piece** Almost always the easiest to find. It's made of a material that stretches as your belly grows, so it can last you your whole pregnancy.
- **The bikini** If the one-piece seems too conservative for you, then why not try a maternity bikini? It allows you to reveal and draw attention to your new cleavage with a supportive, built-in shelf bra, while showing off your belly and legs to boot.
- **The tankini** This is for those who don't like one-piece swimsuits, but feel

reluctant to reveal themselves so much in a bikini. Instead of a bikini bra, the tankini comes with a stretchy cami-style top, which will cover most of your belly.
- **The nursing swimsuit** A nursing swimsuit is perfect if you are breast-feeding and want to start swimming with your baby. The clips on the straps let you open and close the drop cups with no fuss. The adjustable straps and shelf bra also make sure that you can stay comfortable and that there's no chance of your breasts trying to make a great escape!
- **The sarong** This is an essential for every woman who feels self-conscious about her bottom, thighs—or any other wobbly parts. Sarongs come in loads of different colors and fabrics and can be wrapped around you at the beach or while you're lazing by the pool. And there's no need to buy a special pregnancy version—one size fits all!

Working mom

In early pregnancy you might get away with wearing your normal work suit—with a twist!

"I work in PR and need to look put together for meetings with clients and giving presentations. A friend of mine who was pregnant last year gave me a great tip for the office for the first few months of pregnancy. She suggested going for a long-line jacket and wearing it open to cover my belly. Luckily I already had a jacket like that.

Once I began to show, though, I did have to invest in a maternity suit. Some lines can even be altered to fit. They're expensive, but worth it to make me feel business ready. I took a look around, and found quite a few are widely available."

Breasts and bras

A bountiful bust is one of the great things about being pregnant. But your newly expanded bustline needs extra support, so make sure you get measured for some real maternity bras. And don't miss our tips for keeping your breasts healthy and comfortable in pregnancy.

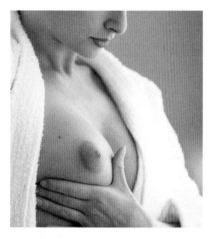

Your breasts will change—you'll need one or two maternity bras as soon as your normal bras start to feel uncomfortable.

How your breasts change

Your expanding breasts can be one of the first signs of pregnancy. They'll get bigger and heavier as your pregnancy progresses and, since your breasts have only ligaments and no muscles, they could be stretched if they are not properly supported.

Most moms-to-be experience an expanding bust, and sometimes sore breasts, well before a growing belly and many outgrow their ordinary bras early in pregnancy. As soon as your normal bra starts to feel uncomfortable you need some maternity bras.

Shopping for a maternity bra?
Look for the following:
● **Support** Look for wide straps, sides, under-bust band, and a deep center at the front. Firm elastic straps eliminate bounce and give you extra support.
● **Coverage** You need as much fabric as possible over the breast area; this will be more comfortable for you as your breasts become more sensitive.
● **Adjustability** A minimum of four sets of back hooks will allow your bra to grow with you.
● **Comfort** Look for bras that are mainly cotton. Many pregnant women find they get hot; cotton lets your skin breathe so you are less likely to sweat.

Make sure you go for professional measuring and fitting either in a store or through a special agency whose staff are specially trained to fit women in pregnancy. They can assess your changing shape and size, ensuring you get bras that fit perfectly and give you the support you need. Make sure you get measured every six to eight weeks.

It's especially important to wear a well-fitting, supportive bra if you are planning to exercise since your breasts are heavier during pregnancy. A special exercise bra will give you support and minimize discomfort.

ParentsAsk...

How do I know when I need a new bra?
As soon as your normal bra starts to feel uncomfortable you should start wearing a maternity bra. It's the best way to support your growing breasts.

Are underwires okay?
Some bra experts and stores advise against underwired bras, believing that the wire interferes with the natural changes in size and shape of the breast. If you do wear one, make sure the wire doesn't press anywhere on the breast and don't sleep in it.

Will I need a bra at night?
If your breasts become very sensitive, a pregnancy sleep bra—a soft, unrestrictive cotton bra available at maternity clothing stores—will help immensely.

When do I need a nursing bra?
Believe it or not, your breasts will get even bigger after the birth, so wait until the last month of your pregnancy, then buy two or three. A good nursing bra needs to be flexible, allowing extra room for when your milk comes in and for when your breasts reduce in size (usually after 12 weeks or so).

Sore breasts

One of the early signs of pregnancy is extremely sensitive, sore breasts. Some women's breasts become so sensitive, in fact, that the sensation of clothing against them is unbearable. This tenderness should get better after the first trimester, once your rising hormone levels have stabilized and your body gets used to them.

A familiar feeling

As your body gears up for the months of pregnancy to come, you produce more of the hormones estrogen and progesterone, just as you do before each menstrual period. In fact, the tenderness you feel is probably an exaggerated version of how your breasts often feel before your period. Along with the hormone surge, your breasts are beginning to increase in size as the fat layer thickens and you add milk glands and extra blood. These changes, though temporarily uncomfortable, have an important purpose: they're preparing your breasts for feeding your baby.

Though your breasts will continue to grow throughout your pregnancy—it's common to go from a B to a D cup, for example—they'll feel more uncomfortable during your first trimester. The size change is most noticeable in first pregnancies.

Tingling and leaking

You may also notice that your breasts throb or tingle during the initial "excitement" phase of lovemaking. In the first trimester, you may also find that you no longer like having your breasts touched. Any pain or discomfort such as this is likely to subside during your second and third trimesters.

Toward the end of pregnancy, you may also find that your breasts start to leak slightly. This is absolutely normal and nothing to worry about. The leaking is a fluid called colostrum, which is your baby's first milk. This rich, high-protein pre-milk is being produced ready for when your baby is born.

If you're experiencing tenderness, your best bet is to find a good, supportive bra (see opposite). Take the time to get fitted by a specialist, perhaps in a department store or maternity store. For leakages, you may want to buy some breast pads to put in your bra.

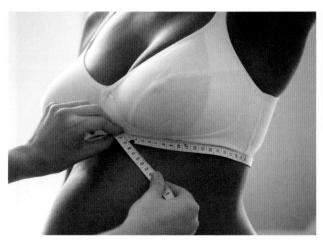

Have a professional fitting for your maternity bras and get yourself re-measured every six to eight weeks since your breasts will keep growing.

Pointers for buying the correct-sized bra

Follow these handy pointers to be sure you buy the right size of bra throughout your pregnancy:

● Make sure the cups fit snugly and smoothly, with no overflow at the top.

● Make sure the center seam lies comfortably against your breastbone.

● Get fitted more than once during your pregnancy, since you may need to change cup sizes several times as your breasts grow.

● Early in pregnancy, ensure that your bra fastens comfortably on to the first set of hooks, to leave plenty of room for your expanding rib cage.

● Late in pregnancy, buy a bra that fastens comfortably onto one of the last set of hooks to allow for your imminent reduction in size.

Dad's **Diary**

The breast issue

"As my partner's breasts became larger, it opened up a whole new can of worms. 'Do my boobs look all right?' she'd ask.
'Yes, they look great.'
'But you always told me that you preferred small breasts?'
'No, yours always look great.'
'But are they better when they're big?'
'Err, no. Yes. Whatever.'

Fiona was actually more sensitive about her changing body shape than I was. Even when she'd wail that she was the size of a house and had the belly of a sumo wrestler, I assured her that she still looked gorgeous all the time. Why, I'd say, you only have to explore the more extreme titles at any magazine store's top shelf to discover how pregnant women trigger the strangest carnal impulses in many men..."

Getting ready for pregnancy

Staying safe and healthy

Your pregnancy diary

Birth and beyond

Beauty treatments

If you're a regular at your local beauty salon, the good news is that being pregnant doesn't mean putting your beauty routine on hold. Your skin may be more sensitive, though, so it's wise to use treatments involving inks, electric currents, and creams and lotions with caution.

ParentsAsk...

Is it okay to have a tattoo done while I'm pregnant?

It's not unusual for people having a tattoo to faint or pass out. Most tattooists wouldn't be prepared to take on the risk of a pregnant woman fainting. Also, not enough is known about any possible effects that the ink, which may be partly absorbed into the body, may have on your baby. So it's sensible to wait to have a tattoo until after your baby is born.

Is it best for me to take my body piercings out now that I'm pregnant?

That depends on where they are. During pregnancy, your abdomen will expand until eventually your belly button protrudes. At this point you may need to remove your navel ring or swap it for a flexible barbell. When it comes to giving birth, if you have to have a cesarean you will be asked to tape your navel ring or possibly remove it.

You don't need to remove jewelry from pierced nipples during pregnancy unless it begins to feel uncomfortable. However, it will need to come out if you want to breast-feed. Your doctor will probably ask you to remove jewelry from any genital piercings when it comes to giving birth. This is because of the risk of them getting caught during the birth or of that area tearing.

The highs and lows

Fabulous and feminine or fat and frumpy? However pregnancy makes you feel, it's bound to change how you feel about your body. It's all too easy to forget about the joys of impending motherhood when you're feeling sick, exhausted, nervous, or just cranky. As your breasts grow, your abdomen swells and your waistline disappears, you may long to have your old shape back.

So while you're reveling in being pregnant, you might not be reveling in looking pregnant. A massage or other treatment can lift your spirits and make you feel better. If you've had a breakout of pregnancy acne, a professional facial might improve your skin and give your confidence a boost. Even a manicure or pedicure can help you feel just a little more glamorous and groomed.

However, before you make an appointment at your local salon for a pampering session, bear in mind that there are certain procedures that you need to be careful with while you're pregnant. Below is a guide to which are safe and which are best avoided:

Tattoos

Little is known about the effects of the ink used during the tattooing process on mother and baby. There's also a small risk that you could get an infection, such as hepatitis B, from unclean equipment. It's best to err on the side of caution and wait until after your baby is born to have that tattoo.

Hair-removal creams

There's no evidence about the safety or otherwise of hair-removal creams during pregnancy, but your skin may be more sensitive than usual. If you're using them at home, always read the instructions on the package carefully first, don't use them on broken skin and always do a patch test first. Remember to tell the beauty therapists you are pregnant if you go to a salon.

Electrolysis

No adverse effects have ever been recorded for electrolysis in pregnancy. However, electrolysists recommend you don't have work done on your breasts or belly during late pregnancy, since both are very sensitive at this stage.

Bikini and leg waxes

The biggest problem with waxing in pregnancy is that, toward the end, it can be difficult to reach, or even see, certain body parts! This is the time to treat yourself to a full salon treatment.

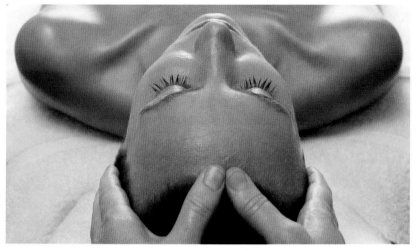

A relaxing facial or gentle massage at your local salon can be just what you need to make you feel great—as well as giving you some time just for yourself!

Oils to avoid

Here are some commonly used aromatherapy oils that should not be used during pregnancy:

- Aniseed
- Angelica
- Basil
- Cedar wood
- Cinnamon
- Sage
- Clove
- Fennel
- Jasmine
- Juniper
- Lemongrass
- Myrrh
- Parsley
- Pennyroyal
- Thyme

Aromatherapy

Many aromatherapists believe that the essential oils—extracts of certain plants and flowers—used in aromatherapy can balance hormone levels, improve your mood and soothe stress.

There is no doubt that the relaxing effects of many of the oils and massage techniques used in aromatherapy can increase your sense of well-being and improve your general health, although there are some oils you shouldn't use while pregnant (see above right).

If you're pregnant, it's best to consult a professional aromatherapist to be sure that you are not using an inappropriate aromatherapy oil or technique. Many complementary therapists can be found in the Yellow Pages (often listed under "Clinics"), but try asking around first for a personal recommendation for a qualified registered practitioner in your area. She should be someone who has plenty of experience of giving aromatherapy treatments to pregnant women. Some practitioners believe that a pregnant woman should not have aromatherapy massages during the first or third trimester, while others take care to use only specialized and light massage techniques.

Create your own mini spa

If you desire a pregnancy pick-me-up, creating your own home spa could be the answer. All you need is a few pampering products.

- **Preparation** Make your bathroom tranquil; dim the lights, and put some scented candles on a safe surface. Pour your favorite bubble bath under warm running water and sink yourself into a deep, luxurious bath.

- **Buffing and exfoliating** Buff your body with an exfoliating brush or use a salt scrub to banish all those dead skin cells. Pay special attention to your elbows and knees, which are usually rougher than the rest of your skin. Use an exfoliating facial wash to get the blood rushing to your cheeks, then relax for a few minutes in the bath with a deep cleansing face mask.

- **Grand finale** When you've finished, wrap yourself in a warm, fluffy towel and when you're dry spend a few minutes moisturizing your body with a super-rich body cream.

- **Time for sleep** By now, you should be feeling so relaxed and soothed that it's time to blow out all those candles, curl up in bed and drift off to sleep. Sweet dreams!

Staying safe in the sun

Many women find their skin is more sensitive to ultraviolet radiation during pregnancy. Even so, the temptation to get a tan may be strong. But is it safe? Here we give the latest advice on the dangers of sunbathing and the risks of using sun beds, sunscreens, and fake tans.

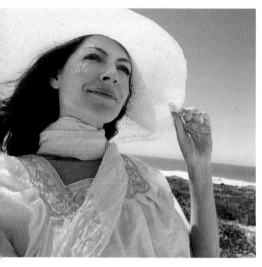

Your skin may be more sensitive now that you're pregnant so always use sunscreen and wear a hat in strong sun.

Is it safe to get a tan?

Many experts advise that getting a tan—whether in a salon or in the sun—isn't a good idea, even if you aren't pregnant. A tan is your skin's protection against the damaging effects of ultraviolet (UV) radiation; evidence suggests that prolonged exposure to UV exacerbates the effects of aging and also increases your risk of developing skin cancer.

Risks of sunbathing

Many pregnant women find they are more susceptible to sunburn. If this applies to you, slap on the sunscreen (see opposite) and avoid the sun where possible. Pregnant women are prone to excessive skin pigmentation because they have higher levels of melanocyte-stimulating hormone than normal. If you get chloasma (see p.69), your skin may react more strongly to sunlight than usual. Be careful: sunbathing may well make it worse.

Also, lying in the hot sun for hours on end increases the risk of overheating and dehydration—neither of which are good for you or your developing baby. Hot weather can make you sweat more, so watch out for the warning signs of dehydration: your nose and mouth may feel dry and your urine may turn dark yellow. However, don't worry if all you want to do is spend a peaceful afternoon in the sun though—just guard against overheating and burning.

The safety of sunscreens

You may find you are more prone to sunburns during your pregnancy, or you

9,500 is the number of cases of malignant melanoma diagnosed in the US.

It's a shocking fact that the incidence of malignant melanoma is about one in 70 and has gone up significantly in recent years.

ParentsAsk...

Supposing I used a tanning bed before I knew I was pregnant?
Regular use of tanning beds is a fairly recent trend and there is little research on their effects in pregnancy. Nor are there any definitive studies about how exposure either to sunlight or to artificial ultraviolet rays affects a developing baby. Some preliminary studies suggest there may be a possible link between exposure to ultraviolet rays and folic acid deficiency. This is because folic acid can be broken down by strong sunlight. In the first few weeks of pregnancy, high levels of folic acid help protect against neural tube defects, such as spina bifida, in the developing baby. While further studies have yet to be done, these studies suggest that intense or prolonged exposure to UV light—as you get on a sun bed—should be avoided around the time of conception and in early pregnancy. After the first 12 weeks, all the developing baby's major organs have been formed so the risks are reduced.

may feel "prickly" after exposure to the sun. That is why it's very important to protect your skin with a high-factor sunscreen (SPF 30 or more) and to wear a hat whenever you go out. Sunscreens are generally safe to use during pregnancy, but you may want to use one for sensitive skin for now. Reapply it regularly and avoid the midday sun.

Remember that both chemical and physical sunscreens can deteriorate over time, so before you use one, check the bottle or tube for the expiration date. If you can't find a date, or if the product seems to have dried up or changed color

or consistency, throw it away and buy some new sunscreen.

You may want to avoid tanning beds (see ParentsAsk, opposite). Lying on a tanning bed could elevate your body temperature to 102 degrees, which could be hazardous to your baby. If you have a skin problem that responds well

to controlled light treatment, ask for a referral to a dermatologist so that your treatment can be properly controlled to keep any damaging effects to a minimum.

If you desperately want to be tan, the current medical opinion seems to be that it's probably safer—and easier—to use fake tanning lotions (see below).

"Sunscreens are **generally safe** but you may prefer to use one for **sensitive skin**."

Fake tans may be safer

Fake tans have become more popular recently. The active ingredient of fake tans is dihydroxyacetone (DHA), which only interacts with the cells in the outer layer of the skin and isn't absorbed into the body's system. The British Medical Association, however, advises pregnant women not to use self-tanning lotions,

since their skin may be more sensitive than usual and may be more prone to having an allergic reaction.

If you do decide to use a fake tan, do a patch test first, even if it's a lotion you have used before. If you have any kind of allergic reaction to the product you should stop using it at immediately.

Tanning pills

If you see advertisements in magazines or websites for tanning pills, don't buy them since the pills can be toxic to an unborn baby. They have also been known to cause hepatitis and eye damage. For these reasons they are banned in the United States.

Solar UV index

The strength of the sun's ultraviolet (UV) radiation is given as the "Solar UV Index". This system has been developed by the World Health Organization (WHO) and is used in many countries alongside weather-forecast maps. Color coding on a map warns of the level of skin-damaging UV radiation in an area. Follow the color coding to make sure you use the correct level of protection.

UV Index		Protect yourself
11+	Extreme	Slip on sun-protective clothing
8, 9, 10	Very High	Slop on SPF 30+ sunscreen. Reapply every two hours
6, 7	High	Slap on a broad-brimmed hat and wear sunscreen
3, 4, 5	Moderate	Seek shade and wear sunscreen
1, 2	Low	Sun protection is generally not needed unless outside for extended periods

Vacations and travel

Once your baby arrives you won't be able to make a move without a mountain of baby gear. That's one good reason to get away for a last romantic break before you give birth. It's usually safe to fly in pregnancy, but give the scuba diving a pass once you're there!

Before you travel

Taking a vacation when you are pregnant is a great idea, especially if this is your first baby. It's likely to be a while before you'll get another chance to really relax.

The time to travel

As long as your pregnancy is going well, it's safe to go ahead and make travel plans. If you have complications, such as high blood pressure, spotting, or diabetes, check with your doctor first.

Most moms-to-be find that the second trimester—weeks 14 to 27—is a perfect time to travel. With nausea and vomiting behind you, your energy levels high and the chances of miscarriage low, you can relax and enjoy your time away.

As long as you don't have medical complications, aren't carrying twins or more, and haven't had a prior premature birth, you can fly on most airlines until 36 weeks of pregnancy. Travel agents

and airlines won't ask if you're pregnant when you book your seat, but you may be challenged at the check-in desk. For this reason, from about 28 weeks of pregnancy, you will need a letter from your doctor confirming your due date and stating that you're unlikely to go into labor on the flight. Check the airline's policy on flying in pregnancy before you leave.

There's no reason to avoid car travel when you are pregnant—don't forget your seatbelt! However, at the end of your pregnancy you may prefer to let your partner drive since your belly will be very close to the steering wheel.

When you are going on a long drive, you should take a bathroom and stretching break at least every 90 minutes. Sitting for long periods can make your feet and ankles swell and your legs cramp. When you are flying, you are at particular risk of your feet swelling and possible blood clots, so remove your shoes. Keep your blood circulating by strolling up and down the aisle and doing simple stretches. Choose an aisle seat so you can easily get to the bathroom without disturbing others. Finally, if there happens to be an empty seat next to you on a plane, train, or bus, take the opportunity to put your feet up.

Tips for safe plane travel

Following the tips below can help you to enjoy safe travel by plane during your pregnancy:

● **Wear support stockings** Keep your circulation flowing and reduce the risk of thrombosis (blood clots).

● **Do some stretches** Stroll up and down the aisle of the plane occasionally and do some simple leg stretches.

● **Don't wear tights** They encourage moist conditions that increase the chances of developing a yeast infection.

● **Drink lots of water** The air on planes can be very dry and you may get dehydrated. Avoid coffee and tea.

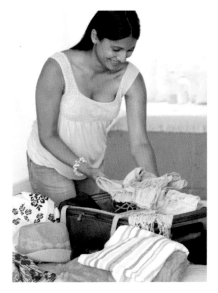

Packing for a last romantic fling? Travel light and take loose cotton clothes so you stay cool and comfortable.

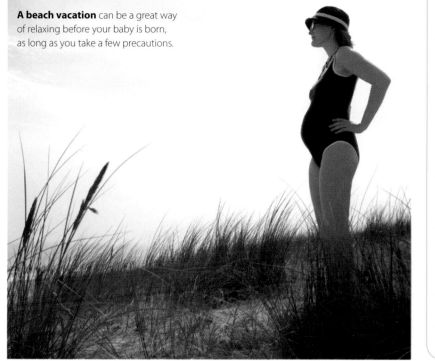

A beach vacation can be a great way of relaxing before your baby is born, as long as you take a few precautions.

Tips for pregnant travelers

Following these tips can help you travel safely during your pregnancy:

- **Reduce stress** Make sure that you schedule plenty of time for traveling and travel light. Relax by reading or listening to music.
- **Maximize your energy** Build quiet times into your routine. Take a bath, take a nap, read on the beach, and spend an evening with room service.
- **Eat smart** Pack healthy snacks in your hand luggage. If you're flying, be aware that these may be removed by security. Drink plenty of extra fluids.
- **Make frequent toilet stops** and carry wet wipes and a hand sanitizer.
- **Avoid yeast** Wear cotton panties and loose cotton layers, especially in hot, humid climates.

While you're there

Vacations taken while you're pregnant are the stuff that memories are made of, so you'll want your special trip to go smoothly. You will need to be a little more careful to keep you and your growing baby safe and to ensure that your time away isn't ruined by illness or accidents.

Sports like waterskiing, snowboarding, skiing, or surfing that carry a risk of falling will have to be put on hold. Scuba diving and other "pressurized" sports are also out, as are amusement park rides.

Wear loose clothes made of natural fibers to help you stay cool, and to prevent rubbing and chafing. Drink plenty of fluids, especially bottled water. To help prevent stomach upsets, always wash your hands before eating, after a visit to the bathroom, and when you get back from excursions. And finally, avoid ice and steer clear of hotel buffets that have been left out of the fridge for long periods or food sold on the street.

Parents**Talk...**

"If you're going to take a vacation during pregnancy, go for all-out relaxation. During my first pregnancy I went to the Caribbean for a week with my husband—we booked a hotel in a lovely resort right next to the beach, with spa facilities, plenty of places to eat, and lots to do and see. Having a week in the sun, taking life at a slow pace and enjoying delicious food and gorgeous surroundings was a truly restorative experience."
Liz, 31, mom to year-old Adam, and two-year-old Shane

"If money's tight, there are plenty of ways to get that much-needed vacation during pregnancy. When I was pregnant with my second baby, we asked my parents to watch our two-year-old daughter for a couple of days and my husband and I had a short break in a country inn. We visited the spa, went for some gentle walks, wined (for him!) and dined, slept late—and came back feeling refreshed, relaxed, and ready to face what lay ahead."
Julia, 34, mom to Paul and Milly

Bonding with your unborn baby

As a mom-to-be it's not hard to bond with the baby inside you. Those little kicks and hiccups give you heart-warming clues to the small person who'll soon arrive. Dads-to-be may take more time, but getting involved with prenatal appointments and choosing names can help.

Single mom

If your partner can't be with you for that first scan, a supportive mom is wonderful to have.

"Mom was with me when I had my first scan. I was so nervous there might be something wrong with the baby, but she kept reassuring me that everything would be okay. It was such a relief to see my fully formed baby on screen with his heart beating strongly. Then he sat bolt upright and that's the picture we got to take home! He'll be her first grandchild. She's been so supportive since I found out I was pregnant, I wouldn't have wanted anyone else there with me."

The importance of bonding

Bonding is the word used to describe the intense attachment that develops between a mom and her baby. Talk about bonding often focuses on the time after your baby is born. But for many moms-to-be, bonding begins much earlier than that, often from the moment you see that line on the pregnancy test telling you you're pregnant.

There are plenty of reasons why bonding with your belly is good for you and your baby. Most important is that making healthy choices about your diet or lifestyle becomes easier because you'll remember why you're doing it.

Pregnancy can be hard work. There are times when you'll feel tired, nauseous, sore, or just plain huge. Feeling a bond between you and your baby will help you see it's all worthwhile. And it will also get your relationship off to the best possible start when you finally meet for the first time.

In the early days, during your prenatal appointments will probably be when you feel closest to your baby. Hearing your baby's heartbeat or seeing your baby on a scan will make her feel so much more real to you.

When you feel your baby move for the first time, somewhere between 16 and 20 weeks, your relationship will develop even further. As those early fluttery butterfly feelings develop into more powerful kicks and slides, try to spend some time each day relaxing and just focusing on your baby's movements. You'll feel like you're beginning to get to know her personality through all her tiny thumps, jabs, and even hiccups.

By this time your baby will be able to feel your touch if you gently rub your hand over your belly. She can also hear your voice and her heart will beat a little faster when she hears it. Some moms find that talking, reading or even singing to their belly is a lovely way to connect with their baby. But don't worry if you

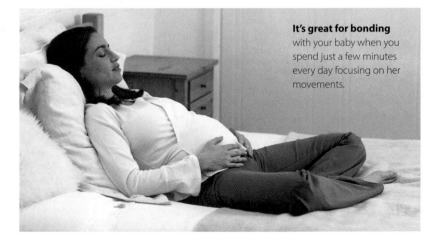

It's great for bonding with your baby when you spend just a few minutes every day focusing on her movements.

don't feel comfortable doing that. Your baby will still hear your voice as you talk to other people.

If you know your baby's sex, giving her a name (or nickname if you haven't yet decided on a name) will help you imagine what she'll be like.

Then, as your due date draws closer you'll spend time preparing the nursery or buying baby clothes. Now you'll probably be imagining her wearing the clothes or sleeping in the crib. And when that finally happens, your relationship will have moved on to its next phase.

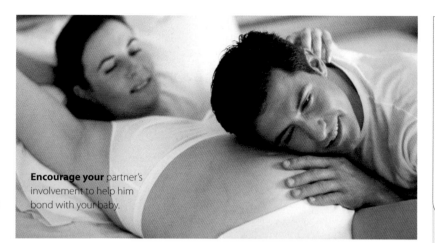

Encourage your partner's involvement to help him bond with your baby.

Involving dad

It's not unusual for dads-to-be to seem a little detached from their partner's pregnancy at first. After all, he's got a lot of thinking to do. Questions that may be running through his mind include: Will he be a good dad? Will labor go smoothly? Will he love the baby?

No dad can possibly relate to the minute-by-minute reality of carrying a baby. But he can be an active observer. Encourage him to take pictures as your belly grows or maybe give you a back massage when you're tired. When the baby's kicking, put his hand on your belly and let him feel the movements.

Go to prenatal appointments together. Be sure he doesn't miss the chance to get a first glimpse of your baby during an ultrasound. And, of course, you should attend childbirth classes together. By the time your baby arrives, you and your partner will have prepared the nursery, installed a car seat (hospitals won't let you drive baby home without one), settled on boy and girl options for your child's name and decided about breast- or bottle feeding.

Dad's **Diary**

The first ultrasound

"Seeing the baby for the first time at the scan—I have to admit, I was speechless. Literally. Reality hit home in a big way, making everything very real all of a sudden. It finally sank in. I was going to be a dad. There was a real baby in there—one that I'd have to care for and provide for over the next 18 years! I didn't know whether to laugh, cry, smile, or what.

Sally was a bit confused by my lack of reaction, but I really couldn't find the words to describe how I felt. Saying I was happy wouldn't have come close to it.

I was surprised by how clear the image was, too. Whenever I'd seen friends' scan pictures, I'd always joked about how all those scan pictures are the same—and how you can't really see what the baby looks like. But seeing my own baby on screen, with his tiny heart beating (strongly thankfully!), his little arms and hands (one hanging onto the umbilical cord), his little legs with his feet crossed and kicking—it was amazing.

It was such a huge relief to know that there were no problems too. Although I know the next scan will be able to tell us more...

We'd decided to wait until we'd had the first scan before we told people our news, so it was great to be able to take our scan pictures and show our tiny baby off to all our friends and family."

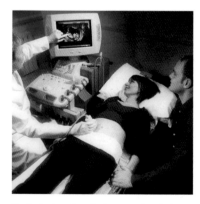

Dads-to-be often find seeing their baby on a scan for the first time very moving.

Getting ready for pregnancy

Staying safe and healthy

Your pregnancy diary

Birth and beyond

Preparing the nursery

Planning your baby's nursery is incredibly exciting and it's something you and your partner can enjoy doing together. Make sure you get the basics covered first—a crib, mattress, and some bedding— and think about safety, heating, and lighting before your little one arrives.

Key nursery needs

Whether your baby's a boy or girl, the basics are always the same. Either sex will need:

- A bassinet, Moses basket, or a full-size crib.
- Sheets and blankets or some sleep sacks.
- Storage (a chest of drawers or wardrobe) for clothing, blankets, and toys.
- A changing mat and a safe, well-positioned place to put it.
- A comfortable chair for feeding.
- A baby monitor and a smoke detector.

Not everything needs to be brand new. Having a baby can be expensive, but with a bit of know-how you should be able to save a lot on your purchases. There are some exceptions, though—most recommendations say not to use a secondhand mattress— but there's no harm in using your niece's crib or finding great decorations such as mobiles in a secondhand shop. Just keep in mind current safety standards for things like the spacing between crib bars (see opposite) and make sure anything secondhand is clean, undamaged, and in good working order.

Starting to plan

Becoming a parent can feel vaguely dreamlike until the crib or rocking chair arrives. But the planning should start before that. Begin with the practicalities, such as whether the radiator will need replacing and how to light the room.

You may have no choice about which room to make into the nursery, but ideally it should be near yours and somewhere quiet. If your home is drafty or damp, can you keep the nursery warm and dry, perhaps with new insulation, double glazing the windows, or damp-proofing? When your baby starts to explore, he shouldn't be able to open windows, lock doors, play with outlets, cords or wires, or get to the stairs. Can you clean the floors easily and is there a place nearby to store dirty diapers or laundry hygienically?

Then there's storage for all his clothing, blankets, and towels, as well as for books and toys. Shelves need to be secured and boxes shouldn't have lids that will slam on little hands or trap your toddler inside. Furniture should be too heavy to tip over if your baby pulls himself up on it, and it shouldn't have loose, sharp, or damaged bits. Beware, also, of lead paint; it's dangerous for pregnant women to remove it and for babies to peel and play with or eat.

Cribs and mattresses

A crib will probably be your baby's bed until he is two or three years old. It should be strong and sturdy without cracked or broken slats, and with no jagged points or edges. You can use your crib from the day your baby is born if you prefer, although many parents choose a Moses basket or bassinet for the first few months, or have their babies in the same bed as them; babies can look and feel a little lost in a big crib.

Cribs can be expensive so you might like to buy one secondhand. If you get a used crib, be careful about safety. Cribs manufactured before 1991 or purchased outside the United States may not meet current regulations. There are many crib styles and some convert into a toddler or full-sized bed, sofa, and more. Bedside cribs are useful for nighttime feedings; they have a removable side so you can put the crib right next to your bed.

Buying a mattress

There are many types of crib mattresses, so you may be confused at first. You may also be concerned to know which is the best and safest mattress to use. Make

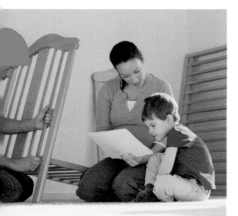

sure your mattress is firm, not soft, and doesn't sag or show any signs of wear and tear. Unless you know the history of a secondhand mattress, buy a new one.

- **Foam mattresses** These are generally the cheapest. They often have an easy-to-clean PVC cover and are available in a variety of thicknesses. But thicker is not necessarily better; density is most important. The better foam mattresses are high-density, about 1.5 pounds per cubic foot. Unfortunately, most foam mattresses don't list density on the packaging, so it's hard to know exactly what you're getting.

Getting the baby's nursery ready can be exciting and gives you the opportunity to involve the whole family.

- **Innerspring mattresses** These consist of coiled springs covered with a layer of foam and soft cotton fabric. One side is usually covered in cotton fabric and the other in wipe-clean plastic. It's a good idea to look for mattresses with a minimum of 150 coils.
- **Natural fiber mattresses** The interior of a natural fiber mattress is usually coconut fiber coated in latex, which is waterproof. The covers are made from soft cotton.
- **Hypoallergenic mattresses** Choose this option if allergies or asthma are a concern in your family. They have a quilted top layer that detaches from the body of the mattress and can be machine-washed in hot water to kill the dust mites that may cause allergies.

Safety in the nursery

When thinking about your baby's nursery, keep these safety tips in mind:
- Make sure crib slats are no more than $2^3/_8$ inches apart (you shouldn't be able to fit a soda can between them) to prevent your baby from slipping or getting caught between the bars. There shouldn't be any missing or broken slats.

- Check that the mattress fits snugly; you shouldn't be able to slip more than two fingers between the mattress and the side of the crib. There should be no corner-post extensions and no decorative cut-outs in the headboard or foot board.
- Don't use a pillow. For safe sleeping,

your baby needs a firm, flat surface.
- Recent findings recommend against using drop-side cribs from any manufacturer because of safety issues. Use a crib without this feature.
- Position the crib away from direct sunshine, windows, heaters, lamps, and wall decorations.

Too hot? Too cold?

It is a natural instinct for you to wrap your baby warmly, especially during the winter, but do not overdo it since overheating is associated with an increased risk of SIDS. A baby will sleep comfortably in a room heated to a temperature between 60° F (16° C) and 68° F (20° C). Our chart will give you an idea of what your baby needs according to the room temperature.

Room temperature	Sleepwear
75° F / 24° C or more	Light one-piece outfit
70° F / 21° C	One-piece footed pajamas or two layers of light clothing
64° F / 18° C	Flannel, footed, one-piece pajamas or one-piece outfit with a wearable blanket or sleep sack
61° F / 16° C	Warm, one-piece pajamas with a wearable blanket or a sleep sack and a hat

Getting ready for pregnancy

Staying safe and healthy

Your pregnancy diary

Birth and beyond

Credit-crunch nursery

If you're smart about it, you can outfit your baby's nursery for next to nothing—great for young couples or anyone on a strict budget.

● Your baby will eventually sleep in a crib, so you could skip the expense of a Moses basket or bassinet and go straight for the crib. The cheapest option is to get one secondhand, then all you need to buy new is a mattress (see p.103) and bedding.

● You don't need a state-of-the-art changing table—just a basic changing mat which won't cost a mint.

● Brighten up the nursery with a coat of paint and a few fun posters.

● Toys and mobiles don't have to cost an arm and a leg—find cheap, cheerful bargains in local discount stores.

● If friends and family want to buy your new baby gifts, ask for specific things or set up a gift registry with a department store.

Decorating

Now for the fun part. If you have a color or theme in mind, build it around the furniture and other pieces you must have in the nursery. Window treatments can create a focal point in an otherwise subtly decorated room, or they can just complement the overall color scheme by pulling together shades or textures that you've used elsewhere in the room. Either way, the window treatment you choose should be able to make the room sufficiently dark for naptime or bright summer evenings and keep the cold out in the winter. Look for materials that won't fade or gather dust, and keep any cords out of baby's reach. You should also make sure that your window treatments—like the bedding or any other fabric in the room—are flameproof.

Why not ask family members for their input on the decorating? Someone may even volunteer to make the curtains or help with the painting!

Color, movement, and music

Infants have limited eyesight at first, but they seem to love black and white patterns. Some babies are even mesmerized by the black beams that run across the white ceiling in traditional old houses.

Young babies also love mobiles with strong colors, music or nightlights, while pictures or mirrors can be a nice addition to the nursery—just be sure they aren't hanging near the crib or changing table, or anywhere an older baby can climb to dislodge them.

You can also add some color with your choice of flooring. It should be comfortable, easy to clean and slip-resistant. Wood or laminate are good choices, and you might consider rubber and bamboo. Sadly, flooring isn't mess-resistant, but as long as books and toys don't cause you to stumble, your baby won't mind a muddle.

ParentsAsk...

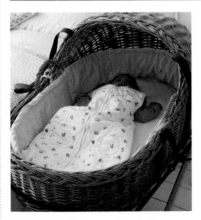

Moses baskets are good for the first couple of months—they are very portable, and small enough to feel cozy.

Will I need a night-light for my baby?

Night-lights can be useful for toddlers who are afraid of the dark but babies don't need them. That's because children don't experience nighttime anxiety until they are two or three years old, when they're capable of imagining scary things lurking in the dark. In the meantime, your baby will sleep better in a dark room.

Should we buy a breathing monitor?

A breathing monitor makes a sound to alert you if your baby stops breathing. Normal, healthy babies do not need one and there is no evidence to show that they prevent sudden infant death syndrome. If at all

possible, your baby should sleep in the same room as you for the first six months. This will help you to keep a closer eye on any changes in your baby's breathing during the night.

Are baby wearable blankets a good idea?

The great thing about baby wearable blankets—warm, one-piece outfits with a bag-style bottom—is that your baby can't kick them off. If you use one, make sure it doesn't have a hood and that it is the right size around the neck so your baby won't slip down inside the bag. These are a good alternative to using blankets, which you should avoid because of the risk of suffocation and making your baby too hot.

Seating and storage

A comfortable chair will be your back's best friend, so invest time in finding one that suits you. You may love the idea of your grandmother's rocking chair, but consider how you will position your baby for feeding and whether it can accommodate both of you. Don't underestimate how much you will come to rely on a sturdy seat at the end of a long day: the last thing you'll want is one that puts you in an awkward, hunched, or twisted position. Some moms couldn't live without a glider chair—a soothing but expensive option—while others are content with the simplest bench. You might even be able to incorporate a seat into an existing space, creating built-in storage.

Storage is such a simple concept, yet so hard for exhausted parents to put into practice. Luckily, there are business empires built on getting organized—just do a quick search online. Try not to be overwhelmed by the options when a few simple baskets, stackable boxes, or shelves could be all you need to minimize the nursery mess.

Convenience is key, but storage can also be designed so it complements the décor. Give baskets the flourish of a ribbon so that they match the curtains or paint wooden boxes to go with the skirting board. Keep diaper supplies on a shelf near the changing table or in a decorative hanging pocket on a peg. You can even display your favorite baby hats or outfits on wall hooks.

Dad's **Diary**

Getting the nursery ready

"We started preparing the baby's nursery this week. When I say we, I mean Emma has chosen the colors, the furniture, the curtains—the tasteful selection of soft toys. I'm doing all the hard work: all the painting and varnishing (Emma's staying out of the way to be on the safe side), putting together the crib and the changing table, building and installing all the shelves, hanging the new blackout blinds, lugging the new rocking chair up the stairs. Phew! When I've finished, all Emma will have to do is arrange the soft furnishings in a decorative manner."

Sharing with a sibling

It is recommended that a baby sleeps in the same room as his parents for the first six months of life. This helps reduce the risk of crib death and is also convenient because babies tend to wake several times a night for feeding in the early part of their lives.

After that time, if your baby and toddler both sleep well, it is fine for them to share a room. Problems only arise if they wake frequently and prevent each other from falling back asleep, although many babies and children aren't bothered by their siblings crying. Also, bedtimes can vary with differing age groups and could potentially cause disturbances. Do make sure, though, that an unchecked toddler is not able to "feed" any inappropriate toys through

the bars of the crib, since these could be a hazard to your baby. Being together at nighttime may enhance your children's relationship and could be a source of

comfort and security to them while they are both young. As they grow, sharing a bedroom will teach important lessons about boundaries and sharing.

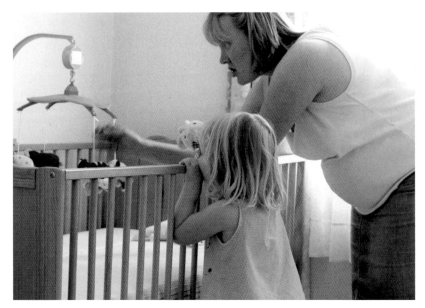

Once your new baby is sleeping well it can be comforting for him and his older sibling to share a bedroom.

Essential baby buys

A stroll around a baby equipment store can be a bewildering and overwhelming experience for parents-to-be. Does your baby really need so much stuff? The truth is that he probably doesn't. Try to stick to the basics—you can always pick up other things you need after he's born.

Clothing for your newborn

When you are buying for your newborn, it's helpful to know what is actually useful—and what you can do without. Here are the essentials:

- One-piece outfits with wide head openings and loose-fitting ankle and leg cuffs; you need four to seven.
- One-piece pajamas or wearable blankets, like the Sleepsack or Lullabag, to keep your baby warm and safe at night; again, get four to seven.
- A soft warm hat for a winter baby, or a wide-brimmed sun hat for a summer baby.
- Socks or booties. Get four to seven pairs to keep his feet warm; he doesn't need shoes.
- A soft blanket or two to wrap and cuddle your baby in.
- A one-piece fleece suit is also useful for a winter baby.
- A sweater or jacket that buttons down the front; most babies don't like having clothes pulled over their heads.

Practicalities

Make sure everything is machine-washable! And where possible, 100 percent cotton so that it's gentle on your baby's skin. Fleecy polyester jackets and blankets can irritate and make your baby too hot. Also, wash all clothing before use in baby detergent free of fragrances and dyes, to avoid irritation.

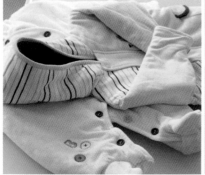

Some warmer clothes are a must for a winter baby. For going out, opt for an all-in-one suit with a cozy hood.

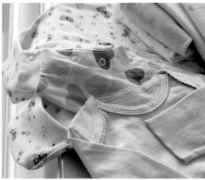

You'll need several little undershirts with envelope necks since new babies don't like having clothing pulled over their faces.

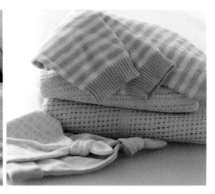

Cellular cotton blankets are great to keep your baby warm and to wrap him in for a snuggle. A couple of soft hats are useful, too.

Bedding and equipment

Use a flannel-backed, waterproof mattress pad, which is safer, cooler, and more comfortable than a plain plastic or rubber cover. Cover the pad with a fitted sheet made of cotton or, in winter, flannel. Make sure the sheet fits snugly around the mattress.

While it's tempting to tuck your infant in with cozy blankets, soft bedding is a suffocation hazard and has been strongly linked to SIDS (sudden infant death syndrome). To keep your baby warm, it's best to use sleepers or pajamas. If you do use a blanket, choose a thin one and tuck it in securely around

The American Academy of Pediatrics (AAP), the Consumer Product Safety Commission (CPSC), and the National Institutes of Child Health (NICHD) recommend that you take all pillows, comforters, quilts, sheepskins, stuffed toys, and other soft objects out of the crib. Don't let your child sleep with a pillow until she's older than age two and has made the transition to a bed.

Other key equipment
In addition to a Moses basket or a crib and mattress (see pp.102–103) there are a number of other essential items:

least the first few days or so. If you're planning to use cloth diapers, have at least one package of disposables handy, too. For cloth diapers, you'll also need diaper liners and waterproof wraps, and a bucket with a lid to store dirty diapers.
● A stroller that has a padded seat and a lie-flat position so it is appropriate for a newborn (see p.109).
● If you have a car, you will need a rear-facing car seat (see p.109).
● If you are planning to bottle feed, you will need bottles, nipples, bottle brushes, and maybe a bottle warmer (see p.108).
● If you are planning to breast-feed, you

"If you are going to **use cloth diapers** have at least **one package of disposables** handy too."

the foot and sides of the mattress, reaching only up to your baby's chest. Tuck it in under her arms, not her chin.

If you decide to use bumper pads, choose ones that are thin and fasten them securely to the crib so they can't come loose. Make sure the bumper ties don't dangle into the crib.

● A baby bath or a newborn bath support that you can put in your own bath (you could use a plastic dish-sink bowl to begin with).
● Diapers (disposable or reusable)—since newborn babies need their diapers changed eight to 10 times a day, buy enough diapers to keep you going for at

will need nursing bras and breast pads. Breast-feeding moms who plan to return to work might need a breast pump.
● Baby wipes, burp cloths, diaper cream.
● A changing mat, or changing table.
● A couple of small towels and some mild baby bath.
● A changing bag.

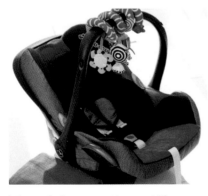

A rear-facing car seat is essential for a new baby. You must make sure it is properly installed and fits your car perfectly.

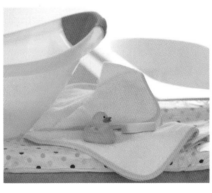

A baby bath is useful, although you could start with a plastic bowl. A changing mat or changing unit is a must have.

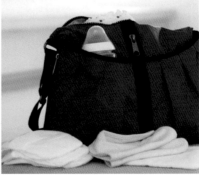

You'll definitely need a changing bag with lots of pockets to hold all your baby's supplies when you go on outings.

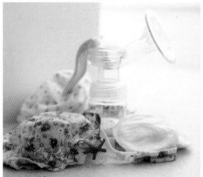

If you plan to breast-feed, you will need a nursing bra and breast pads, and a breast pump will be useful for expressing milk.

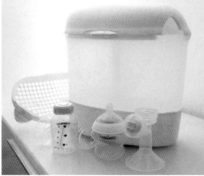

A sterilizer isn't necessary for bottle-feeding, but if you want to sterilize your bottles you might want to invest in one.

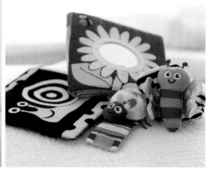

In the first few months, your baby will appreciate small brightly colored soft toys, such as rattles, and soft books with a mirror.

Baby goes green

The greenest choice is not to buy much baby equipment at all and borrow where possible. But here are some unusual green buys:

● A natural crib mattress made from coir with an organic cotton cover. It's more expensive than a traditional mattress but lasts longer.

● Hooded bamboo baby towels: they're extra-absorbent.

Sometimes you don't have to buy anything—or very little! Try the following:

● Join a toy library.

● Take baby in the bath with you.

● Raid the pantry for vegetable oil —great for dry skin and baby massage.

● A sling or front carrier (you won't need a car seat if you're walking everywhere), and a borrowed carriage.

● Washable breast pads and a couple of breast-feeding bras (organic cotton if possible).

● Secondhand or borrowed baby clothes. If you want to buy new, choose organic Fairtrade cotton.

● Choose long-lasting toys that can be passed down to the next generation.

Feeding

All you really need in order to breast-feed are your baby and your breasts. For bottle-feeding moms, though, there are some products and accessories that will make life easier.

● **Breast pumps** If you're going to be expressing at work and want to make your pumping time as short as possible, get an electric pump that is reliable, quiet and fast. If you only plan to express once or twice a week, a hand pump will probably do just as well.

● **Nursing bras** A good nursing bra needs to be comfortable and adjustable, should give good support and must be easy to get in and out of. It's worth being fitted for one after you have reached 36 weeks of pregnancy.

● **Feeding bottles** If you're planning to bottle feed, basic bottles are inexpensive and available in wide-neck or standard. Each bottle generally comes with a nipple and a lid. Anti-colic bottles claim to reduce the amount of air a baby takes in while feeding, which is thought to be a possible cause of colic. If your baby is unsettled after feedings and suffers with gas, it might be worth investing in one of these systems, but be aware that they don't work for every baby.

● **Breast milk storage supplies** If you're pumping, you'll need plastic or glass feeding bottles with secure caps to seal in freshness. Or you can use plastic bags made especially for storing milk.

● **Bottle warmer** There's no health reason to feed a baby warmed milk, but your baby may prefer it. You could buy a bottle warmer, or simply warm a bottle in a pan of hot—not boiling—water, or by running it under the tap.

● **Nipples** These come in various "flow" sizes, in different types of material— latex or silicone—and in different shapes, including standard and "natural," which mimic the shape of a nipple. Generally, you should start with slow flow for newborn babies.

● **Other supplies** You might find it helpful to use a dishwasher basket for nipples, rings, and bottle caps, and a bottle-drying rack. These are available at most baby supply stores. If you plan to routinely sterilize bottles, you may want to invest in an electric sterilizer or one that goes in the microwave.

Entertaining your baby

When it comes to entertaining your baby, you'll find that, in her first months, she will most appreciate things she can look at and listen to. She might enjoy:

● **Mobiles** Look for ones with high-contrast colors (black and white is good) and patterns as well as those that play music. For safety's sake, keep the mobile out of your baby's reach.

● **Mirrors** Although she won't realize it's herself she's seeing at this stage, your baby will find her own reflection fascinating. By three months, she may begin smiling at it. Look for a mirror that you can hang near a changing table.

● **Soft books with high-contrast patterns** There are plenty of these for sale. Lie down next to her so she can watch you as you read aloud to her.

● **Rattles** Give your baby a soft rattle to hold and shake. That way she can enjoy and experiment with sounds that she makes herself.

● **Wind chimes** Hang a set of these in a place where she can watch them move and listen to the sound.

● **Black, white, and red toys** These high-contrast toys and playmats will help your child pick out the differences in shapes and patterns.

Taking your baby out

You may want to have the coolest stroller on the block. Maybe you like keeping your baby cuddled up next to you in a sling. Perhaps you have an older child to bring along. Whatever your needs, there's a system that's just right.

● **Convertible strollers** These have multiple positions and can grow with your baby. Some have a removable bassinet for newborns and adjustable, upright seats for older babies.

● **Umbrella strollers** These are lightweight and compact, but are best for older babies and toddlers, who don't need as much head support.

● **Multiple occupancy strollers** Tandem models seat children one behind the other; some replace the rear seat with a jump seat/standing platform. Side-by-side strollers let two children communicate with each other.

● **Jogging strollers** Thick rubber wheels give a smooth ride everywhere. They're especially good for moms who

like to go running with their baby. When your baby's under six months old, use an adapter to attach your baby's car seat to the stroller. This will keep your baby's head and neck stable.

● **Car seat strollers** A travel system is a type of stand-alone stroller on which you can snap an infant car seat. There are also lightweight stroller frames; you simply snap the car seat into it.

● **Car seats** Choosing the right car seat for your child's age and weight, and installing it correctly, is very important. Some child seats work better in some models of car than others, so try before you buy if possible.

● **Carriers** Baby carriers, backpacks, and slings are simple, lightweight systems that allow you to keep your baby close to you, but still have your hands free for other activities. When using a sling, be sure your baby's face is visible (not covered by fabric) at all times, and check on her frequently.

Laid-back mom

If you want to be able to get up and go without messing around with a stroller, then try a sling.

"With my first baby I found using a stroller really cumbersome so I ended up mostly using a sling. It was so easy. It was really just a long piece of stretchy fabric but it was very comfortable to wear. And my baby loved it—and often went right off to sleep in it, too.

Sometimes I would use the sling around the house when I wanted to do something and needed my hands free, but it was absolutely fantastic when we were out and about. It was a really nice feeling to be able to go where I wanted without worrying about how I was going to get there. I'm pregnant again now and I know that having a sling is going to help me take care of the new baby and my toddler at the same time. Sounds silly but I can't wait to start using it again."

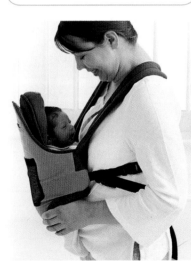

A front pack carrier is a convenient way of taking your baby out and about, and many babies just love the closeness a carrier gives.

Getting ready for pregnancy

Staying safe and healthy

Your pregnancy diary

Birth and beyond

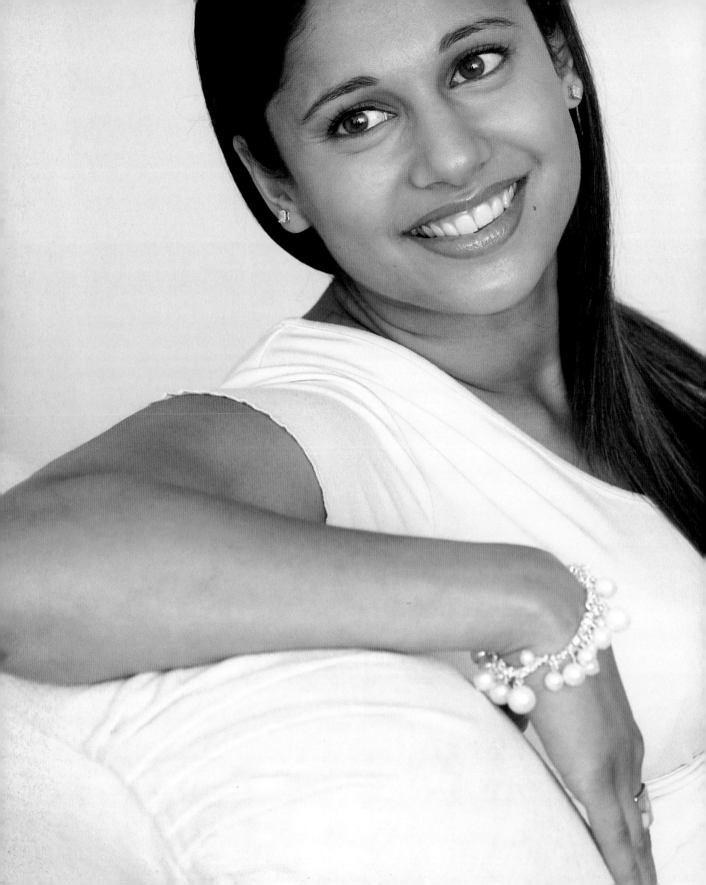

Your pregnancy diary

A week-by-week guide

The first trimester

All change

There are many changes to get used to in the first trimester, so take things one step at a time. Remember to eat well, rest when your body tells you to, and remind yourself that women have been growing babies for thousands of years, so your body knows what it should be doing.

The start of the journey

The first trimester (or three months) lasts to the end of week 13. This is when you may be experiencing some of the most unpleasant pregnancy symptoms, such as nausea and fatigue. It's an emotional time, too, because you flit between excitement and joy, anxiety, and uncertainty. Try to enjoy these early weeks as much as you can. You're at the beginning of an incredible journey.

From cell to tiny human

During the first trimester, your baby develops from a microscopic single cell to a fully formed tiny human being with all the major organs in place and ready to grow. At 12 weeks, your baby will have grown to around 2¼ inches long from crown to rump (about the size of a lime) and will weigh around ½ ounce. She'll even have toothbuds and finger nails. Her heart will start beating during week six, and will beat 150 times a minute—roughly twice the rate of an adult heart.

You'll experience a lot of physical changes too. Your uterus will expand to accommodate your growing baby. Before pregnancy it was the size of a clenched fist; by six weeks it will be as big as a grapefruit. You may experience some aching in your lower abdomen as

your muscles and ligaments stretch to support it. You'll find you need to urinate more often too, as your uterus presses on your bladder. Your breasts may feel sore and they may grow large enough for you to need a bigger bra by the end of this trimester. By seven weeks, you'll have 10 percent more blood than you did before you were pregnant (by the end of your pregnancy, you'll have 40 to 45 percent more blood running through your veins and arteries to meet the demands of your full-term baby).

Once you know you are pregnant, make an appointment to arrange prenatal care. It's usual to be seen at around seven to nine weeks. This allows time to arrange any first trimester screening tests (see pp.128–9). You'll be offered your first ultrasound when you're 16 to 20 weeks pregnant, or earlier if you are unsure of your dates or are suspected of carrying multiples. This scan will also tell you if you're carrying more than one baby. If you've decided to have a nuchal translucency (NT) scan (see p.137) to screen for Down syndrome, it needs to be done at 11 to 13 weeks. Sometimes an early scan is needed, for example, if you are feeling pain or are bleeding, or if you've had a miscarriage in the past.

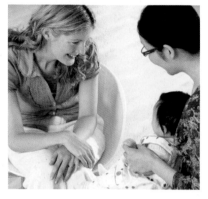

Once you know you're pregnant, take the opportunity to learn from your friends about their experiences of pregnancy.

Laid-back mom

Staying relaxed about becoming pregnant can help you keep calm when your test's positive.

"I'd been on the pill for five years, but a couple of months ago, my partner and I decided I should come off it and we'd let nature take its course. I've just taken a pregnancy test and I'm thrilled that it's positive. I thought I'd feel a bit panicked when it actually happened, and I certainly didn't expect to get pregnant so quickly, but I think because we've been so relaxed about the whole thing, I still feel perfectly calm. I'm just ridiculously happy now!"

Getting ready for pregnancy

Staying safe and healthy

Your pregnancy diary

Birth and beyond

▼ Your body at **03** Weeks

03 Weeks

✳ A momentous meeting has taken place inside you—a single sperm has broken into and fertilized your egg.

✳ You probably don't know you're pregnant yet, but you may see a little spotting by the end of this week.

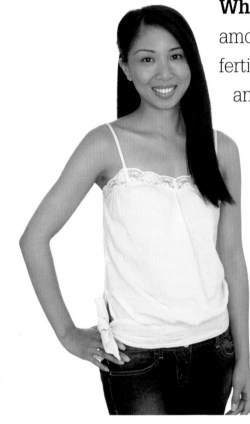

While you're waiting for your period a huge amount of activity is going on in your body. Your fertilized egg is busy implanting itself in your uterus and your hormone levels are going crazy.

I think I may be pregnant

A momentous meeting has taken place inside you—a single sperm has broken through the tough outer membrane of your egg and fertilized it, triggering conception. Several days later, the fertilized egg has burrowed into the lining of your uterus and has started to grow. A baby is in the making! You probably don't know you're pregnant yet, but you may notice a little spotting by the end of this week. This so-called implantation bleeding may be caused by the egg burrowing into the blood-rich uterine lining (a process that began last week at six days after fertilization), but no one knows for sure. In any case, the spotting is very light and only a minority of pregnant women experience it at all.

Hormonal changes
What's going on in your uterus now? A lot. Your baby-in-the-making is just a tiny ball, or blastocyst (see pp.34–5), consisting of several hundred cells that are multiplying wildly. Once the blastocyst takes up residence in your uterus, it is called an embryo (see pp.34–5). The part of the embryo that will develop into the placenta starts producing the pregnancy hormone human chorionic gonadotropin (hCG), which tells your ovaries to stop releasing eggs and triggers increased production of estrogen and progesterone. These keep your uterus from shedding its lining—together with its tiny passenger—and stimulate placental growth. The hormone that turns a pregnancy test positive is hCG; by the end of this week, you may be able to take a pregnancy test and get a positive result. (If your test is negative and you still haven't had your period in two or three days, then try again.)

While all this is going on, amniotic fluid is beginning to collect around your multiplying ball of cells in the cavity that will eventually become the amniotic sac. This fluid will cushion your baby during the weeks and months ahead.

Right now, your little embryo is receiving oxygen and nutrients (and discarding waste products) through a primitive circulation system made up of microscopic tunnels. These connect your developing baby to the blood vessels in your uterine wall. By the end of next week, the placenta will be well enough developed to take over this task.

▼ Your baby at **03** Weeks
....
Amazing things are happening, perhaps even before you know you're pregnant.

✳ This week, a rush of activity occurs. In the 12 to 24 hours after you ovulate and an egg is swept into a fallopian tube, that egg can be fertilized if one of 300 million sperm (an average ejaculation) manages to swim all the way to the fallopian tube—from the vagina through the uterus—to penetrate it.

Pregnant again?

Many of us find that second and subsequent pregnancies pass in a flash and suddenly the birth is approaching, without you having gone through any of the emotional preparation or made any of the practical arrangements that you did first time.

It's different

You will probably find that you start to show much earlier than last time, and that you feel the new baby moving several weeks before you did with your first. For a lot of women, nausea and vomiting are not as bad in their second pregnancy, but this isn't universal. Some of the symptoms you had during your first pregnancy, such as varicose veins and hemorrhoids, may well recur, but you'll know better how to deal with them this time.

If you had a medical problem in your first pregnancy, such as gestational diabetes (see p.229) or obstetric cholestasis (see pp.230–31), it may recur in your second. If you had preeclampsia (see p.233) in a first pregnancy, you have about a one-in-five chance of it recurring. However, you now know the kind of diet you need to have, the medication you should take, and the specialists you have to see, so both you and your doctors can manage the condition much more effectively.

Recurring worries

You may find yourself worrying about problems you had during your first pregnancy or labor. Perhaps you pushed these bad experiences to the back of your mind once they were over, but now they are resurfacing because you're pregnant again. Don't struggle along without talking to someone.

Ask to have a talk about them with your doctor, or talk to a friend or your childbirth teacher. Or you might arrange to get a copy of your medical records from your previous pregnancy and read through them.

Most pregnant women have 10 to 15 prenatal visits. You may feel that you're not receiving the same level of attention as you did before, but this is because second pregnancies are generally straightforward. If there is anything worrying you, give your doctor a call.

Shared experiences

Perhaps you are pregnant with your second child at the same time as your friends are pregnant with their second. You can share experiences with them, sympathize with each other over

If you're pregnant for the second time, take every opportunity to spend time with your first child before your new baby arrives.

pregnancy symptoms, and grab a quick cup of coffee while your toddlers play together! If there is a big gap between your pregnancies, perhaps contact the hospital where you plan to deliver; they often run "refresher" courses for women who are expecting their second or subsequent babies.

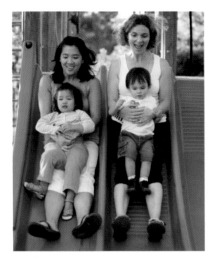

ParentsAsk...

I've had some light bleeding. Is that a period or something else?

It's impossible to say for sure at this stage. If your period is usually right on schedule and you are now late, you may well be pregnant. On the other hand, it's not uncommon for women to get their period a few days late sometimes.

It's thought that implantation (when the embryo attaches itself to the lining of the uterus; see pp.34–5) can sometimes cause spotting. However, one small study in the United States found that nine percent of women had at least one day of bleeding during their early pregnancy, and this was more likely to happen when a woman's period was due than around implantation.

If you have other symptoms, such as a one-sided pain low down in your abdomen, see your doctor immediately; you could have an ectopic pregnancy (when the embryo has implanted in the fallopian tube rather than in the uterus; see pp.44–5). Bleeding with abdominal pain may also be a sign of an impending miscarriage, but that certainly isn't true in every case.

Finally, it's possible that the blood you saw may have nothing to do with pregnancy. Your cervix could be inflamed and bleed easily, especially after pap smears, internal examinations, or sex. Or you may have an infection. Either way, it's always important to report any bleeding between periods or after sex to your doctor.

Getting ready for pregnancy

Staying safe and healthy

Your pregnancy diary

Birth and beyond

Your body at **04** Weeks

04 Weeks

❉ You may not feel pregnant yet, but your body is already going through enormous changes.

❉ Feeling queasy yet? If not, brace yourself—nausea and vomiting (morning sickness) can strike anytime.

If finding out you're pregnant brings mixed feelings, listen to those feelings and talk them through. Remember, you have another eight months or so to get used to the idea of becoming a mom.

Feelings of anticipation

The two layers of the embryo form organs and tissue

Excitement, joy, anticipation—all of these emotions run high once you find out you're pregnant. But pregnancy brings out the worrier in us, too. And for good reason: you're growing a life inside of you. It's natural to worry about what you eat, drink, think, feel, and do because you don't want anything to hurt your baby. You may also worry about how this new person will change your life and personal relationships.

Pregnancy can be a stressful and overwhelming time. You may be overjoyed at the thought of having a baby one day, and then the next day start wondering what you've got yourself into. You may be worried about whether you'll be a good mom, whether the baby will be healthy, and how the cost of having a child will affect your family's future finances. And you may worry about how your relationship with your partner and your other children will be affected—whether you'll still be able to give them the attention they need. As

unsettling as this is (especially if you pride yourself on being in control), try to remind yourself that emotional upheaval is normal at this stage. Mood swings are thought to be caused partly by fluctuating hormones (see p.71 and p.76). They tend to be most pronounced in the first 12 weeks of pregnancy. They should gradually diminish as you figure things out and as your body adapts to its new role. To help with mood swings if you're feeling low, you could try the following suggestions:

● **Talk it over** Air your worries about the future with your partner or with understanding friends. Just putting your concerns into words often helps dispel them or helps you find solutions.

● **Do something that makes you feel good** This might mean carving out some special time for you and your partner. Or it might mean taking some time alone for yourself: curl up for a nap, go for a walk, go for a massage, or go to see a movie with a friend.

● **Take care of yourself** Get plenty of sleep, eat well, exercise, and try to have some fun. If you still find anxiety creeping in, try taking a pregnancy yoga class, or practicing meditation, or other relaxation techniques.

▼ Your baby at **04** Weeks

Your ball of cells is now officially an embryo (see pp.34–5). It is changing fast.

❉ It is now divided into two layers that will form your baby's organs and tissues. It is attached to the developing placenta by a stalk that will soon form part of the umbilical cord. The embryo also starts changing from a disk to an upside-down pear shape with a line—the primitive streak—down the center.

My cluster of cells

This week marks the beginning of the embryonic period, when the blastocyst has implanted and become an embryo. From now until 10 weeks, all of your baby's organs will begin to develop and some will even begin to function. As a result, this is the stage when he'll be most vulnerable to anything that might interfere with his development.

He is now the size of a poppy seed and consists of two layers: the epiblast and the hypoblast. All his organs and body parts develop from these.

The primitive placenta is also made up of two layers at this point. Its cells are busy tunneling into the lining of your uterus, creating spaces for your blood to flow so that the developed placenta will be able to provide nutrients and oxygen to your growing baby when it starts to function at the end of this week.

Also present now are the amniotic sac, which will house your baby, the amniotic fluid, which will cushion him as he grows, and the yolk sac, which produces your baby's red blood cells and helps deliver nutrients to him until the placenta has developed and is ready to take over this duty.

If you're taking any medications—prescription or over the counter—ask now whether it's safe to keep taking them. And be sure to alert your doctor to any other issues of concern.

The next six weeks are critical to your baby's development. The rudimentary versions of the placenta and umbilical cord, which deliver nourishment and oxygen to your baby, are already functioning. Through the placenta, your baby is exposed to what you take into your body, so make sure it's good for both of you.

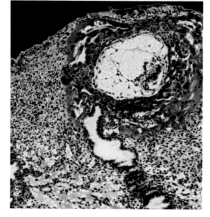

Eleven days after fertilization the inner cells of the embryo start developing into two layers—the epiblast and the hypoblast.

If you haven't already tried a home pregnancy test, taking one now will confirm your pregnancy. Once you get confirmation, you can call your doctor and make an appointment. Good consistent prenatal care is one of the best ways to ensure that you and your baby are healthy throughout pregnancy.

Dad's **Diary**

From pharmacy to father

" 'Can I help you?' the pharmacist enquires. I blush bright red. 'Condoms?' she second guesses. 'Actually, I need a pregnancy test.'

'Oh! Any preference for the type?'

The pee-on-a-stick type? The words form in my mind, but somehow I resist saying them. I shake my head. I don't have a preferred pregnancy-testing method.

The pharmacist passes me a box with a reassuring warm smile. 'This one should be fine.' I hurriedly exit the store, feeling like some naughty schoolboy. But at nearly 40 years old, I am anything but.

Now back at home with Jo, I supervise a controlled test under strict laboratory conditions; we have to do it properly. 'Two minutes.' I begin a countdown as if

commentating on a space-shuttle launch. My stopwatch bleeps. It's the moment of truth. We stare at each other in silence for a moment before I flip the test over. 'Well?' Jo begs.

Through the gaps in my fingers I am staring at the test window. I'm staring at the very faint blue line which is starting to appear. I can hear Jo's voice somewhere in the distance, but I daren't take my eyes off that line. Come on! You can do it! I will it on as if we have just fast-forwarded nine months to the birth.

'Yes!' At last I can afford to look up at Jo. 'Yes. I'm going to be a Dad!' "

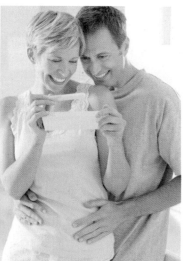

If you've decided to start a family, the joy of discovering you're pregnant is one that you'll want to share with your partner.

Getting ready for pregnancy

Staying safe and healthy

Your pregnancy diary

Birth and beyond

Your body at **05** Weeks

05 Weeks

❊ Pregnancy symptoms continue or start this week. Most women notice nausea, fatigue, and sore breasts.

❊ Hormonal changes this week will start to expand your kidneys, making you need to urinate more often.

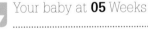

You're thrilled to be pregnant, but not so thrilled by the effect it has on your party animal lifestyle. But remember, giving up the booze, cigarettes, and recreational drugs is the best way to protect your baby.

Time to kick those bad habits

We all have our vices, but while you're pregnant it pays to put the partying on hold—at least for a while!

I'm a smoker…

Even if you haven't been able to stop smoking in the past, you can do it this time. About 40 percent of all pregnant women who smoke manage to quit the habit. Different people take different approaches to giving up smoking.

Most successful quitters set a "giving-up date" and make it public by telling friends, family and colleagues. Once you've established the "when,"

bite to eat; others go for a walk. Find something to distract your mind for a few minutes. Quiting smoking can be much easier if you don't try to do it by yourself. Support from friends and family can increase your chances of success. Ask the people close to you for help.

I take drugs

Getting off any drug is never easy when you are addicted, even when you are pregnant. Although it may take courage, it is always better to let your maternity care providers know if you are taking a particular drug. Then they will be able

Your baby at **05** Weeks

You may not look pregnant yet, but plenty of changes are happening inside you.

❊ At this early stage you may not even have had any pregnancy symptoms but your baby is growing rapidly. The embryo still looks more like a tadpole than a human, but by the end of this week the tiny S-shaped heart may have begun to beat and the eyes and ears will have started to develop.

"Binge drinking **is dangerous** for your **developing baby**."

it's time to think about the "how." Ask yourself if you're ready to go cold turkey or if you'd prefer to use nicotine replacement therapy (NRT). You'll need to plan ahead for cravings, too. These last only two or three minutes on average so your plan can be a simple one. Some people chew gum or grab a

to make sure you and your baby receive the specific help and care you need. Remember: you won't be the first mom-to-be in this position that they've ever met, and they will do what they can to help. By asking for help you will be demonstrating your willingness to put your baby's health first. If you take just

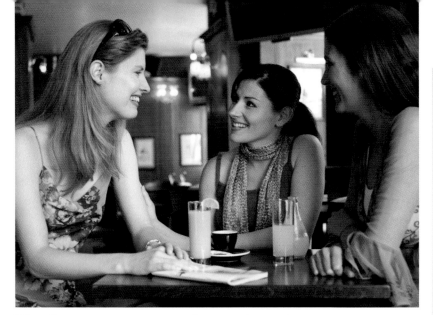

Now that you are pregnant you can still enjoy a night out with your girlfriends at a bar or restaurant, but have juice instead of alcohol.

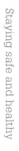

Organized mom

Keeping a pregnancy diary can have practical uses as well as being part of your family history.

"I haven't kept a diary since I was a teenager, but as soon as I discovered I was pregnant, I really wanted to make a record of all the weird and wonderful things that are happening to me. Whenever I ask my mom about when she was pregnant with me, she can never quite remember. I don't want to forget a thing—and I'd like my baby to be able to read my pregnancy journal one day, too. I make a note of changes to my body, how I'm feeling, all my anxieties. It's great to get things off my chest, even though no one else reads it. It's also quite practical. I note what I've eaten so I can keep track of my calorie intake and make sure I'm getting all the right nutrients."

recreational drugs occasionally or on the weekends, these will still harm your baby, so now is the time to stop.

I like a drink or two

Binge drinking or getting drunk during pregnancy is dangerous for your developing baby. Binge drinking is drinking five or more units of alcohol on one occasion. Alcohol is a toxin. When you drink, it rapidly reaches your baby through your bloodstream and across the placenta. Too much alcohol can cause permanent damage to the cells of a developing baby. It can also cause problems during pregnancy, such as miscarriage and premature birth. Experts are less sure whether drinking at moderate levels is dangerous or not. Several scientific reviews of the research have found no consistent evidence of adverse affects of drinking at low (under two units a day) to moderate levels (two to five units a day). But there is no known "safe" level of alcohol either, so it's best to steer clear of alcohol.

All public health officials in the United States, along with the American Academy of Pediatrics and the American College of Obstetricians and Gynecologists, recommend you give up drinking before getting pregnant. But if you didn't, try not to worry. Thousands of women have a few drinks before they know they are pregnant, or conceived around the time of a binge drinking session, and their babies have been fine.

Recreational drugs and pregnancy

Recreational drugs can be harmful to you and your baby during pregnancy. Here's an idea of how they affect you:
- **Marijuana** Several studies have associated regular use of marijuana during pregnancy with fetal growth retardation and low birthweight.
- **LSD** One study showed that the pure form of LSD did not cause any fetal abnormalities or an increased risk of miscarriage. However, there have been reports of congenital abnormalities in the babies of women who use LSD and other drugs. As we do not know exactly what effect these drugs have on unborn babies, it's wise to avoid them.
- **Cocaine** This drug can cause serious problems. If used in the early months, it can increase the risk of miscarriage. Used later, it could trigger premature labor. It may also cause the placenta to separate from the wall of the uterus before labor begins.
- **Ecstasy and amphetamines** These substances have been linked to birth defects, mainly of the limbs and heart.
- **Heroin** This can cause growth restriction, premature delivery—around half of the babies who are born to heroin-addicted mothers are born early—and stillbirth.

Diet in the first trimester

If you live on tuna sandwiches and coffee, it's time to spruce up your diet. Not only will this help you cope with early pregnancy symptoms like fatigue and nausea, but it will ensure that you and your baby get all the vital nutrients you need while you're pregnant.

The perfect pregnancy diet

You may not have much of an appetite at the moment, especially if you're suffering from nausea and vomiting. On the other hand, you may be packing away more food than you ever dreamed possible. However you find that pregnancy is affecting your appetite, it's important to try to eat healthily when you can. A healthy diet will make you feel better, and give your baby all the nutrients she needs to develop.

Small, regular meals and frequent (noncaffeinated) drinks, can combat any nausea or fatigue. Contrary to popular belief, you need only about 300 extra calories a day when you're pregnant, less in your first trimester, so you definitely should not feel that you have to try to eat for two.

Fruit and vegetables

Try to eat seven or more servings of fruit and vegetables a day as part of a healthy pregnancy diet. If you're not a fan of fruit and vegetables make a start by eating more of those you do like. Add sliced bananas or apple to your breakfast cereal, grate carrots onto your lunchtime wrap, drink a lunchtime glass of pure fruit juice (this counts as one portion) or have two different vegetables with your main meal instead of your usual one.

Folic acid is a particularly important nutrient during the first trimester (see opposite). Overcooking destroys folates, so try to eat your vegetables lightly steamed, microwaved, or raw.

And finally, eat when you feel hungry. As long as you are eating wholesome, fresh foods and gaining weight at the appropriate rate, relax!

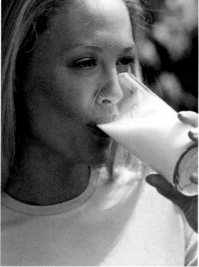

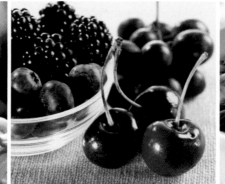

Seven servings of fruit or vegetables (above) should be a regular part of your diet. A handful of grapes or two handfuls of cherries or berry fruits make up a portion. **Milk and dairy products (left)** such as cheese and yogurt are sources of calcium.

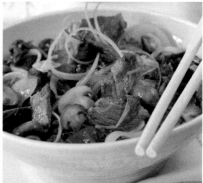

If you're suffering from nausea and vomiting in the early months of your pregnancy, eating small, regular meals will be better than infrequent, large ones. You'll probably feel better if you eat lightly cooked food. Stir-fries are better than deep-fried food.

Essential vitamins and minerals

In some circumstances it can be difficult to get all the nutrients you need through diet alone—if you are suffering badly with nausea and vomiting, for example. In this case, your doctor may advise you to take a vitamin and mineral supplement especially designed for pregnant women.

There are no hard and fast rules as to what has to be in a multivitamin in order for it to be called an prenatal supplement, but a good supplement generally contains more folic acid, iron, and calcium than a general multivitamin. It also must not contain the retinol form of vitamin A, which can be harmful to your growing baby.

Folic acid

Folic acid is a B vitamin, which is also found in a number of foods. These include lentils, chickpeas, leafy greens, broccoli, asparagus, peas, brown rice, fortified breakfast cereals, wheatgerm, citrus fruit and juice, and papaya. Experts recommend that all women of childbearing age take 400 micrograms (mcg) of folic acid a day, and once they find out that they are pregnant, they should increase that amount to 600 mcg. Doing this can reduce your risk of having a baby with a neural tube defect, such as spina bifida.

Fact: Riboflavin, found in milk, eggs, and mushrooms, not only promotes good vision and healthy skin in you—it is also essential for your baby's bone, muscle, and nerve development.

Iron

Iron is needed to make the extra blood required to support your growing baby. Your body makes so much extra blood when you're pregnant that you need about 27 milligrams (mg) of iron every day—that's more than the recommended daily allowance of 18 mg. Good sources of iron include lean red meat, fish, poultry, fortified bread and cereals, dark green leafy vegetables (such as spinach and arugula), beans and lentils, and dried fruits such as figs. Although liver is a good source, you should avoid eating it when pregnant because a buildup in your body can harm your unborn baby.

Calcium

Before, during, and after pregnancy, a woman needs about 1,000 mg of calcium per day. Calcium is found in milk products, dark green leafy vegetables, tofu, and canned salmon and sardines (you should eat the bones).

Other nutrients

Besides folic acid, iron, and calcium, a good prenatal supplement should also contain vitamin C, vitamin D, B vitamins, such as B6 and B12, potassium, zinc, and vitamin E. Once you have found the right supplement, you should never take more than the recommended daily amount (usually one multivitamin a day). Taking megadoses of certain vitamins can be harmful both to you and your baby.

Strict vegetarians and women who suffer from conditions such as diabetes, epilepsy, gestational diabetes, or anemia, should talk with their doctor about any special supplements they might need.

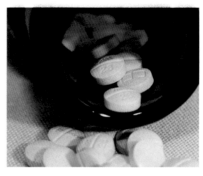

If your diet doesn't give you all the nutrients you need, you may need to take a multivitamin supplement for pregnancy.

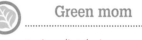 **Green mom**

A vegetarian diet during pregnancy can provide all the nutrients you need.

"Now that I'm pregnant, I've been eating lots of legumes, nuts, seeds, and soy products to make sure I'm getting enough protein. And I know that iron and calcium are two nutrients that are particularly important during pregnancy. I've read up about it and discovered that the iron is important for the extra blood I'll need, and the calcium will protect my bones. As a vegetarian, I've had to make sure I'm getting enough in my diet. For iron I've been eating more whole-wheat bread, legumes, fortified cereals, and green vegetables, and for calcium I've been having plenty of cheese and milk, although one of my pregnant vegetarian friends who doesn't eat dairy products has been taking a calcium supplement."

Nuts are a good source of protein and many contain calcium, too.

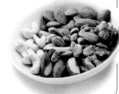

FIRST TRIMESTER	SECOND TRIMESTER	THIRD TRIMESTER

Your body at **06** Weeks

06 Weeks

✳ Sore breasts and frequent trips to the bathroom may start to disturb your sleep about now.

✳ It's common to feel tired or even exhausted as your body becomes used to changing hormone levels.

As soon as you suspect that you're pregnant, call your doctor. She can confirm your pregnancy, answer any questions you may have, and begin providing you with your prenatal care.

Prepare for your first appointment

You'll see a lot of your doctor during your pregnancy—so it's important to choose someone you like and trust. Most pregnant women have between 10 and 15 prenatal visits, beginning about their eighth week. Typically, a mom-to-be will visit her doctor every four weeks during the first and second trimesters, once every two weeks until 36 weeks, then weekly until the baby is born. But if you have had any medical problems in the past or develop any new problems during this pregnancy, you may need more prenatal visits than average.

If you have a partner or labor coach, you may want that person to come to some appointments with you.

During the weeks before each of your visits, jot down any questions or concerns in a notebook. Of course, if you have any pressing questions or develop any unusual symptoms, don't wait for your appointment—call your doctor right away.

Your doctor will start by asking how you're feeling, whether you have any complaints or worries, and what questions you may have. She'll have other questions as well, which will vary, depending on how far along you are and whether she has specific concerns.

The goal of prenatal visits is to see how your pregnancy is proceeding and to provide you with information to help keep you and your baby healthy. Your doctor will check your weight, blood pressure, and urine; measure your abdomen; check the position of your baby; listen to your baby's heartbeat;

A large head and developing organs can now be seen

Your baby at **06** Weeks

At this stage, your baby has reached about the size of a small bean.

✳ If you could see inside yourself at the end of this week, you'd see that your baby has a large head with dark spots where the eyes are beginning to form, and tiny ears just appearing. The liver, lungs, stomach, and pancreas are starting to develop and his blood-circulation system continues to become more sophisticated.

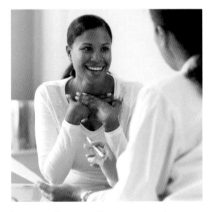

At your first appointment, your doctor will calculate your due date and answer any questions you may have.

perform other exams and order tests, as appropriate; and monitor any complications you have or develop, and intervene if necessary.

At the end of the visit, your doctor will review her findings with you, explain what normal changes to expect before your next visit and what warning signs to watch for, counsel you about lifestyle issues (such as nutrition and avoiding tobacco, alcohol, and drugs), and discuss the pros and cons of optional tests you may want to consider.

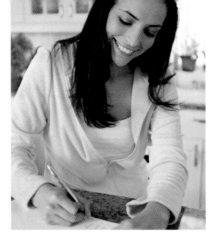

Making a list of questions that you'd like to ask your doctor can help you to focus during your prenatal appointment.

Health-care professionals

As soon as you decide to start trying to conceive, you should begin looking for a practitioner who can care for you during your pregnancy. Below are your primary options:

● **Family physician** If you already have a good relationship with a family practitioner who provides prenatal care, you may not need a new practitioner.

● **Obstetrician-gynecologist** Most US women choose an obstetrician. If you're having multiples or develop certain complications, you'll probably need to see an ob-gyn or a perinatologist, who specializes in high-risk pregnancies.

● **Midwives** Midwives usually offer a more holistic approach to your care. They often work in conjunction with a birthing center or a hospital, and can assist you if you choose to give birth at home.

If you do decide that you want a home birth, you can choose a certified nurse-midwife (CNM) or a direct-entry midwife. For a hospital birth, you can choose an ob-gyn, a family physician, or a certified nurse-midwife.

Organized mom

If you never shop without a list, you're sure to have a list ready for that first prenatal appointment.

"I'm so excited about being pregnant but, since this will be my first baby, I don't want to forget to ask the doctor anything important. I've prepared a list of questions for when I get to see her at my first prenatal appointment. Here they are:

● Is there anything special I can do to make sure I stay healthy?
● Do I need to take any supplements?
● Which foods should I avoid?
● Which screening tests can I have?
● When will I have my first scan?
● Do I have any other options for giving birth besides at my local hospital (for example, at home)?
● How far in advance do I need to arrange childbirth classes?
● What exercise can I do, and are there any pregnancy exercise classes I can join?
● Which over-the-counter and prescription drugs should I stop taking now that I'm pregnant?"

The role of the amniotic sac

The amniotic sac is the bag of fluid inside your uterus that contains your baby. It's made up of two membranes called the amnion and the chorion. The amniotic sac is filled with amniotic fluid (also known as "the water"), which helps to cushion your baby from bumps and injury, as well as providing him with fluids that he can breathe and swallow. This clear, slightly yellow fluid maintains a constant temperature for your baby and provides a barrier against infection.

The amniotic sac begins to form and fill with fluid within just a day or two of conception. The amount of fluid in the sac will increase gradually until around week 38, when it will reduce slightly until your baby is born.

The membranes which make up the sac occasionally rupture as labor begins, but they usually remain intact until the end of the first stage of labor. The membranes may also be broken by a doctor to induce or to speed up labor.

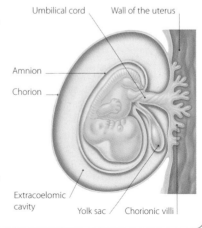

Umbilical cord Wall of the uterus

Amnion

Chorion

Extracoelomic cavity

Yolk sac Chorionic villi

▼ Your body at **07** Weeks

07 Weeks

✽ Your uterus has doubled in size in just two months but you're unlikely to look pregnant yet.

✽ Emotions run high in the early weeks so you're bound to feel fragile or irritated occasionally.

If you are one of the unlucky moms-to-be who is suffering from nausea and vomiting, be gentle on yourself, accept all offers of help and see if any of our tried-and-tested tips work for you.

Nausea and vomiting

The small tail of the embryo will soon disappear

No one knows why the first sign of pregnancy for many moms-to-be is an early morning dash to the bathroom. With around eight out of 10 pregnant women feeling sick, and half of them actually vomiting, many women spend the early weeks of pregnancy feeling awful rather than "blooming."

How badly affected you may be varies widely from woman to woman. You may get the occasional bout of mild queasiness when you first wake up, or you may endure weeks or even months of feeling or actually being sick.

Pregnancy sickness used to be known as "morning sickness" but this name is misleading. It may be worse in the morning, but most sufferers get it throughout the day and into the evening. It can take over your life for a time. If you get it badly you may find yourself unable to work, to care for your toddler or other children, to cook, shop, or run your home.

The cause is unknown, but nausea and vomiting are thought to be connected to the effects of the hormone hCG. Although it won't help your nausea, feeling sick is actually a good sign since it means that your pregnancy hormone levels are high enough. Other hormones, such as estrogen and the thyroid hormone thyroxine, are also thought to play a part.

Nausea and vomiting usually start at around five or six weeks of pregnancy but most women find that they improve by 14 weeks. Some suffer until 16 weeks, whereas others experience varying degrees of it for the whole nine months. Luckily, this is unusual, and there may be support available.

The most severe form of pregnancy sickness is called hyperemesis gravidarum (literally "excessive vomiting in pregnancy"). If you are vomiting frequently, are unable to eat and drink without vomiting, or are losing weight, then you are probably suffering from hyperemesis. This can affect your health and that of your baby, so talk to your doctor about it as soon as you can. There are certain treatments that can help you at home, or you may need to go to the hospital.

▼ Your baby at **07** Weeks

Your baby's growing fast now. She has doubled her size since last week.

✽ In theory, your baby is still an embryo because she has the remains of a small tail, which will disappear in the next few weeks. Her heart and brain are becoming more complicated, her eyelid folds are forming, and her nostrils may be visible. Her arm buds are starting to look more like arms and curve slightly over her heart.

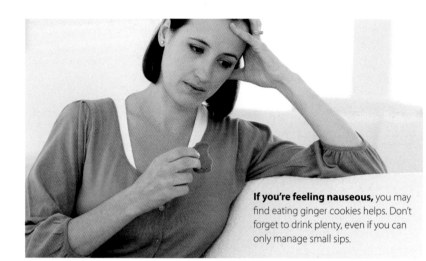

If you're feeling nauseous, you may find eating ginger cookies helps. Don't forget to drink plenty, even if you can only manage small sips.

It is a good idea to tell your partner, family, and friends how you're feeling, and what you need, since they may be struggling to know how to help you. You may also have to tell people at work about your pregnancy (and about your nausea and vomiting) earlier than you were planning, so you can get the support you need. Try not to get overly tired and to minimize any stress. If necessary, take some time off work. Eat little and often, and try to figure out which foods work for you and which make you worse. Rich, fatty, highly spiced foods are often the culprits. Most importantly, keep well-hydrated, sipping iced water, ginger ale, tea, or whatever you can manage.

Safe remedies for nausea and vomiting

If pregnancy sickness is making your life a misery, hopefully one of the remedies below will help.

Ginger Steep fresh, grated ginger in boiled water, let cool and sip it throughout the day.

Acupressure You could try wearing wristbands that stimulate an acupuncture point (the Pericardium 6, or PC6, point), which can relieve sickness. Try putting the bands on first thing in the morning before you even get out of bed. During the day, if you experience a wave of nausea, press on the button (one wrist and then the other) about 20 to 30 times at one-second intervals.

Mint Sip peppermint or spearmint tea. Sugar-free chewing gum or peppermint candy may also help.

Fetal development

Big news this week. Hands and feet are just starting to emerge from developing arms and legs—although they look more like paddles at this point than the tiny, pudgy extremities you're daydreaming about holding and tickling. Technically, your baby is still considered an embryo and has something of a small tail, which is an extension of her tailbone. The tail will disappear within a few weeks, but that's the only thing that is getting smaller. Your baby has doubled in size since last week and now measures ½ inch long—about the size of a blueberry. Developing muscles mean she's also becoming a jumping bean, moving in fits and starts.

Your baby now has eyelid folds partially covering her eyes, which already have some color, and tiny veins are visible beneath parchment-thin skin. Right now, the teeth and palate are forming, and the ears continue to develop.

Both hemispheres of her brain are growing, too, and her liver is making red blood cells. This continues until her bone marrow forms and takes over this role. She also has an appendix and a pancreas, which will eventually produce insulin to aid in digestion. A loop in her growing intestines is bulging into her umbilical cord, which now has distinct blood vessels to carry oxygen and nutrients to and from her tiny body.

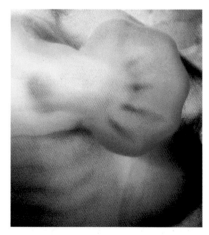

Identifiable hands and arms are starting to develop in this six- to seven-week embryo, although the hands look a bit like paddles.

▼ Your body at **08** Weeks

08 Weeks

❉ Although you're unlikely to have gained much weight, parts of you, like your breasts, are certainly growing.

❉ As your uterus grows, you may feel cramps in your lower abdomen as your ligaments stretch.

Your first visit will probably be the longest one you have with your doctor unless you encounter problems along the way. Don't forget to raise any issues you've been wondering about.

Your first prenatal visit

Now officially a fetus

▼ Your baby at **08** Weeks

Your baby is constantly moving and shifting, though you still can't feel it.

❉ He now measures approximately ½ inch. His embryonic tail is gone, and all his organs, muscles, and nerves are beginning to function. His hands now bend at the wrist, and his feet are starting to lose their webbed appearance. Eyelids are beginning to cover his eyes and taste buds are starting to form on his tongue.

Even if you've confirmed your pregnancy with a home test, it's wise to follow up with a physical examination so you can begin getting prenatal care. Most doctors won't schedule a visit before you're about eight weeks pregnant unless you have a medical condition, have had pregnancy problems in the past, or have symptoms such as vaginal bleeding, abdominal pain, or severe nausea and vomiting. If you're taking any medications or think you may have been exposed to a hazardous substance, ask to speak to the doctor as soon as possible.

Your doctor will want to know the day your last period started so she can determine your due date. She'll ask about any symptoms or problems you've had, whether your menstrual cycles are regular and how long they usually last, and details about any gynecological problems you have now or have had in the past. She'll also want details about any previous pregnancies.

She'll review your medical history and ask about issues such as smoking, drinking, and drug use that could affect your pregnancy. Take some time to think about any exposure you might have had to other potential toxins (bring a list of possible "suspects," especially if you live or work near toxic materials). Let her know if you've recently had any rashes or viruses, or other infections.

Your doctor will also ask whether you or any of your relatives have had any chronic or serious diseases, chromosomal or genetic disorders, or birth defects. She'll also offer you various screening tests that can give you some information about your baby's risk for Down syndrome as well as for other chromosomal problems and possible birth defects.

She'll give you a thorough physical, including a pelvic exam, and will order routine blood tests and ask for a urine sample to test for urinary tract infections UTIs) and other conditions.

She will also give you advice about eating well, foods to avoid, and the kind of weight gain to expect. She'll describe common discomforts of early pregnancy and warn you about any symptoms that need immediate attention.

Your emotional health is very important, too. If you're feeling depressed or overly anxious, your doctor can refer you to someone who can help. She'll also talk to you about the dangers of smoking, drinking alcohol, using drugs, and taking certain medications. If you need help quitting smoking or any other addiction, ask for a referral to a program or counselor.

Finally, she'll go over some do's and don'ts of exercise, travel, and sex during pregnancy; discuss environmental and occupational hazards that can affect your baby; and explain how to avoid infections such as toxoplasmosis. If it's flu season or the season is near, she should tell you about getting a flu shot.

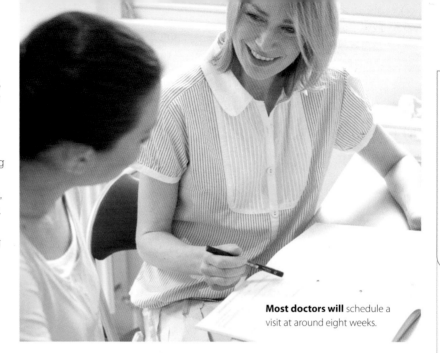

Most doctors will schedule a visit at around eight weeks.

Single mom

Planning your prenatal care can help you feel more in control of your pregnancy.

"Despite the fact that I've progressed from feeling nauseous to actually being sick, I'm starting to feel positive about my pregnancy. I was a little nervous about my first appointment with the doctor. I was worried he might be judgemental about me being single and pregnant, but he wasn't at all. He explained what prenatal care is available where I live, when I'll have my scans, and what will happen at my appointments. It all feels very real now and I feel much more confident now that I know I'll have total control over what happens in the next seven months.

So, I've stopped worrying so much about how I'll cope alone, and how I'll manage financially, and I've started worrying about all the usual things that bother pregnant moms—and that actually feels quite good!"

Blood tests

At your first prenatal visit, your doctor will run several blood tests. Common tests include:

- **Blood type, Rh factor** This determines your blood type, and whether it's Rh-negative (see p.233). A complete blood count will tell if you have too little hemoglobin in your red blood cells (a sign of anemia; see p.229).
- **Rubella (German measles) immunity** Caught during pregnancy, this can lead to miscarriage, stillbirth, or serious birth defects (see pp.227–8).
- **Hepatitis B testing** If you are a carrier of the hepatitis B virus, this may put your baby at risk (see p.227).
- **Syphilis screening** This is relatively rare today, but all women should be tested because it can cause serious problems for you and your baby.
- **HIV testing** The Centers for Disease Control and Prevention, the American College of Obstetricians and Gynecologists, and other organizations recommend that pregnant women be tested for the human immunodeficiency virus (HIV),

the virus that causes AIDS (see p227). If you test positive, you and your baby can get treatment to help maintain your own health and greatly reduce the chance that your baby will be infected.

- **Other blood tests** All women should be offered first-trimester screening for Down syndrome and some other chromosomal abnormalities.

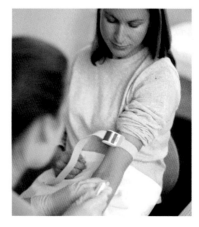

Your doctor will run a number of blood tests when you go to your first prenatal appointment.

▼ Your body at **09** Weeks

09 Weeks

❊ By now you'll find that hormonal fluctuations are really making your emotions yo-yo.

❊ At this stage, pregnancy hormones in your body may be causing some painful headaches.

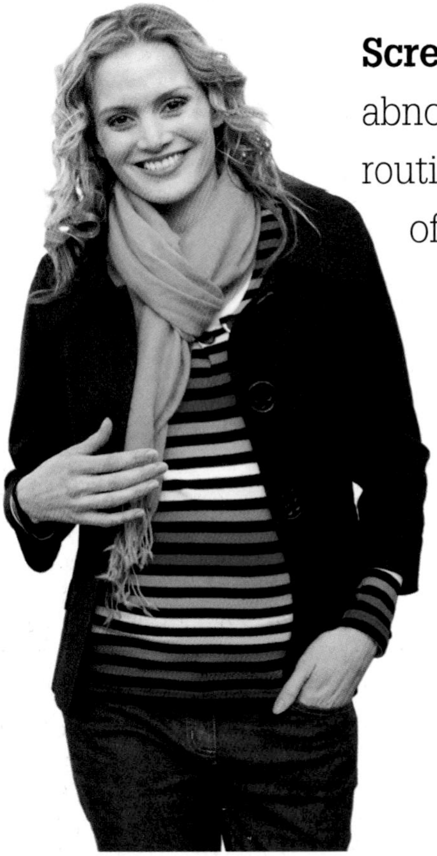

Screening tests can identify birth defects and abnormalities fairly early in pregnancy. Some tests are routine, and others are offered to women at higher risk of problems. Here's what to expect.

Genetic testing

At your first prenatal appointment, your health-care provider should explain your options for prenatal genetic testing. She'll offer you various screening tests that can give you information about your baby's risk for Down syndrome (see pp.214–15) and other chromosomal problems and birth defects.

During your first trimester, you may be offered a blood test that is carried out between 9 and 13 weeks. You may also be offered a nuchal translucency (NT) screening (see p.137). Together,

the blood test and the NT ultrasound are known as the first-trimester combined screening.

First-trimester screening may be done in conjunction with the multiple marker screening (sometimes referred to as the triple or quadruple screen), a blood test done between 15 and 20 weeks that can tell whether your baby is at an increased risk for certain problems. It screens for Down syndrome and trisomy 18, as well as neural tube defects such as spina bifida.

▼ Your baby at **09** Weeks

Your baby weighs under ½ ounce—but she is poised for growth.

❊ All of her body parts are now present and correct, including arms, legs, eyes, genitals, and other organs. Her eyelids are fused and won't open until 27 weeks. Her wrists are more developed, her ankles have formed, and her fingers and toes are clearly visible. Her arms can even bend at the elbows now.

Understanding doctor lingo

Mystified by pregnancy shorthand? Here's what all those abbreviations mean:

Length of pregnancy 8+3 (8 weeks and three days pregnant)

Blood pressure 120/70 (the lower figure should not be higher than 90)

Urine PGO—contains Protein, Glucose or anything else (Other); NAD—no abnormalities detected

Height of uterus The height of your uterus (in centimeters) usually corresponds to the number of weeks you've been pregnant. So, at 20 weeks, the height should be 18 to 22 centimeters.

Position of your baby (see p.197)
Vertex (VTX)—head-down
Br—bottom down or breech

Heartbeat FHH: fetal heart heard; FHNH: fetal heart not heard

Depending on your ethnic background and medical history, you may also want to have carrier screening (see p.223) to see whether your baby is at risk for certain genetic disorders such as cystic fibrosis, sickle-cell anemia, thalassemia, and Tay-Sachs disease. Risk factors include having a family member with the disorder (or a family member who's a known carrier) or being part of an ethnic group at increased risk for the disease.

Finally, you'll be offered genetic diagnostic tests that can tell if your baby has Down syndrome or other problems. These tests include chorionic villus sampling (CVS; see p.136), generally done at 11 to 12 weeks, and amniocentesis (see p.147), usually done at 16 to 20 weeks. Women who have CVS or amniocentesis are usually at increased risk for genetic and chromosomal problems, in part because these tests are invasive and carry a small risk of miscarriage. The tests can determine with greater than 99 percent certainty whether your child has a chromosomal abnormality. Some women choose to wait for the results of screening tests before deciding whether to have one of these diagnostic tests.

If you need more information, your practitioner will be able to refer you to a genetic counselor.

Telling everyone you're pregnant

When you tell people you're pregnant is entirely up to you. Many moms-to-be wait until they're at least 13 weeks pregnant and the risk of miscarriage drops. Some wait until they've had their first scan, while others, particularly first-time parents, can't wait to share their news with everyone.

Keeping your baby news a secret is understandable in the first trimester, particularly if you've had a miscarriage in the past. But if your pregnancy ends and no one knows, it can be hard to deal with your loss by yourself.

If you have children already, their age may help you decide when and how to tell them. If you have an older child, you'll probably want to tell her at around the same time as you tell other family members. Once she knows, she'll want to share the news.

It's best to tell your older child your news when you tell the rest of the family.

A toddler won't really understand that you're having a baby until you start to show—or even until you have your baby. Don't forget that it's important to check with your employer to find out how far in advance they need to be notified of your taking leave (see pp.64–5).

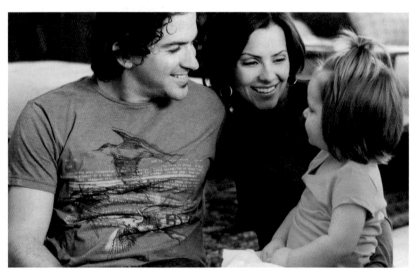

Getting ready for pregnancy

Staying safe and healthy

Your pregnancy diary

Birth and beyond

Sleep in early pregnancy

If you can't remember when you last had a good night's sleep, don't despair. In early pregnancy, high levels of pregnancy hormones can leave you feeling exhausted during the day and tossing and turning at night. But this should pass once you enter your second trimester.

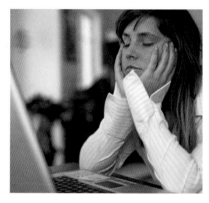

Exhaustion in the early days is normal. Listen to your body and get as much rest as you can for your sake and your baby's.

Bedtime ritual for a good night's sleep

If you're suffering from disrupted sleep now that you're pregnant, try some or all of these useful tips:

● Cut down on caffeinated drinks, such as tea and coffee, and avoid them completely during the afternoon and evening.

● Keep your bedroom cool.

● Use your bed for sleep and sex only.

● If your chores aren't done by dinnertime, leave them for tomorrow.

● Finish exercising at least three or four hours before you go to bed.

● Regulate your body clock by going to bed at the same time every night.

Tired all the time

At this stage you'll probably be feeling very sleepy during the day. This is caused by raised levels of progesterone in your body. Although this hormone makes you drowsy, it can also disrupt your sleep at night. Sadly, there's no real way around this problem other than to rest when you can, even if you can't actually sleep.

Your newly tender breasts may make it hard for you to find a comfortable sleeping position also, especially if you normally sleep on your stomach. Your first trimester is the perfect time to get used to sleeping on your left side. This improves the flow of blood and nutrients to your baby, and helps your kidneys to get rid of waste and fluids.

Another sleep stealer is your growing uterus, which puts pressure on your bladder and sends you scrambling to the bathroom seemingly endlessly. You may find that it helps if you drink plenty of fluids during the day, but cut down in the late afternoon or evening.

If you feel caught in a vicious circle of wakefulness at night and exhaustion during the day, you're not alone. More than half of all pregnant women take at least one nap during weekdays, while 60 percent take at least one weekend nap. You should expect this first three months to be the most tiring time of your pregnancy, so remember to listen to your body when it's telling you to slow down or rest.

ParentsAsk...

Am I too tired? Could I be anemic?
Fatigue is a common sign of anemia (see p.229)—but it's also experienced by many pregnant women who are not anemic. Breathlessness, headaches, tinnitus, and palpitations are other symptoms of anemia, along with unusual food cravings. Your eyelids, fingernails, and tongue may also look paler than usual.

How will I know if I'm anemic?
The routine blood tests that you will have at your doctor's office will check whether your hemoglobin levels are satisfactory or not. It's normal for the levels to drop a little during pregnancy because there's far more fluid in your blood to dilute the red blood cells. Only if your levels drop very low indeed will your doctor prescribe iron supplements for you.

In your dreams...

First your husband sleeps with your best friend. Then you sleep with an old boyfriend from your school days. Now you're trying to make a quick getaway—but from what? As you travel down the highway, you have a nagging feeling that you've forgotten something. Suddenly you remember: you've left your baby at the gym!

Have you lost your mind? No—not your waking mind, anyway. During pregnancy, your dreams have more twists and turns than ever before. It's all down to your surging hormones, perhaps entwined with mixed feelings about your changing shape, and maybe the added ingredients of anxiety and excitement about becoming a mother.

Another reason why your dreams may have changed in style is that you are more likely to interrupt a dream-filled cycle of REM sleep by frequent waking during the night to go to the bathroom, ease a leg cramp, or change to a more comfortable position.

Some common images

Although it's impossible to predict what dreams you may have, there are some images that can often appear at certain stages of pregnancy. It's common to dream about birth and motherhood, sex, tall buildings, and water.

You could record your dreams and what you think they mean in a journal. Share your weird and wonderful tales with your partner, and don't forget to ask him what expectant father's dreams he's having. As a dad-to-be, his feelings of excitement, anticipation, anxiety, and worry may open a floodgate of dreams, too. Sharing your dreams and feelings throughout your pregnancy will help you both feel loved and needed.

Working mom

Usually on top of things at work? Now finding you can hardly keep your eyes open? It's just normal.

"I'm 10 weeks pregnant and the worst pregnancy symptom I'm suffering right now is the fatigue. I can barely stay awake while I'm at work sometimes. This week, I've been going back to the car at lunchtimes for a 20-minute cat nap to recharge my batteries. I feel a bit better afterward, but it's been very difficult to concentrate. The hardest time is mid-afternoon—I could literally fall asleep at my desk around that time. None of my colleagues know that I'm pregnant, and my workload hasn't changed, so I guess I just have to struggle on as best I can. When I finally manage to get home, I'm usually asleep in front of the TV by 7:30 pm."

Raised levels of progesterone can disrupt your nighttime sleep and make you crave a daytime nap. You're not alone!

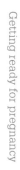

Getting ready for pregnancy

Staying safe and healthy

Your pregnancy diary

Birth and beyond

FIRST TRIMESTER	SECOND TRIMESTER	THIRD TRIMESTER

▼ Your body at **10** Weeks

10 Weeks

❋ Your uterus is now about the size of a grapefruit—almost big enough to fill your pelvis.

❋ Strange dreams are common during pregnancy and could also contribute to disrupted nights.

It's natural to be concerned about twinges in your tummy when you are pregnant. They're common and usually nothing to worry about. You do need to be on the look out for certain warning signs, though.

Aches and pains in the early weeks

Pains in the stomach are fairly common in early pregnancy and, on their own, are rarely a sign of a serious problem. Carrying a baby puts a great deal of pressure on your muscles, veins, ligaments, and the rest of your insides, so it's not surprising that you feel some discomfort, around your abdomen.

The fetus swallows and starts to have taste buds

Pregnancy cramps

Some common causes of cramps in early pregnancy include:

● **Ligament stretching** You might experience mild cramps on one or both sides of your abdomen. This is caused by the ligaments stretching so that they can support your growing uterus. It might occur from early through to late pregnancy. To help alleviate this, try sitting down, or lie down and put your feet up. Resting comfortably when you get any pain will usually alleviate it.

● **Orgasm** You may find that you get cramps during and after an orgasm, sometimes combined with a backache.

This may be because the veins of your pelvis are congested. Or you may be tense: some people feel nervous about having sex during pregnancy. This can occur any time during pregnancy.

Although you don't have to avoid sex during a normal pregnancy, you may want to take it soft and slow. A gentle post-orgasm back rub may help soothe the pain. However, if you experience cramping along with spotting, heavy bleeding, fever, chills, vaginal discharge, continuous tenderness, and pain, or if the cramps don't subside after several minutes, call your doctor.

Could it be more serious?

Some of the conditions that can cause cramps during the first trimester are ectopic pregnancy (see pp.44–5) and early miscarriage (see pp.42–3). If your symptoms match the symptoms of either of these conditions, you should call your doctor immediately. If you think you may be having an early miscarriage, you should lie or sit down with your feet up, and try to relax as much as you possibly can.

If your cramping is accompanied by heavy bleeding, call 911 or go to the nearest emergency department.

▼ Your baby at **10** Weeks

Congratulations—your embryo is now called a fetus, which means "offspring."

❋ He is now swallowing and kicking, and all his major organs are fully developed. The external sex organs are just starting to show and, in a few weeks' time, they will be developed enough to reveal whether you're going to be the mom of a boy or a girl. More minute details are appearing, too, like fingernails and peach-fuzz hair.

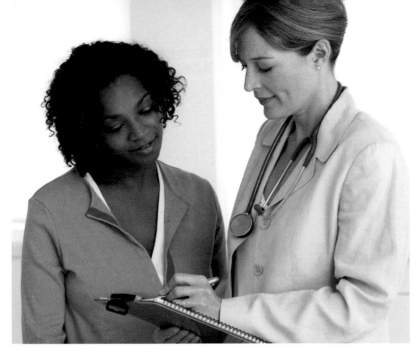

Your doctor should be able to help you with any questions you have—don't be afraid to ask, even if you think they're silly.

Getting the most out of your prenatal appointments

Many women look forward to their prenatal appointments but are disappointed to find that, with the exception of the first visit, they're in and out of the office in 10 minutes. A quick visit is usually a sign that everything is progressing normally. If you feel like you don't have enough time to voice your concerns, though, take these steps before your next appointment:

● **Write down your concerns** Between visits, jot down your questions. Bring the list to each appointment so you can run through it with your doctor. And if anything else is bothering you, speak up. Your doctor isn't a mind reader and won't be able to tell what you're thinking just by performing a physical examination.

● **Mention everything, no matter how small** In addition to any physical complaints you may have, let your doctor know if you have any emotional concerns or fitness or nutrition questions.

● **Ask about the administrative stuff** Save questions about insurance and directions to the hospital for the office staff so your doctor has more time to answer what's important.

● **Be open-minded** When talking with your doctor, you should feel comfortable speaking freely, but remember to listen, too. And keep in mind that some days are busier than others. That doesn't mean your doctor doesn't have to answer your questions, but sometimes a discussion can be continued at the next visit if it's a really busy day or she needs to head to the hospital to deliver a baby. But don't tolerate a doctor who won't give you thorough answers, doesn't show reasonable compassion, or barely looks up from your chart. You and your baby deserve more than that.

If you aren't satisfied with your obstetrician, you might want to look for someone new. Most women work with an obstetrician, but certified nurse-midwives have become more and more popular. Midwives generally take a more holistic approach and will often have more time to answer all of your questions. In 2003, certified nurse-midwives attended just over 7 percent of deliveries in the United States and over 10 percent of vaginal births.

The most important thing is to choose someone you feel completely comfortable with, who's appropriate for your individual needs, who'll respect your wishes, and who practices in the right setting for you.

FIRST TRIMESTER   SECOND TRIMESTER   THIRD TRIMESTER

Your body at **11** Weeks

11 Weeks

❉ Leg cramps and heartburn may be annoying you during the day and keeping you up at night.

❉ A dark vertical line of pigmentation, called the linea nigra, may appear on your belly.

You're nearly at the end of the first trimester and, if you haven't yet paid attention to your fitness, remember that it's not too late. Staying active offers a multitude of benefits for pregnant women.

Keeping fit

Giving birth is akin to running a marathon—it requires stamina, determination, and focus. Keeping physically active during the months of your pregnancy is good preparation for the hard work of labor.

Weight-bearing exercise throughout pregnancy may reduce the length of labor and lessen the risk of delivery complications. Weight-bearing exercise can mean simply using the weight of your body when you exercise, for instance when you walk briskly, jog, or dance. Or it can involve weight training, using free weights or a machine. If you already do weight-bearing exercise you may well be able to continue now that you're pregnant, but check with your doctor first. If you are new to exercise, ask your doctor what's safe for you. If you join an exercise class, always tell the teacher that you are pregnant.

Other reasons for keeping fit

You may not have a belly yet, but you'll soon reach the stage where your body's not the svelte thing it used to be. Although you know it's for a good cause, watching the scale creep its way up to numbers you've never seen before can be extremely disheartening. Staying active can make you feel less frumpy. It can also help you shed weight faster postpartum. What is more, some research has shown that babies of women who exercised during pregnancy may do better during labor than those of the non-exercisers.

And if that weren't enough, exercise also strengthens your cardiovascular system so you don't tire as easily—which is a real plus now that you're pregnant. It also helps you deal with stress and can give you a better night's sleep. Read pp.56–7 to learn more about the types of exercise that are appropriate for you to do during pregnancy and about how to exercise safely. What are you waiting for?

Tips: Kegel exercises help to prevent stress incontinence later in life and help ensure that your sex life is as good after your baby is born as it was before; they are often called "sexercises."

Your baby at **11** Weeks

Your 1½-inch baby now has all her parts, from tooth buds to toe nails.

❉ She is now really busy kicking and stretching; her movements are so fluid that, if you could watch them, you would think it was a sort of water ballet. Her fingers and toes have fully separated, too. Now her main task is to grow larger and stronger until she can survive on her own outside your uterus.

The benefits of Pilates

The abdomen and pelvic floor muscles (see below) are known in Pilates as the "stable core." Pregnancy can weaken these muscles, leading to poor posture and back pain. Pilates exercises are useful for pregnant women since many of them strengthen the core muscles. Some exercises are performed in a hands-and-knees position, which lessens the weight on your back and pelvis. The Wall Slide strengthens your core muscles and also improves the mobility of your hips, so it is a sound pregnancy investment.

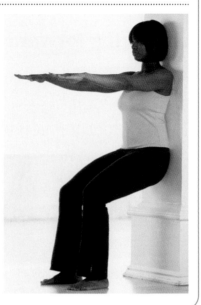

Press your back against a wall, feet hip-distance apart. Raise your arms as you bend your knees and slide gently down the wall. Go as far as you can, then slide back up.

Your pelvic floor

Your pelvic floor muscles form a broad sling between your legs from the pubic bone in front to the base of your spine at the back. Being pregnant can place a lot of stress on those muscles. They can become weak and stretched, which increases your risk of stress incontinence (urine leaks when you laugh, cough, sneeze, or exercise) after you have given birth. To strengthen these important muscles, try doing Kegel exercises:

● Place one hand at the top of your belly and the other on one of your shoulders. Breathe normally for four or five breaths.
● The hand on your belly should move up and down more than the hand on your shoulder. If this isn't happening, try to stop your shoulders from moving, but don't try to make your belly move.

● Gently pull up and in "down below" as you breathe out. Imagine that you're trying to stop yourself from passing gas and trying to stop the flow of urine midstream at the same time.
● Then try to hold a contraction for a few seconds while you breathe in and out as normal.
● Make sure that you're squeezing and lifting without pulling in your tummy, squeezing your legs together, tightening your buttocks, or holding your breath.
● When you've done all this, go back to the beginning and start again.

You should aim to be able to hold a pelvic floor contraction for 10 seconds while breathing normally. If you lose your breathing control, stop and start again. Try to do sets of 10, with three to four sets three times a day.

Active mom

When you've always exercised, it can be a shock to realize you may need to try a gentler routine.

"I'm a bit of a gym bunny. Before I got pregnant I'd go at least five times a week after work. I did weight training, an aerobics class, spinning. You name it—I'd give it a try.

During that first trimester, though, I started feeling so unbelievably tired. There was no way that I could keep up the routine because after work all I wanted to do was go home and crawl right into bed.

I felt so guilty for abandoning my fitness regimen and started to panic about just how much weight I was going to put on. I spoke to my doctor about it, and she said that while the routine I did at the gym might be a bit too much for me now, there was no need to give up exercise entirely. So now I've started a gentle routine that includes swimming, yoga, and lots of walking. I feel just great and ready for the months ahead!"

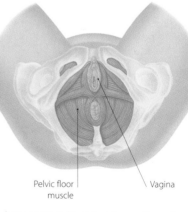

Pelvic floor muscle | Vagina

Your pelvic floor muscles are like a sling or hammock running from front to back. During pregnancy they stretch, which can cause stress incontinence.

Getting ready for pregnancy

Staying safe and healthy

Your pregnancy diary

Birth and beyond

Ultrasounds and CVS

Around now, you may be looking forward to your first ultrasound. It's an amazing moment in your pregnancy, and one to share with your partner or a friend. Bear in mind, though, that ultrasounds occasionally pick up problems—speak to your doctor if you are worried.

Your first ultrasound

Most moms-to-be have an ultrasound (also called a sonogram) when they're between 16 and 20 weeks pregnant (see p.156). You might have one as early as four weeks if there's any sign of a problem, and many women have one between 11 and 13 weeks as part of the nuchal translucency test.

An ultrasound uses sound waves to create a visual image of your baby, placenta, and uterus, as well as other pelvic organs. It allows your doctor to gather valuable information about the progress of your pregnancy and your baby's health, including measuring your baby's size and setting your due date, checking to see if there's more than one baby, and checking for any abnormalities. If you would like to find out whether your baby's a boy or a girl, you usually can when you have your midpregnancy ultrasound.

Although about 70 percent of pregnant women in the United States have an ultrasound, if you're having a low-risk pregnancy, you might not be offered one at all. In fact, the American College of Obstetricians and Gynecologists recommends ultrasounds only when there's a specific medical reason.

Chorionic villus sampling (CVS)

Chorionic villi are tiny projections on the placenta that reveal the chromosomal makeup of your baby. CVS involves extracting a fragment of chorionic villi to detect chromosomal abnormalities such as Down syndrome. You will be able to discuss the pros and cons before you decide to have the test. It can be done using one of the following methods:

● **Transabdominal CVS** You may be given a local anesthetic before a needle is inserted through your abdomen into your uterus to the placenta.

● **Transvaginal CVS** Your doctor inserts fine forceps or a small tube through your vagina and cervix into the uterus. You should have the results of the CVS in seven to 10 days.

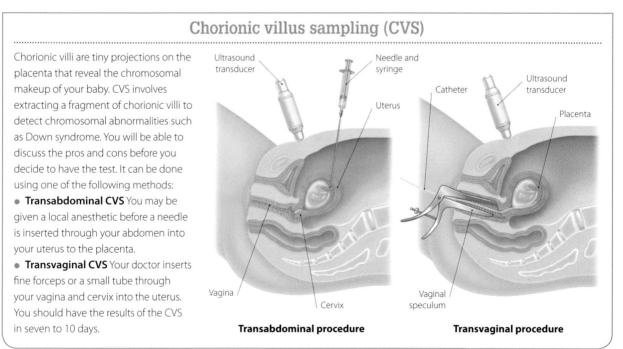

Transabdominal procedure — Ultrasound transducer, Needle and syringe, Uterus, Vagina, Cervix

Transvaginal procedure — Catheter, Ultrasound transducer, Placenta, Vaginal speculum

Transabdominal procedure   **Transvaginal procedure**

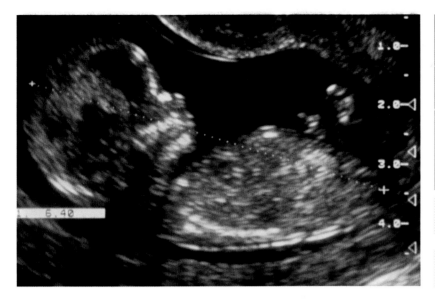

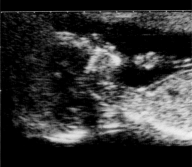

The nuchal fold (red) of this fetus is narrow and clear. With a more opaque fold, the baby is at higher risk of having Down syndrome.

At the age of 12 weeks, an ultrasound scan clearly shows the profile and part of the body of the fetus (left).

Getting ready for pregnancy

Staying safe and healthy

Your pregnancy diary

Birth and beyond

The nuchal translucency scan

A nuchal translucency (NT) scan assesses whether your baby is likely to have Down syndrome. Nuchal translucency refers to the collection of fluid under the skin at the back of your baby's neck. All babies have some of this fluid, but many babies with Down syndrome have an increased amount.

What the results can tell you

The NT scan can't tell definitely if your baby is affected, but it can help you decide whether or not to have a diagnostic test, such as CVS (see opposite) or amniocentesis (see p.147). The NT scan must be done between 11 weeks and 13 weeks and 6 days of pregnancy. It's usually done through your abdomen, but occasionally a vaginal scan, which will give better views, is required.

To date your pregnancy accurately, the sonographer measures your baby from the top of his head to the bottom of his spine. She then measures the width of the nuchal translucency. An NT measurement of up to 2 millimeters (mm) is normal at 11 weeks, and up to about 2.8 mm is normal by 13 weeks and 6 days. An increased NT doesn't definitely mean there's a problem. However, since the NT increases, so does the risk of Down syndrome and other chromosomal abnormalities.

Your scan measurements are combined with your age to generate your individual risk for this pregnancy. This may be higher or lower than your background risk (the average risk that applies to all women of your age). You'll get the results right after your scan.

Most women given a high risk (a one-in-150 chance, or less) of having a baby with Down syndrome will go on to have a normal baby. Even with a risk as high as one in five, your baby has four chances out of five of NOT having Down syndrome. The only way to know for certain if he has Down syndrome or another chromosomal abnormality is to have a CVS test or amniocentesis.

The decision to have invasive tests can be very difficult, but you don't have to decide in a hurry. Sometimes, a screening test can suggest that a normal baby has a high risk of Down syndrome. This is called a false positive. Combining an NT scan with a blood test, which is usually offered at the first trimester combined screening (see p.128), will give a more accurate result. The NT scan alone will detect about 70 to 80 percent of babies with Down syndrome. The detection rate for the first-trimester combined screening ranges from 79 to 90 percent.

75% of babies with Down syndrome are picked up by an nuchal translucency scan and another five percent of women are given a false positive. This means that one in 20 women are wrongly given a high risk.

▼ Your body at **12** Weeks

12 Weeks

❊ With luck your nausea will be on the wane and you'll soon be feeling more energetic.

❊ This is roughly the stage when your raging hormones should start calming down.

If you're over 35 you may be wondering how your age will affect your pregnancy. The good news is that the vast majority of pregnancies for women in this age group are uneventful and lead to healthy babies.

Concerns of older moms

Organs grow quickly and eyes move closer

Overall, the risks faced by women over 35 during pregnancy tend to be exaggerated. Many recent studies have shown that, in healthy women, the risks of delaying pregnancy are low, even though being over 35 is associated with an increased risk of certain complications.

It appears that it's not just your age that matters: the state of your health before you conceive matters, too. There is evidence that older women are more likely to develop diabetes, high blood pressure, or placenta previa during pregnancy. But both mother and baby still usually do well. And, although the risks of stillbirth are higher for older women, the rates are still very, very low.

Modern maternity units are able to take older women's complications in their stride. By working with your maternity care team and, for example, controlling your diet if you are diabetic, you can help reduce the risks for yourself and your baby. An increased rate of induced labor, forceps delivery, and cesarean has been found for women over 35 in the United States, although the exact reasons for this aren't clear. It may be that obstetricians are more likely to intervene in older women's deliveries.

Genetic defects

The odds of having a baby with a genetic defect such as Down syndrome increase dramatically as you get older. Figures from the Office of National Statistics for 2005 show that the risk rises from about one in 759 births for women at age 30, to one in 302 at age 35, and one in 82 at age 40.

If you're almost, or over, 35 you should consider genetic testing (see pp.222–3) because the risk of genetic problems increases significantly as you age. And since genetic abnormalities are the most common reason for miscarriage, the risk of miscarriage also increases with age.

Whatever your age, if you are considering pregnancy, see your doctor for a preconception checkup (see p.16). The doctor will take a detailed medical and family history for both you and your partner to identify any conditions that might adversely affect the health of you or your baby.

▼ Your baby at **12** Weeks

Now your baby's tissues and organs begin to grow and mature rapidly.

❊ Starting with your baby's face, his eyes, which began to form on the sides of his head, have moved closer together, and his ears are now almost in their normal position. His intestines, which started out as a large swelling in the umbilical cord, will begin moving into his abdominal cavity about now.

How the placenta works

The placenta develops in the lining of the uterus. It is fully formed, with two arteries and a vein, and functioning by about 10 weeks after fertilization.

Your baby's blood flows into the placenta through the arteries. Oxygen and food from your blood are carried into the baby's blood in the placenta. The baby's blood returns through the vein, taking waste products and carbon dioxide back to the placenta for disposal. Although the circulation of your blood and your baby's blood come close, there is no direct connection.

Another of the placenta's functions is to produce hormones, such as estrogen and progesterone. These help your baby to grow and develop, and cause many of your body's changes during pregnancy.

The placenta also protects your baby from infections and harmful substances. What's more, its large surface area, plus the amount of blood flowing through it, provides the perfect mechanism for dispersing heat and helping control your baby's body temperature.

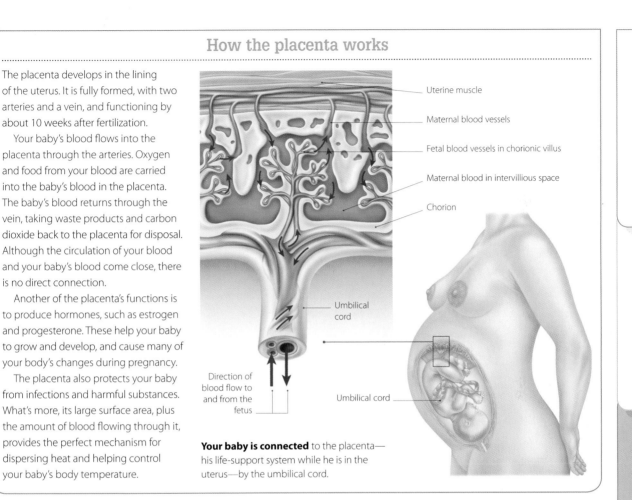

Uterine muscle

Maternal blood vessels

Fetal blood vessels in chorionic villus

Maternal blood in intervillious space

Chorion

Umbilical cord

Direction of blood flow to and from the fetus

Umbilical cord

Your baby is connected to the placenta—his life-support system while he is in the uterus—by the umbilical cord.

Fetal development

The most dramatic development this week: reflexes. Your baby's fingers will soon begin to open and close, his toes will curl, his eye muscles will clench, and his mouth will start to make sucking movements. In fact, if you prod your abdomen, your baby will squirm in response, even though you won't be able to feel it.

His intestines, which have grown so fast that they now protrude into the umbilical cord, will begin to move into their proper place in his abdominal

cavity at about this time. His kidneys are developing, too: they begin excreting urine into his bladder.

Meanwhile, nerve cells are multiplying rapidly, and in your baby's brain, synapses—where two nerve cells connect—are forming furiously. His face looks unquestionably human: his eyes are now at the front of his head, and his ears are almost where they should be. From crown to rump, your baby-to-be is just over 2¼ inches long (about the size of a lime) and he weighs ½ ounce.

Now your doctor can feel the top of your uterus (the fundus) low in your abdomen, just above your pubic bone. You may already be wearing maternity clothes, especially if this isn't your first pregnancy, but if you're still small and not yet ready for maternity clothes, you've no doubt noticed that your waist is thickening and that you're more comfortable in loose, less restrictive clothing. You may now find that, once the feeling of sickness has passed, your appetite returns.

Your body at **13** Weeks

13 Weeks

❋ If you are lucky, you may find that your sex drive is making a comeback this week.

❋ Your breasts may have already started making colostrum, the first milk that nourishes your baby.

You're almost in the second trimester now

and you may soon find your energy levels returning to normal. Use your newfound energy to get some exercise, but don't forget to get some rest, too.

Feeling better now?

By the end of your first trimester, you will hopefully be over the worst of any nausea and vomiting. Once it has passed, you may even feel ravenous. By 16 weeks you may have gained as much as 10 pounds and by week 22 you may put on about 8 ounces a week, though if you're carrying one baby you should end up gaining no more than about 35 to 40 pounds. You may have sudden cravings for weird and wonderful foods. So satisfy your heightened sense of taste and smell! Now is not the time to be worrying about your weight. Eat healthily, especially if you're hungry, but don't deprive yourself—remember that gradual weight gain is a positive sign of a healthy pregnancy. So why not meet a friend for a leisurely lunch?

Exercise and rest

Take advantage of your revived energy levels to strengthen and prepare your body for the physical demands of labor, birth, and motherhood that lie ahead. Yoga (see p.59) and Pilates (see p.57) exercises can help relieve aches and pains in your back and pelvis and, toward the end of pregnancy, can even

help position your baby for delivery. Regular, gentle exercise also makes it easier to get your body back in shape once the baby's born. You will find useful tips on exercising on pp.56–7 and on p.134.

Although you'll soon be feeling livelier, make sure you set aside a few quiet hours to relax. Your physical and emotional well-being are important right now, so put your feet up—or better still, take a cat nap—whenever you get the chance. If your feet are sore and swollen, have a long, luxurious soak in the bath and massage them afterward with your favorite moisturizing lotion or foot balm.

A key moment

One of the most exciting moments of the second trimester is feeling your baby move. In a first pregnancy, most women notice this "quickening" some time between 16 and 20 weeks. You may feel these first wiggles as a flutter low down in your abdomen.

Around this time you'll probably be offered a midpregnancy ultrasound—a prenatal test to screen for any possible birth defects (see pp.156–7).

▼ Your baby at **13** Weeks

Amazingly, although your baby is still really tiny, she already has fingerprints.

❋ Your baby is now nearly 2¾ to 3¼ inches long and weighs nearly ¾ ounce. When you poke your stomach, she may start rooting (searching for a nipple). If you're having a girl, she now has approximately 2 million eggs in her ovaries, although she will have only half this number by the time she's born.

That loving feeling

As the fatigue of early pregnancy lifts, you may feel your libido return, which is sure to please your partner. In fact, some women find that their libido is at a high in the second trimester but, with any stage of pregnancy, there is a wide variety in how women feel and how sexually active couples are.

Meanwhile, for your partner, your pregnant physique is a constant reminder of his virility—he may well find your blossoming breasts and soft curves irresistible. Why not celebrate your sensuality with some new, sexy lingerie? Or plan a romantic evening

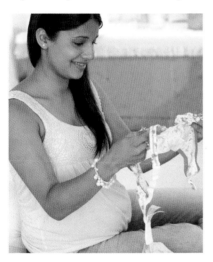

with your partner—at the theater, movies, a favorite restaurant, or somewhere else where you can appreciate each other's company before you become Mom and Dad! If you can't afford to go out, get your partner to cook an intimate dinner for two, or turn your bedroom into a romantic hideaway, with candles and soft music. Turn off your phones and hide anything that reminds you of work.

Going shopping

Last but by no means least, there's shopping. Although at 13 weeks many women "make do" with their existing wardrobe, soon it will be worth buying some maternity clothes. As your breasts expand with extra milk ducts, you'll need to make sure you're regularly measured for a good maternity bra (see p.92).

If your feet tend to swell it might be wise to invest in a pair of shoes a size bigger than normal. Switch to flat styles as you begin to carry more weight. Your growing belly alters your center of gravity—which makes balancing on high heels even trickier than usual.

As well as being functional, maternity bras come in all sorts of shapes and colors—you can find some very attractive designs.

ParentsAsk...

Now that I'm at 13 weeks, is my risk of miscarriage over?

About 15 percent of known pregnancies end in miscarriage. More than 80 percent of women who miscarry do so in the first 12 weeks, but occasionally a woman will miscarry much later.

What causes miscarriage?

Probably at least half of all miscarriages in the first trimester of pregnancy are the result of chromosomal abnormalities that prevent the baby from developing normally. Later miscarriages—after 20 weeks—may be the result of an infection or an abnormality of the uterus or placenta, or a weak cervix that is not strong enough to keep the uterus tightly closed until the baby is ready to be born.

Is it true that some tests can cause miscarriage?

Unfortunately, two of the tests used to detect abnormalities in babies—amniocentesis (see p.147) and CVS (see p.136)—can make you miscarry. Amniocentesis results in miscarriage for around one percent of women. CVS may cause miscarriage in between one and two percent. Discuss the risks and how you feel about them with your doctor.

Twins and more

If you are carrying twins or more, chances are you'll already have had a scan and you'll be coming to terms with your amazing news.

During the rest of your pregnancy, you will have more prenatal appointments and ultrasound scans than you would in a single pregnancy. If you are expecting twins, your appointments will be more frequent: You can expect to see your doctor once a month for the first

24 weeks, every other week until 32 weeks, and then weekly (or more often if necessary) after that.

And because a multiple pregnancy is considered higher risk, even if you are young and healthy, you may need to see a perinatologist as well as your regular obstetrician. Also known as a maternal-fetal medicine specialist, a perinatologist is an obstetrician who specializes in high-risk pregnancies.

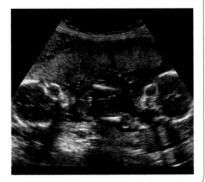

Getting ready for pregnancy

Staying safe and healthy

Your pregnancy diary

Birth and beyond

The second
trimester

The time of your life

The second trimester is an exciting time. With nausea and vomiting and miscarriage worries behind them, most women feel full of energy and excited about their growing belly. Why not treat yourself to a few new clothes and maybe even a romantic pre-baby break?

Making the most of it

Most women find the second three months the easiest stage of pregnancy. They can sleep sounder and their belly isn't too big to impede their movements. Make the most of these middle months to enjoy low-impact exercise (see p.57) and maybe arrange a last-minute vacation too, while you can still move around easily—and before you need to worry about the possibility of baby arriving early. You may also notice a distinct improvement in your libido as the nausea and fatigue recede and your energy levels rise!

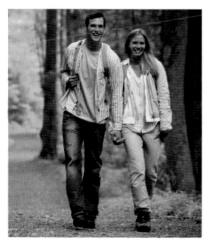

At this stage of your pregnancy you'll probably be feeling your best and looking forward to the arrival of your new baby.

Your growing belly

At the start of the second trimester your uterus may be big enough to show the world that you're expecting, but your baby is still tiny—only about the size of half a banana.

Over the next few weeks she will sprout hair—not only on her head and brows but all over her body—in the form of ultrafine hair called lanugo. Some of her muscles are starting to work, too— she will soon be grasping, frowning, grimacing, and even sucking her thumb.

From 17 weeks her eyes will look forward instead of to the sides and the rubbery cartilage that will become her skeleton is about to start hardening into bone. By 18 weeks she can both feel and hear. Admittedly, all she can hear at the moment is your heartbeat and the flow of your digestive system, but soon she'll be able to detect noise outside the uterus and identify your voice.

After you reach the halfway stage of pregnancy your baby will start to gain weight rapidly—at the rate of about an ounce a day. By 21 weeks she could measure about 10½ inches from crown to heel. Her eyebrows and eyelids are fully developed and fingernails now cover her fingertips. She is really starting to look like a miniature newborn.

At 24 weeks your baby becomes "viable"—meaning that if she were born prematurely now, she might survive, with special care. At 26 weeks, her eyes begin to open and, toward the end of the seventh month, her response to sound grows more consistent. As you approach the final stage of pregnancy— your third trimester—your baby is really starting to grow and fill the available space in your uterus.

Active mom

Most women experience a massive improvement in the way they feel in the second trimester.

"The first trimester was an absolute nightmare for me, what with all that nausea and vomiting, plus the exhaustion. I genuinely don't think I've ever felt so horrible in my whole life. The good news is that, once I entered the second trimester, everything got way better. I stopped feeling nauseous, the overwhelming fatigue vanished, and I could get back into an exercise routine. I try to swim or go for a walk every day. I'm definitely rocking the pregnancy glow now!"

Getting ready for pregnancy

Staying safe and healthy

Your pregnancy diary

Birth and beyond

FIRST TRIMESTER	SECOND TRIMESTER	THIRD TRIMESTER

▼ Your body at **14** Weeks

14 Weeks

✳ Some women find that nausea drags on. If you're still very sick, consult your doctor.

✳ You may notice that your hair is now more lustrous—becoming thicker and fuller.

Your baby is beginning to look like a real person now, and is practicing different facial expressions. Meanwhile, your uterus is starting to show above your pelvis—a reassuring sign that he is growing.

How your baby's growing

You've reached 14 weeks and your baby is stretching out and starting to look like a real little human. He's about the size of a lemon and has nearly doubled his weight in just the last week. His body's growing faster than his head right now, and his head sits upon a neck that's starting to look more like a real neck. By the end of this week, his arms will have grown so that they're more in proportion to the rest of his body. His legs still have some lengthening to do, though.

Your baby's skin is extremely sensitive now, and he's starting to develop an ultra-fine, downy covering of hair all over his body known as lanugo. It usually disappears before birth. Although his eyebrows are beginning to grow and the hair on top of his head is sprouting, this hair may change in both texture and color once he is born. He now has sockets in his gumline ready for 20 little teeth to form, and he even has tiny vocal cords, although he won't actually make any sounds until he's born. Thanks to impulses from his brain, your baby's facial muscles are getting a really good workout as his tiny features form one

expression after another. He can squint, frown, and grimace. Although you can't feel his tiny punches and kicks yet, your little boxer's hands and feet measure about ½ inch long and are quite flexible and active. Tiny fingernails are starting to grow. He can grasp, too, and if you have an ultrasound scan, you may catch him sucking his thumb.

Your baby's organs

Crucially, your baby's liver starts making bile this week—a sign that it's doing its job properly—and his spleen starts helping in the production of red blood cells. His intestines have moved into his abdominal cavity from the umbilical cord, and the muscles in his digestive tract are already contracting. His kidneys are producing urine, which he releases (urinates) into the amniotic fluid around him—a process that he'll keep up until birth.

And last but not least, your baby's genitals are starting to take on male or female characteristics. This won't be visible on scans just yet. You'll have to wait until your mid-pregnancy scan to know if it's a boy or a girl.

▼ Your baby at **14** Weeks
....

This week, your baby's parchment-thin skin is starting to cover itself with lanugo.

✳ This will disappear by the time he is born unless he's born prematurely. He can now grasp, squint, frown, and grimace. He may even be able to suck his thumb. His movements probably correspond to the development of impulses in the brain. Crown to rump, he's now about 3¼ inches long and weighs 1½ ounces.

How your body's changing

The top of your uterus is peeking above your pubic bone now, which may be enough to push your belly out a tad. Starting to show can be quite a thrill, giving you and your partner visible evidence of the baby you've been waiting for. Take some time to plan, daydream, and enjoy this amazing time. It's normal to worry a bit now and then, but try to focus on taking care of yourself and your baby.

Birth is still months away, but your breasts may have already started making colostrum, the first milk that's designed for your baby immediately after birth. Even if your breasts are small or you have inverted nipples, you should still be able to breast-feed if you want to.

Pregnancy is a challenge for your immune system so you may find that you have more coughs and colds than usual.

Your immune system is slightly impaired when you're pregnant so you may have noticed that you've had a few more coughs and colds recently than you normally would. Although they are annoying and tiring, these sniffles won't harm your baby.

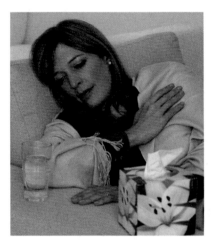

ParentsAsk...

Why are my hands and feet always warm?

It is quite common to feel warmer than normal when you are pregnant, and many women say they find that their hands and feet become particularly hot. This is probably due to the hormonal changes that occur during pregnancy and to an increase in blood supply to the skin. Do not despair. There are measures you can take. It might help if you:

- Fill a foot spa or small tub with cool water and soak your feet.
- Buy a mini battery-operated fan and carry it with you everywhere.
- Wear clothing and shoes that are made of natural fibers, which allow the skin to breathe.
- Run your hands and wrists under a cold tap to cool your pulse points, and use a cool wet washcloth on your forehead and the back of your neck—this should help cool you down quickly.

Getting ready for pregnancy

Staying safe and healthy

Your pregnancy diary

Birth and beyond

Dad's **Diary**

So Dad, your life is about to be turned upside down by the latest addition to your family. But how up to date on baby information are you? Take our quick quiz to see how much you know, and what you still need to learn about life as a dad. Then turn to p.320 for the correct answers.

1 How long should you let your newborn cry at night before picking him up?
(a) Less than one minute
(b) Five to ten minutes
(c) Ten to 15 minutes
(d) Until he stops.

2 How many times a day does the average newborn eat?
(a) Three meals a day
(b) Every four hours
(c) Eight to ten times
(d) On the hour every hour.

3 What's the standard advice on how long after childbirth you should wait until you and your partner can have sex again?
(a) One week
(b) Six weeks
(c) Until your partner says so
(d) Until her doctor gives the green light.

4 What's the number one never-leave-home-without-it item you should bring for an afternoon at the park with your 6-month-old?
(a) Your cell phone
(b) A burp cloth or other soft cloth

(c) The video camera
(d) A diaper.

5 What should you always bring your partner if you're around when she is breast-feeding?
(a) A glass of water
(b) A magazine
(c) Her favorite beer
(d) The TV remote.

6 What's the recommended position for a sleeping baby?
(a) On his tummy
(b) On his side
(c) On his back
(d) In his car seat.

▼ Your body at **15** Weeks

15 Weeks

❋ You may feel your baby's first wiggles as a flutter low down in your abdomen.

❋ Your immune system is slightly impaired so you may suffer from coughs and colds more easily.

You may have discovered that you're a sensitive soul now that you're pregnant. We're not just talking about crying over soppy movies either. Your skin can be more easily irritated than usual, so be extra careful with it.

Skin changes

Minor skin problems during pregnancy are common and most won't cause any harm. However, talk to your doctor if your skin is inflamed or blistered, or if you have a rash, irritation, or itchiness that lasts more than a couple of days.

Chafing

As you put on weight, chafing can take place between your thighs or under your breasts, resulting in red, moist skin. Your skin may then become inflamed and blistered and you may notice an odor. This is a condition known as intertrigo.

Keep the affected area as dry as possible and try to keep your skin cool by wearing cotton clothes and avoiding wearing hose. See your doctor, as intertrigo may cause yeast (see p.239).

Sensitive, irritated skin

Skin tends to become more sensitive during pregnancy, not only because of the higher levels of hormones in your body, but because the skin has become more stretched and delicate. Soaps and detergents may suddenly cause irritation, and conditions such as eczema may become worse.

Try to identify what could be causing the irritation—could it be your laundry detergent or a perfume that you use? Choose loose, cotton clothes and keep your body well moisturized. Long soaks in a warm bath will dry out your skin, so keep these to a minimum.

Rashes and itchiness

It's pretty common for rashes and itchiness to come and go during pregnancy, without any obvious cause. Dabbing on calamine lotion should help to reduce any itching.

Intense itching all over—particularly at night and on the palms of your hands and the soles of your feet—can be a sign of a rare pregnancy-related liver disorder called obstetric cholestasis (see pp.230–31). As with any itching, report it to your doctor if it doesn't go away within days.

75–90% of pregnant women will be affected by stretch marks but they will fade closer to your own skin color after your baby is born.

▼ Your baby at **15** Weeks

Her legs are now growing longer than her arms and her fingernails are fully formed.

❋ You may not know it, but your tiny tenant frequently gets hiccups now. Babies don't make any sound, though, because their trachea is filled with fluid rather than air. Your baby now weighs around 2½ ounces and measures nearly 4½ inches long. All her joints and limbs are now able to move.

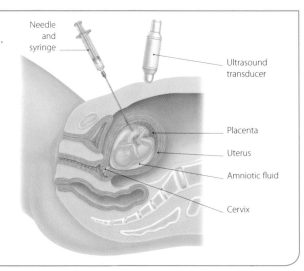

Amniocentesis test

Amniocentesis is a diagnostic test that involves taking a sample of amniotic fluid from your uterus to see whether your baby has any serious abnormalities. It is usually used to detect chromosomal disorders in your baby, such as Down syndrome (see pp.214–15).

Amniocentesis is usually performed in the second trimester, after 16 weeks of pregnancy. Your doctor will insert a long, thin, hollow needle through your abdominal wall and extract some of the fluid around your baby. You may not get the results until two to three weeks after you have the procedure.

Sadly, it's estimated that about one in 200 to one in 400 women miscarries as a result of amniocentesis. If you're uncertain whether or not to have an amniocentesis, or if you're very anxious about the procedure, talk through your concerns with your doctor.

Needle and syringe
Ultrasound transducer
Placenta
Uterus
Amniotic fluid
Cervix

Prenatal care in the second trimester

During the second trimester, you'll see your doctor once every four weeks. Here's what to expect:

● **The basics** She'll weigh you, check your blood pressure, and test your urine for protein. She'll measure the distance from your pubic bone to the top of your belly to check that your baby is growing well, and she'll listen to the baby's heartbeat. She'll also want to know how you're feeling. If it's near flu season, she may advise you to get a flu shot.

● **15 to 20 weeks** You may have a multiple marker screening (see p.128) to assess your baby's risk for certain chromosomal problems and other birth defects. Your doctor will also offer you amniocentesis (see above), which can diagnose Down syndrome as well as other chromosomal abnormalities, genetic disorders, and neural tube defects. If you're not having the multiple marker test or amniocentesis, you'll be offered the alpha-fetoprotein (AFP)

blood test, an ultrasound, or both to screen for neural tube defects. This includes either the AFP blood test or ultrasound or both.

Most doctors order an ultrasound between 16 and 20 weeks to check for physical abnormalities and to verify the baby's due date. This may also be a chance to find out your baby's gender.

● **24 to 28 weeks** You'll be given a glucose screening test to check for gestational diabetes, and possibly another blood test for anemia. If you're Rh-negative, an extra tube of blood may be drawn to check for Rh antibodies before you're given an injection of Rh immune globulin at 28 weeks (see p.233).

● **Education and counseling** Sometime during this trimester, your doctor should talk to you about childbirth education classes. You may want to look into breast-feeding and baby-care classes to take during your third trimester.

Organized mom

Noticing your baby move for the first time is very special. You're sure to want to record it.

"I felt my baby kick for the first time when I was 19 weeks pregnant. I was at work, in a meeting. At first, I wasn't sure if I'd imagined it or if it was my stomach rumbling because I was hungry. Then a few minutes later it happened again, and it was different than anything I'd felt before—like butterfly wings flapping. I was so excited and wanted to share it with my colleagues. They all gathered round to try and feel it, but it was so gentle they couldn't.

As soon as I could, I called my partner to tell her and she was excited too. In fact, she sat all evening with her hand on my stomach, hoping to feel the movements. It took a week or so before they were really strong enough for that, though. The next day I wrote about it in my pregnancy diary. I don't want to forget a thing."

Getting ready for pregnancy

Staying safe and healthy

Your pregnancy diary

Birth and beyond

Diet in the second trimester

Your baby grows rapidly during this trimester and your appetite may start to grow too. Try not to snack on junk food. Instead, prepare healthy snacks like raw veggies and humus for when the munchies strike. And be careful to eat a diet that gives you all the necessary nutrients.

Healthy essentials

You should now be getting some of your energy back. On the other hand, you may find that you are suddenly more susceptible to coughs and colds and to minor infections.

Antioxidants

Fresh fruit and vegetables are rich in antioxidants, which can help you fight off infections, so try to get plenty of fruit and vegetables into your diet. (At least seven portions a day is the recommended intake anyway, whether you are pregnant or not.) Some experts believe that a diet rich in antioxidants may also help to prevent preeclampsia.

Omega 3 essential fatty acids

These are important in pregnancy for your baby's brain, eye, and vision development. Oily fish, such as mackerel, herring, and sardines, are good sources. If you are a vegetarian, try linseed or flax seed oil instead. The US Food and Drug Administration recommends that you should eat no more than 12 ounces of fish a week. This is because oily fish can contain environmental pollutants that may affect the development of your unborn baby (see p.53). However, oily fish is still a good source of omega 3 fats and is rich in other nutrients.

Four healthy pregnancy snacks

Now that you're in the second trimester, hopefully you should feel that you are getting some of your energy back—and your appetite, if you suffered from nausea and vomiting. However busy your life is, make the time to eat well. Try these healthy snacks to help satisfy those hunger pangs.

Cranberry and soft cheese wrap with arugula

Mix some dried cranberries and cream cheese together. Spread over a tortilla wrap and arrange some arugula on top. Roll up and serve with cherry tomatoes or a green salad with balsamic dressing, and a glass of cranberry juice.

Papaya smoothie

Take half a small, ripe papaya, and remove all the seeds and skin. Chop roughly and place in a blender. Add one cup of chilled apple and mango juice and blend together until smooth.

Melon with blueberries and yogurt

Mix some cubes of cantaloupe with a handful of fresh blackberries or blueberries. Serve with a spoonful of Greek-style yogurt and a drizzle of honey.

Humus with pita

Drain a 14-ounce can of chickpeas and blend it in a food processor together with 1 tablespoon tahini, the juice of half a

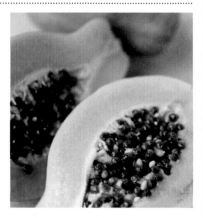

lemon, and a clove of garlic. Drizzle in 1 tablespoon olive oil and a little water to make the mixture creamy. Serve with slices of pita bread.

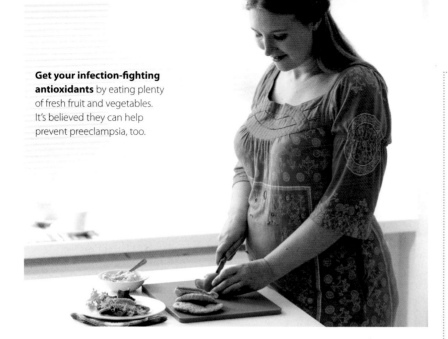

Get your infection-fighting antioxidants by eating plenty of fresh fruit and vegetables. It's believed they can help prevent preeclampsia, too.

ParentsAsk...

I've just been told I have gestational diabetes. What is it and what can I do about it?

This is diabetes that develops for the first time during pregnancy (see p.229). You can usually manage it by changing your diet and getting regular exercise. Your obstetrician will advise you on how to control your blood sugar levels by cutting down on sugary foods and drinks. You will be helped to look at your eating patterns, and advised to choose a balanced diet of whole-grain carbohydrates, lean proteins, and healthy fats.

You will also be asked to monitor your blood sugar levels to check whether the changes you've made are making a difference—your doctor or diabetes specialist will show you how to do this. You should be offered extra ultrasound scans every four weeks from 28 to 36 weeks of pregnancy to see how your baby is growing and how much amniotic fluid you have.

Vitamin A

Our bodies need vitamin A for vision, the skin, and to stay healthy in pregnancy. Vitamin A comes in two forms—retinol and beta-carotene. Both are needed, but too much retinol can harm a developing baby by causing birth defects. Liver and liver products are very high in the retinol form of vitamin A and should be avoided when you are pregnant. Other foods, such as egg yolk, butter or margarine, and milk, also have retinol in them, but at levels that are safe. Good sources of beta-carotene are carrots, sweet potatoes, papaya, oranges, and green vegetables, especially broccoli, watercress, spinach, and spring greens.

Getting your iron

Before you conceived, you needed about 18 mg of iron a day. That's a lot and many of us probably don't get the recommended daily amount. During pregnancy, you need extra iron—27 mg a day—to help keep you and your baby healthy. The iron helps your blood to transport oxygen around your body.

If you don't have enough iron to fuel hemoglobin production (to make red blood cells) for both you and your baby, you may develop iron-deficiency anemia (see p.229). This is the most common type of anemia in pregnancy. A surprisingly high proportion of women—about one in five—develop iron-deficiency anemia when they are pregnant, so it is something that you need to be on your guard about.

As with most vitamins and minerals, food is the best source of iron. You shouldn't need iron supplements if you are careful to have a diet that's rich in iron. This means eating lots of dark green leafy vegetables, whole-wheat bread, iron-fortified cereals, lean red meat, dried fruit, and legumes.

Vitamin C helps your body absorb the iron in your diet. Try drinking plenty of orange juice or eating fruit or vegetables that are rich in vitamin C when you have an iron-rich meal. Tea and coffee make it difficult for your body to absorb iron, so it's best not to drink them at mealtimes. If you do have to take iron supplements, the drawback is that they have some unpleasant side effects. They can cause constipation and other stomach upsets, such as nausea, diarrhea, and stomachache. Increasing the fiber in your diet can help prevent constipation, and taking the supplements with a meal can help the other side effects.

If the side effects become a serious problem, ask your doctor to prescribe you another brand or to reduce the dose. Taking less is probably better than not taking any at all.

16 Weeks

✳ Your uterus has expanded so much that the ligaments in your abdomen are stretching to make room.

✳ You've probably gained at least five pounds by now, and maybe as much as 10 pounds.

The effect of pregnancy hormones and your extra weight can lead to back problems. Help keep backaches at bay by watching your posture, ditching the high heels, and getting some regular exercise.

Protecting your back

The muscles of your back, lower abdomen, and pelvic floor help to move and stabilize the joints of your back and pelvis. As your uterus and baby grow, it can become more difficult for the muscles to do this, which can give you back pain.

Tips for avoiding back pain

● **Avoid heavy lifting** If you have to lift or carry anything, hold it close to your body, bend your knees rather than your back, and try not to twist. If you have a toddler, see if they can climb onto a chair or sofa before you pick them up.

● **Exercise regularly** You can reduce the risk of developing back pain if you exercise regularly. See pp.57, 134 and 184–5 for advice on the best forms of exercise during pregnancy.

● **Wear shoes that are comfortable for you** Some women will only be comfortable in flat shoes, but other women need a bit of a heel to take the pressure off their back.

● **Improve your posture** When standing, imagine that someone is making you taller by pulling a string attached to the top and back of your

head. Tightening your pelvic floor muscles (see p.135) and your stomach muscles will help support your back in this posture.

● **Try pelvic tilting** Stand with your back against a wall, feet a few inches away from the wall, and knees slightly bent. Put one hand in the hollow of your back and tilt your pelvis backward so that your back squashes your hand. Now tilt your pelvis the other way to take the pressure off your hand. Continue to tilt forward and backward in a rhythmical fashion. (See also Back exercises for pregnancy, opposite.)

● **Get into a good sitting posture** When sitting, ensure that your back is well supported. Try placing a small towel rolled into a sausage shape in the hollow of your back.

● **Kneeling on your hands and knees** This reduces pressure on your back from your baby. Round your back up into a hump shape (tucking your tailbone under you), then gently arch your back in the opposite direction so you stick your bottom out (humping and hollowing). Repeating this in a rocking motion helps relieve back or pelvic pain.

▼ Your baby at **16** Weeks

Your baby has now grown to about the size of a large avocado.

✳ He weighs approximately 3½ ounces now and, in the next three weeks, he will double his weight and add quite a bit to his length. In or out of the uterus, babies are playful creatures. Yours may already have discovered his first toy— his umbilical cord. He'll have fun pulling and grabbing it.

Planning a break

If you're having a final fling with your partner before settling down to the delights of family vacations, opt for comfort over adventure as well as good standards of hygiene and medical care. Choose shortish flights (north to south rather than east to west to minimize jet lag) and look for a place with a pleasant rather than baking temperature.

Make sure you have the following packed in your hand luggage:

● **Your driver's license or photo ID** It sounds obvious, but double check if you're suffering from pregnancy-related

forgetfulness! Also, don't forget your passport if you are traveling abroad.

● **A letter from your doctor** If you are flying in late pregnancy, this must give your due date and confirm that you are fit to fly. Most airlines won't let you fly near your due date without a note.

● **Your medical records** If you do have a pregnancy-related problem while you're away, the local doctor can see your records and can also fill in details of any treatment you have.

● **Any prescribed medication** If you are traveling abroad, it's wise to carry

a note from your doctor explaining what the medication is and why you need it.

● **Copies of your travel insurance** It is worth writing this number, and the helpline number on several postcards and keeping them in different places.

● **Details of how to contact a local doctor or hospital** Take these as well as the number for your doctor at home. If you are traveling abroad, check the US Centers for Disease Control and Prevention website for vaccination recommendations, including which are safe for pregnant women.

Back exercises for pregnancy

Kneeling pelvic tilt
Done on all fours, this strengthens the abdominal muscles and eases back pain.

● Get down on your hands and knees, arms shoulder-width apart and knees hip-width apart, keeping your arms straight but not locking the elbows.

● As you breathe in, tighten your abdominal muscles, tuck your buttocks under, and round your back.

● Relax your back into a neutral position as you breathe out.

● Repeat these movements, following the rhythm of your breath as you do so.

Tailor or cobbler pose
This yoga position helps open your pelvis and loosen your hip joints in preparation for birth. It can also improve your posture and ease tension in your lower back.

● Sit up straight against a wall with the soles of your feet touching each other (sit on a folded towel if that's more comfortable for you).

● Gently press your knees down and away from each other, but make sure you don't force them.

● Remain in this position for as long as you feel comfortable. Release, take a few breaths, then repeat.

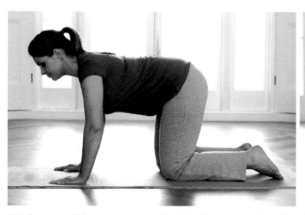

Get down on all fours to do your pelvic tilts. Follow the rhythm of your breath by breathing in and tightening your abs. On the out breath, relax your abs and return your back to a neutral position.

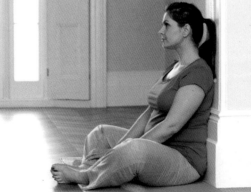

Sit in tailor or cobbler pose to open your hip joints and prepare them for the birth ahead. Gently press your knees down without forcing them. Hold as long as it's comfortable, then relax and repeat.

Getting ready for pregnancy

Staying safe and healthy

Your pregnancy diary

Birth and beyond

FIRST TRIMESTER	SECOND TRIMESTER	THIRD TRIMESTER

Your body at **17** Weeks

17 Weeks

❋ If you are a first-time mom, you may well start to feel your baby's movements around now.

❋ You may be gaining weight rapidly at this point as your baby grows, even if you're not eating much.

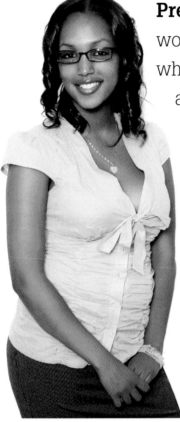

Pregnancy is mostly seen as a woman's thing. Few women believe that their partner really understands what's involved. But dads-to-be can participate. You'll also need to think about childbirth classes soon.

How partners get involved

Partners—you may not be pregnant, but you can be an active observer. Let your partner know you're enjoying seeing her pregnant body. Take pictures to record her growing belly. Give her a back massage. Feel the baby kick. If you read the week-by-week pregnancy diary in this book, you'll know just what's happening, and what needs doing.

Be there

Try to make it to some of your partner's many prenatal appointments. And don't miss the chance to get a glimpse of your baby during a scan. If your partner has an amniocentesis or other procedure, make sure you're there to support her. And, of course, attend childbirth classes, and work on the breathing and relaxation exercises together.

As your partner tries to improve her diet, give up alcohol, and drink more fluids, you can support her by sharing these lifestyle changes. Eliminate from the house and shopping cart any bad-for-baby foods that might tempt her. Cut down or cut out alcohol yourself. Don't smoke. Treat yourselves to some healthy pastimes too—a walk in

the park, a swim, or even surprise her with a stay at a spa with treatments for pregnant women.

Love her changing body

Understand that your partner may feel unattractive now that she's pregnant. So do your best to compliment her on how nice she looks, and tell her what you love about her pregnant body. You may also find that, what with hormone changes, back pain, and nausea, your sex life takes a back seat for a while.

Your partner may also be pretty demanding. Go with it. She's doing most of the hard work. The least you can do is deal with the food shopping, send her flowers, and indulge her demands for cream cheese and jelly sandwiches.

75% of partners-to-be experience pregnancy

"sympathy symptoms." Strange as it may sound, some men start to feel pregnant while their partner is expecting—even to the point of exhibiting similar symptoms.

Your baby at **17** Weeks

With a bit of luck and technology, your doctor may be able to hear your baby's heartbeat now.

❋ There's almost nothing more exciting than knowing your baby's heartbeat can be heard. She is now nearly 5 inches long and weighs about 5 ounces. Her skeleton is mostly rubbery cartilage, which will harden later. A protective substance, myelin, begins to wrap around her spinal cord.

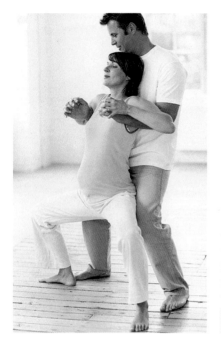

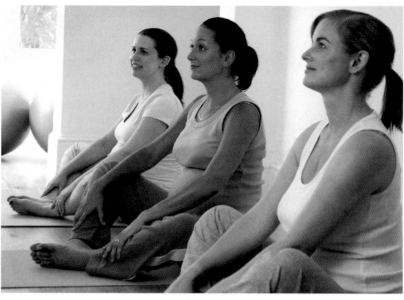

Going to childbirth classes gives you the opportunity to practice positions for labor and birth as well as the breathing exercises. It's also a social occasion.

Childbirth classes

Childbirth classes help to prepare you for labor, birth, and early parenthood. Classes range from intensive courses that begin early in pregnancy and last until after your baby is born, to one-shot refresher sessions. All should be led by a trained childbirth instructor. BabyCenter's online birth class lasts for three hours and can be watched anytime. To see what a childbirth class should cover, refer to p.78. Most classes also cover some of the more common childbirth complications and how they might be handled, as well as the basics of breast-feeding and general newborn care. Some specific types of childbirth classes include:

● **Lamaze** These classes aim to "increase women's confidence in their natural ability to give birth," teaching simple coping strategies including breathing techniques.

● **Bradley Method** This embraces the idea that childbirth is a natural process and that, with the right preparation, most women can avoid pain medication and routine interventions during labor and birth.

● **HypnoBirthing** Women are taught how to use deep relaxation, visualization, and self-hypnosis so they can have a calm, comfortable birth even when medical intervention is necessary.

● **ICEA** Some childbirth instructors are certified by the International Childbirth Education Association (ICEA), an organization that provides education and training programs for instructors. If you're thinking of using an ICEA-certified instructor, ask what information and which techniques for coping with labor will be covered in class.

Other options to consider include Birthing from Within, a spiritually focused approach; BirthWorks, which encourages women to have faith in their bodies' knowledge of labor; and the Alexander Technique, a movement-awareness method that focuses on alignment, balance, and coordination.

Organized mom

Childbirth classes prepare you well for your baby's birth and are great for involving your partner.

"When I found out I was pregnant, I couldn't wait to start my childbirth classes. I hate feeling out of control and knew that they would teach me what to expect and how to make pregnancy and birth as enjoyable and healthy as possible. As soon as I could, I booked myself and my partner into a couples' class. I thought it would be a great way to make the whole thing seem more real for my partner, too."

Getting ready for pregnancy

Staying safe and healthy

Your pregnancy diary

Birth and beyond

▼ Your body at **18** Weeks

18 Weeks

❋ Bigger, more comfortable clothes are a must now. You may even need bigger shoes as your feet swell.

❋ Nose bleeds are common as your increased blood supply puts pressure on the delicate veins of your nose.

With your belly growing rapidly it's probably obvious that you're pregnant. Strangers may smile at you or even start a conversation. You need to be prepared for well-meaning but unwanted advice.

Time for rapid growth

A boy's genitals are visible; a girl's are in place

Your baby is now about 4¾ inches long and weighs almost 6¾ ounces.

He's busy flexing his arms and legs—movements that you'll start noticing more and more in the weeks ahead. His blood vessels are visible through his thin skin, and his ears are now in their final position, although they're still standing out from his head a bit.

A protective covering of myelin is beginning to form around his spinal cord and nerves, a process that will continue for a year after he's born. If you're having a girl, her uterus and fallopian tubes are formed and in place. If you're having a boy, his genitals are noticeable now, but he may hide them from you during an ultrasound! His chest moves up and down to mimic breathing but he's not taking in air, only amniotic fluid.

Because your baby's growing so rapidly, an increase in your appetite is pretty common about now. Make it count by choosing meals and snacks that are nutrient-rich instead of empty calories. Bigger, more comfortable clothes are a must now as your appetite and waistline grow.

Your cardiovascular system is going through significant changes, and during this trimester your blood pressure will probably be lower than usual. Don't spring up too fast from lying or sitting or you might feel a little dizzy.

From now on, it's best to lie on your side—or tilted to one side. If you're flat on your back, your uterus can compress a major vein, which can decrease the blood return to your heart and your baby. Try a pillow behind you or under your hip or upper leg for comfort.

Mid-pregnancy ultrasound

This scan is often done sometime in the second trimester (usually between 16 and 20 weeks) to assess fetal growth and development, screen for certain birth defects, check the placenta and umbilical cord, and determine whether the gestational age is accurate. During this scan, you might see your baby kick, flex, reach, roll, or even suck his thumb. Bring your partner along, and whether or not he's able to accompany you, make sure you ask for printouts of the baby in various poses.

▼ Your baby at **18** Weeks
....

Your baby's chest moves up and down, but he's taking in amniotic fluid, not air.

❋ The amniotic fluid protects him as he grows inside the amniotic sac. He is now about 4¾ inches long from crown to rump and weighs about 6¾ ounces. If you're having a girl, the vagina, uterus (womb), and fallopian tubes are already in place. If it's a boy, the genitals are distinct and recognizable.

Feeling baby's first movements

Pregnant women usually feel the first movements of their fetus around 16 to 20 weeks, although this can vary from woman to woman. At first, the movements feel like a gentle fluttering, and it can often be mistaken for "gas." As your baby grows, these sensations change so that you start to feel thumping or kicking movements which become stronger as your pregnancy progresses. First-time moms often feel movements later than moms who have been pregnant before as they are not exactly sure what to expect. Women who are very active may also miss the subtle feelings of early movement.

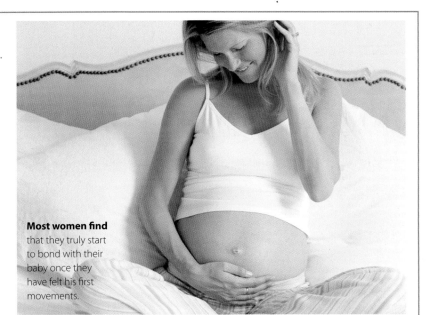

Most women find that they truly start to bond with their baby once they have felt his first movements.

Dealing with unwanted or unhelpful advice

Now that you're pregnant, you'll probably find you're given lots of advice by friends and relatives—and even complete strangers—especially once you start showing. Some of it will be helpful: "try sleeping with a pillow under your legs" or "make up lots of freezer meals before the baby arrives." And some of it not so helpful: "sleep while you can now—you'll get no sleep when the baby's born!" or "you look small for seven months—are you sure your dates are right?"

Dealing with unwanted advice and tactless comments can be tricky—especially when you're battling with pregnancy hormones. Remember, most people offer you advice with the best of intentions and, in the case of friends and family, it's because they care about you.

It's a good idea to have some stock responses prepared for those moments when you're given unsolicited—or even questionable—advice. Politely thank the giver for their concern and tell them you'll think about their suggestion, or that you'll ask your doctor when you go for your next appointment. If Grandma tells you to stock up on beer to help you to breast-feed successfully, it might be worth updating her on current alcohol guidelines.

When people give you unasked-for advice, or advice that makes you worry, try not to get angry or upset. It's really not worth it. If you're having a particular problem with a friend's or relative's intrusive comments, and you don't feel able to confront them, ask someone to mediate for you.

Working mom

You may have to compromise on the shoe front, but you can still look stylish and be comfortable.

"I finally caved in and bought some new work shoes. All my work shoes have really high heels, but I've had some lower-back pain lately. I'm told the ligaments in your back soften during pregnancy and I don't want to cause any lasting damage. So I bought a couple of pairs of ballet flats. They're very comfortable and very stylish. I'm sure they'll be great as I get bigger. I'll still wear my killer heels—but only for special occasions."

Wearing flat shoes can help prevent lower-back pain.

Getting ready for pregnancy

Staying safe and healthy

Your pregnancy diary

Birth and beyond

Screening at the halfway stage

You'll probably have your mid-pregnancy ultrasound around this time. It's an exciting moment in your pregnancy and one you'll want to share with your partner. Occasionally, problems do get picked up, but chances are your baby will be absolutely fine.

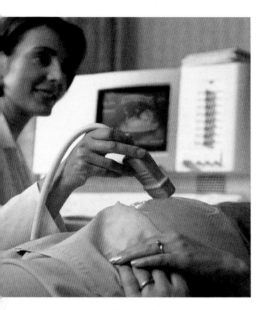

Partners are usually welcome when you have a scan and you can normally watch what's happening in your uterus on a screen.

Mid-pregnancy ultrasound

Most women are offered a mid-pregnancy ultrasound, or sonogram, at 16 to 20 weeks to check that their baby is developing normally. It is done in order to look for any abnormalities in your baby's development and growth, and also to check the position of the placenta in the uterus.

Seeing your baby on a screen is an exciting and emotional time. Most sonographers welcome your partner and your other children to share the experience with you. Many couples want to know the sex of their baby and get some photos. It's important to remember, though, that this scan's main purpose is to look for abnormalities.

You are usually allowed to watch the ultrasound as it is being performed. If you haven't already had an ultrasound, the sonographer will check that there is only one baby and will confirm your due date. She will point out your baby's heartbeat, face, and hands before looking at him in detail. The scan normally takes about 15 to 20 minutes.

ParentsAsk...

Will I be able to find out the sex of my baby at the mid-pregnancy ultrasound?

By 16 to 20 weeks, when the ultrasound is usually done, your baby's sex is often clearly visible. Be sure tell the technician if you don't want to know the baby's gender so she doesn't ruin the surprise. You can bring home pictures of your baby from the scan. These will probably be on thermal paper: it is heat sensitive, so don't laminate them. If you want copies, it's best to scan them into a computer or photocopy them.

What happens next if they find a problem at the ultrasound?

Don't panic. Often, a follow-up test shows that there is no cause for concern. But in the unlikely event that your baby has a health problem, the information from the ultrasound can help your doctor determine how to give your baby the best possible outcome.

What support will we have if something's seriously wrong?

If you are one of the few unlucky ones and a scan reveals a serious problem, you should be given plenty of support to guide you through all the options. Although such serious problems are rare, some families are faced with the most difficult decision of all—whether to end the pregnancy. Other problems may mean that a baby needs surgery or treatment after birth, or even surgery while it is still in the uterus. There will be a whole range of people to support you through any painful times, including midwives, obstetricians, pediatricians, physical therapists, and the hospital chaplain.

The technician will check the location of the placenta. If the placenta is covering the cervix (placenta previa; see pp.231–2), it can cause painless but severe bleeding later in the pregnancy. If your practitioner detects this condition, she'll most likely order a follow-up ultrasound early in your third trimester to see if the placenta is still covering the cervix. Only a small percentage of placenta previas detected on an ultrasound before 20 weeks are still there at delivery.

If the ultrasound shows that you have too much or too little amniotic fluid, there may be a problem. You'll have a complete workup to see if the cause can be identified. Your doctor may then monitor you with regular ultrasounds.

Your doctor looks closely at your baby's basic anatomy (see Anatomy scan checks and measurements, below). If you've had any suspicious results from a multiple marker or first trimester screening (see p.128), or if there's any other cause for concern, the technician will do a more thorough (level II) scan to check for birth defects or Down syndrome.

Sonograms carried out at state-of-the-art academic centers can detect abnormalities up to 80 percent of the time, while at sites such as doctor's offices, the detection rate can dip as low as 13 percent. So consider requesting a "registered medical diagnostic sonographer" to administer your ultrasound and a radiologist or obstetrician who specializes in ultrasound to interpret the results, especially if other tests have raised suspicions about possible problems.

New 3-D ultrasounds that use special equipment to show a view of your baby that's almost as detailed as a photograph are becoming popular. The new technology requires a more skilled sonographer and isn't available yet in many places. Some centers offer 3-D ultrasounds solely to create keepsake photos or videos for parents. Remember that the personnel at these places may not be qualified to counsel you if your ultrasound reveals a problem. And since the scan is for "entertainment only," the results may be falsely reassuring.

Anatomy scan checks and measurements

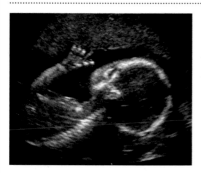

Head The shape and size of the head are usually checked first.

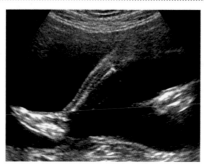

Legs and feet These will be checked in case there are any abnormalities.

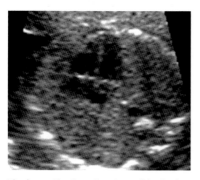

The heart The four chambers of the fetal heart can be clearly seen and checked.

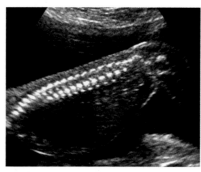

Spine The vertebrae will be counted and checked to make sure they are aligned.

The sonographer will check the various parts of your baby's body that show how well he is growing.

● The head is usually examined first, to check its shape and internal structures.
● The spine is checked to make sure that all the vertebrae are aligned and that the skin properly covers the spine at the back.
● The baby's abdominal wall is also checked to make sure it covers all the internal organs.
● The heart is looked at to check its size and shape.
● The stomach should be visible below the heart.
● The sonographer will check that your baby has two kidneys, and that urine flows freely into the bladder.
● The arms and legs will be checked in case of abnormalities.
● Your baby's hands and feet will be examined.
● The placenta, umbilical cord, and amniotic fluid will all be checked.

Getting ready for pregnancy

Staying safe and healthy

Your pregnancy diary

Birth and beyond

▼ Your body at **19** Weeks

19 Weeks

❋ Your uterus has grown well into your abdomen—the top of it probably reaches your belly button.

❋ You may ache in your lower abdomen as muscles and ligaments stretch to support your belly.

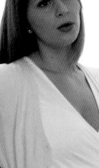

Congratulations—you're at the halfway mark!

You may be suffering from some aches and pains in your back and lower abdomen now. There's no need to worry. Most of these pains are perfectly normal.

Aches and pains

It's common to get aches and pains in your lower abdomen during this stage of pregnancy. Aching (as opposed to cramping) is usually caused by the stretching of the muscles and ligaments area. It is often confused with, or misdiagnosed as, sciatica.

If you have pain on or around the front of your pubic bone, you may be suffering from separation of the

"Sitting with **your feet up** will help **alleviate your symptoms**."

supporting your uterus. You'll probably feel it most when you're getting up from a bed or chair, when you cough or when you get out of the bath.

Sitting comfortably with your feet up should alleviate your symptoms. These are perfectly normal and give you an excuse to get off your feet—and even be waited on! However, don't hesitate to call your doctor any time abdominal aching is accompanied by severe pain or cramping, bleeding, fever, chills, or a feeling of faintness.

Backaches are also common during pregnancy (see p.150). Pain at the back of the pelvis is known as pelvic pain (see p.231). The pain is often one-sided and may be concentrated in the buttock

pubic bone (see p.231). With this, it's common to feel a grinding or clicking in your pubic area and the pain may travel down the inside of the thighs or between your legs. The pain is usually made worse by separating your legs, walking, going up or down stairs, or moving around in bed.

Hip pain is also common. It can be particularly problematic in bed, and can make sleeping difficult. Sleeping on your side with your legs bent and a pillow between your knees may help. If any of these conditions are a problem, talk to your doctor. Alternatively, your doctor can refer you to a physical therapist who will be able to help differentiate between these conditions.

▼ Your baby at **19** Weeks

At this stage of your pregnancy your baby's five senses are starting to develop.

❋ The nerve cells serving each of her senses—taste, smell, hearing, sight, and touch—are now developing in their specialized areas of her brain. She now measures around 6 inches, and weighs about 8½ ounces. If you are carrying a girl baby, she now has roughly six million eggs in her ovaries.

What's happening to your breasts?

By now you have no doubt noticed the huge changes taking place in your bra cups: larger breasts and darkened nipples and areolas (the circles of skin surrounding your nipples). You may also have noticed the appearance of tiny bumps around your areolas. These are called the glands of Montgomery. They produce an oily substance that cleanses, lubricates, and protects the nipples from infection during breast-feeding.

Perhaps even more remarkable than this visible transformation are the extensive changes taking place on the inside. Your breasts are made up of supportive tissue, milk glands, and protective fat. Amid the fat cells and glandular tissue is an intricate network of channels or canals called milk ducts.

Pregnancy hormones make the milk ducts increase in number and size. Each one branches off into smaller canals near the chest wall called ductules. At the end of each ductule is a cluster of small, grapelike sacs called alveoli. A cluster of alveoli is called a lobule; a cluster of lobules is called a lobe. Each breast contains 15 to 20 lobes.

Milk is produced inside the alveoli, which are surrounded by tiny muscles that squeeze the milk out into the ductules. These ductules converge and lead to bigger ducts that end at your nipple. Your milk-duct system becomes fully developed sometime during your second trimester. This means that you can breast-feed your baby even if she's born prematurely.

You'll begin full-scale milk production within 24 to 48 hours of giving birth. The estrogen and progesterone levels in your body start to drop. The hormone prolactin then signals your body to make lots of milk to nourish your baby.

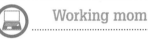

Working mom

Finding a comfortable pair of maternity hose can prove to be an unexpected challenge.

"It's taken me ages to find a pair of maternity hose that I like. None of them look particularly sexy before you put your clothes on top of them (my other half laughed his head off when he saw me try the first pair on), but then hose never do look that great!

Some are more comfortable than others—and the prices range from cheap and cheerful to pretty pricey. It's much more comfortable to wear hose with a high cotton content—the last thing you need is hot, sweaty legs when you're pregnant. I may invest in a more expensive pair when my belly gets bigger—some of them have built-in support around the belly, which sounds like a good idea."

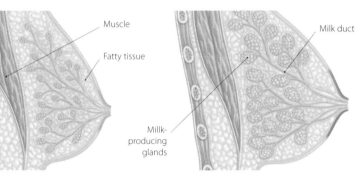

Before pregnancy your breasts consist of fatty tissue on top of a layer of muscle.

During pregnancy milk-producing glands are stimulated. Ducts take milk to the nipple.

Getting ready for pregnancy

Staying safe and healthy

Your pregnancy diary

Birth and beyond

Parents**Talk...**

"I was really worried when doing nothing more energetic than getting out of bed or up from a chair made the lower part of my stomach ache. I called my doctor and she reassured me that it's nothing to worry about, as long as it's not a severe pain or cramp. She said it's just my muscles stretching as my baby grows."
Fritha, 27, first-time mom

"Whenever I start to feel uncomfortable, if possible I'll sit down and put my feet up. After a few minutes, I usually find that the aching eases or stops entirely. I must admit that I do sometimes milk the situation though. My husband has brought me many a cup of tea while I've been exaggeratedly sighing in my chair."
Dee, 33, pregnant for the second time

▼ Your body at **20** Weeks

20 Weeks

✳ Some breathlessness is normal and may get a little worse as your uterus pushes up against your lungs.

✳ You can probably feel your baby move around now. Those flutters are one of the joys of pregnancy.

You may be feeling a little heavy now, especially if you're carrying twins. It's not just the weight of your baby that's the problem, but your uterus becoming increasingly muscular as it starts preparing for birth.

Pregnant with twins

When you are expecting twins, you might suffer more from some of the usual symptoms of pregnancy. Anemia (see p.229) is more common with twins, for example, and can make you feel very tired. You are also likely to gain more weight than mothers expecting one baby. As in any pregnancy, try to eat a healthy, balanced diet and also to ensure that you gain enough weight to help your babies to grow well.

Later on in pregnancy there is more strain on your muscles because you are carrying extra weight, so back pain (see p.150) might be a problem. Another problem is breathlessness (see opposite); having two babies pushing up against your diaphragm can make it worse.

Extra care

You should be offered extra scans to see how your babies are positioned in the uterus, how well they are growing, and whether any complications are developing. Regular blood pressure and urine tests are especially important, too, as you have a higher-than-usual risk of developing gestational hypertension (see pp. 229–30), preeclampsia (see p.233), or

Fact: If it were possible, more than two-thirds of moms-to-be said they would choose to have twins. They love the idea—you only have to be pregnant once to have a big family right away.

gestational diabetes (see p.229). Bed rest isn't often recommended these days, just because you're pregnant with twins. However, you will still need extra rest. If you have older children, arrange more child care if you can. And snatch daytime naps whenever possible.

If you are at work, weigh the pros and cons of taking maternity leave early. Carrying twins is hard work and premature birth happens in about half of twin pregnancies. One of the most important lessons to learn when you have twins is to ask for help. If people offer to lend a hand, let them; if not, ask them. You could also contact a multiple-birth support group for advice and that is a good way to make friends who also have twins. Ask your doctor for details.

▼ Your baby at **20** Weeks

This week your baby will be swallowing more of the amniotic fluid.

✳ Any excess water will move into his large bowel. He now measures about 6½ inches from crown to rump. A whitish coat of a slick, fatty substance called vernix caseosa is beginning to cover him. This helps to protect his skin during its long immersion in the amniotic fluid. It also helps to ease delivery.

Breathlessness

About seven out of 10 pregnant women feel breathless at some point. It can start in the first or second trimester, and is probably due to your respiratory system adapting to the effects of pregnancy hormones. In addition, your rib cage moves up and outward. This gives you a greater lung capacity and helps your body to process oxygen and carbon dioxide more efficiently.

Later on, as your uterus pushes your diaphragm toward your lungs, you'll probably have some breathlessness too, especially if you're expecting twins or carrying your baby high.

Most women in their first pregnancy find that their baby engages, or drops down into the pelvis, from around 36 weeks (see p.205). You may well find that this helps to relieve the

breathlessness. In later pregnancies your baby may not engage until the very end. If you've still got a while to go, try doing some light exercise. If you are out of shape, you are more likely to feel breathless, which is why a gentle workout can help.

Although breathlessness is normal during pregnancy you should always call your doctor if you notice other alarming symptoms, such as chest pain, palpitations, or a racing pulse. Breathlessness can also be a sign of anemia (see p.229). Ask your doctor to check for this with a blood test if it hasn't been done recently.

There is no need to worry about your baby. You may fear that you're depriving him of oxygen, but rest assured that he is getting what he needs.

"Rest assured that **your baby** is getting the **oxygen he needs**."

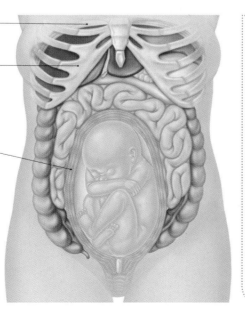

Diaphragm is pushed toward the lungs

Rib cage moves up and out to make extra space for your lungs

Expanding uterus pushes the diaphragm up

You'll probably be feeling breathless whichever way up your baby is now (most turn head down in readiness for birth). That's because your expanding uterus squeezes your other organs up, especially your diaphragm and rib cage.

ParentsAsk...

I'm having twins. Will I be able to have a normal delivery?
Many women carrying twins are able to have a vaginal birth, although around six out of 10 twin births are by cesarean section. Talk to your doctor about the policy in your local hospital and talk through your options. It may depend in part on the position your babies are in when you go into labor. If your first twin is in a head-down position and the placenta isn't in the way of the cervix, a vaginal birth is often possible. Also, ask your doctor about the amount of experience she has of delivering twins vaginally.

Getting ready for pregnancy

Staying safe and healthy

Your pregnancy diary

Birth and beyond

Sleep in the second trimester

By now your body will be adjusting to the huge hormonal and physical changes of pregnancy, and you can sleep more peacefully as a result—barring a few minor sleep disturbances, such as leg cramps, weird dreams, and a stuffy nose, of course!

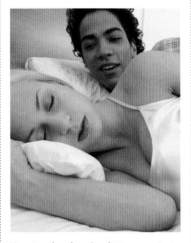
Sleeping in comfort

Chances are that you're sleeping better now than you have in months. That's because the influx of progesterone that started when you became pregnant has tapered down to a steady drizzle.

> "You won't be **scurrying to the bathroom** as often as **before**."

So although your hormone levels are still rising, it's happening more slowly now, and you'll probably be feeling less tired than you did during the early months.

The other good news is that your baby is now positioned above your bladder, rather than next to it, so you won't be scurrying for the bathroom as often as you have been.

Keep in mind, though, that the quality of your sleep, as well as the amount of time you spend asleep, still won't be as good as it was before you were pregnant and you may at times be affected by snoring and congestion, leg cramps (see opposite), and vivid dreams.

You are more likely to snore because the increase in progesterone can make your nasal passages swell slightly, causing congestion. Try sleeping on your side rather than your back, or try wearing a nasal strip to keep your nostrils wide open (these are available at most pharmacists) .If you are having problems getting comfortable, you can use pillows to support both your belly and your back in bed. Tucking a pillow between your legs supports your lower back and may make sleeping on your side more comfortable. You can also get pillows that are made especially for pregnancy, although you may need to scour the classified ads in baby magazines or surf the net to find them.

Bizarre dreamworld

If you are having strange dreams, which may or may not include pregnancy and baby-related images, it may be that your sleep and dream patterns are being affected by your hormones, your changing shape and mixed feelings of anxiety and excitement about becoming a mom. All you can do is try to enjoy your new technicolor dreamworld. You could also record your dreams and what you think they mean in a journal.

Leg cramps and other nighttime miseries

Your leg muscles are now bearing your increasing weight and can sometimes seize up during the night in protest. Too little calcium and potassium circulating in your blood can also cause spasms, as can your expanding uterus pressing on the nerves leading to your legs.

To prevent nighttime cramps, eat a banana for a potassium boost or drink a glass of milk before bed for a calcium boost. Rotate your ankles and wiggle your toes whenever you can. Try stretching your calf muscles several times before you go to bed.

If you do get a cramp, straighten your leg, heel first, and gently flex your ankles and toes. You can also relax the cramp by massaging the muscle or warming it with a hot-water bottle. Walking around for a few minutes may help, too.

Your sleep may also be disturbed by restless legs—crawling, creeping, or tingling sensations inside your foot and calf. Nearly all sufferers report an overpowering urge to move their legs. No one knows exactly what causes restless legs, but it may be inherited.

Medication is available for the problem but none is safe during pregnancy. Try keeping a journal of what you eat and drink, what you do, and your emotions. After a few weeks, you may be able to tell if diet, stress, or even environmental factors are causing your symptoms.

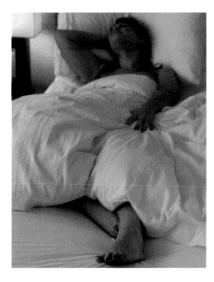

If you get a leg cramp at night, straighten and stretch your leg, then flex your ankles.

How exercise can help you sleep

Regular exercise during pregnancy makes you healthier, both physically and mentally, and it can help you sleep more soundly, too—provided you do the right amount at the right time of day.

For one thing, exercise helps you work off any excess energy, and will tire you enough to lull you into a deeper, more restful slumber. Gently stretching your muscles helps ward off sleep-disturbing aches and pains, such as leg cramps.

On the other hand, if you exercise shortly before you go to bed, you may feel revved up instead of ready to wind down. Some experts say that working up a sweat too close to bedtime can interfere with your natural sleep cycle and rob you of restorative deep sleep. So it's important to set aside the late afternoon or early evening for exercise and give yourself at least four hours to unwind before you hit the sack.

Natural sleep remedies

If you're having trouble getting to sleep now that you're pregnant, ask your doctor about natural remedies that will be safe for you and your baby.

Herbal remedies A hop pillow may help if you want to use herbal remedies, but avoid drinking hop teas unless prescribed by a qualified medical herbalist and after asking your doctor.

Aromatherapy Lavender, chamomile or ylang ylang essential oils may help when used for a massage, but use occasionally and only two to three drops in two teaspoons of a base oil such as almond oil.

Flower remedies Remedies containing a mixture of flower essences are specifically designed to ease general stress and tension and may help you sleep. Again, ask your doctor before taking any remedy.

Homeopathy Some restless sleepers say they've been helped by certain homeopathic remedies such as coffea and aconite, but there's no systematic research to prove these remedies work. If you want to try homeopathy, see a professional homeopath who can prescribe a remedy and dose based on your symptoms. Strong tinctures can be dangerous.

The occasional aromatherapy massage with lavender oil can help with sleeplessness.

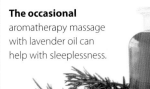

Getting ready for pregnancy

Staying safe and healthy

Your pregnancy diary

Birth and beyond

▼ Your body at **21** Weeks

21 Weeks

✳ It's hard to be graceful when you're pregnant. Don't be surprised if you find you're more clumsy now.

✳ You're carrying more weight, your center of gravity has changed and all your joints are loosening up.

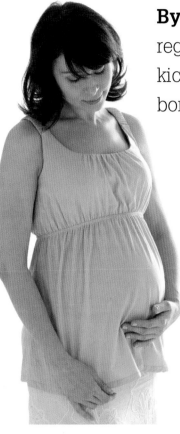

By now you should be feeling your baby moving regularly—often when you are trying to rest! Those kicks and nudges will help you and your partner to bond with the little person growing inside you.

Your baby's movements

If this is your first pregnancy you will probably first be aware of your baby's movements at around 18 to 20 weeks. For subsequent pregnancies, when you are already familiar with the telltale signs, you will probably first feel her movements a bit earlier, at around 15 to 18 weeks.

After the initial vague stirrings, which some women say feel like a butterfly's wings flapping, your baby's movements become stronger and more regular. Later, you will start to feel thumping or kicking movements, though not all the time because she sometimes just wants to rest.

While you are busy you will probably be less aware of the movements your baby is making. It's more likely you'll start to notice them when you sit down and relax. Every baby has his or her own individual pattern of waking and sleeping. By late pregnancy you will probably have become tuned into your baby's particular pattern of movements. This is what you might expect as your baby grows.

● **From 20 to 24 weeks** As the weeks go by, you'll notice how your baby's

activity will gradually increase. From now onward, over the next 10 weeks, your baby will be having a very busy period, with plenty of kicking and turning somersaults.

● **From 24 to 28 weeks** Baby hiccups are common at this time but start earlier in pregnancy. This explains the jerking movements you may feel. The amniotic sac now contains up to 1½ pints of fluid. This helps your baby move about freely. At around this time, you may notice her jump at sudden noises.

● **At 29 weeks** At this stage in your pregnancy, your baby will begin to make smaller, more definite movements. She is starting to get more cramped inside your uterus.

● **At 32 weeks** Your baby's movements will reach a peak of activity and, from now on, you will notice an increase in the frequency and type of movements as your baby gets bigger and stronger.

● **From around 36 weeks** Your baby may take up her final (usually head-down) position at about this time, particularly if this is your first pregnancy. That is because, in a first pregnancy, the

---

▼ Your baby at **21** Weeks

From now on, watch what you say since your baby can probably hear you!

✳ Now you can communicate with her by talking, singing, or reading aloud. Studies even suggest a newborn will suck more vigorously when feeding if you read aloud from a book that you've read aloud from during pregnancy. Your baby now measures about 10½ inches and has real eyebrows, eyelids, and fingernails.

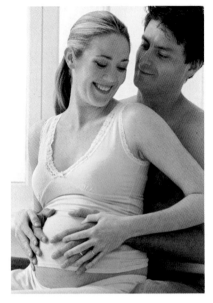

As your pregnancy progresses your baby's movements get stronger and your partner should be able to feel them, too.

muscles of your uterus and abdomen are still firm and will help to keep her in place. The main movements you are likely to feel now are jabs from her arms and legs, and possibly a few painful kicks to your ribs.

If this isn't your first pregnancy, your abdominal muscles are likely to be weaker. This gives your baby the chance to keep changing her position and she could continue to do so even right up to your due date.

● **From 36 to 40 weeks** Now you are in the last weeks of your pregnancy and your baby will be getting larger and her roll-over movements will become less frequent. If she's sucking her thumb and "loses" it, you may feel quick, darting movements. This is her head turning from side-to-side while she tries to find her thumb again.

During the last two weeks of your pregnancy, the movements are likely to slow down and your baby's growth rate will decline slightly. This is all completely normal and nothing to worry about.

Avoiding excess weight gain

If you are worried about how much weight you are putting on, keep a food diary for a few days. This will quickly show you how balanced your diet is. If you're eating plenty of fruit and vegetables, lots of multigrain foods, and some good proteins and dairy products, then there is less need to worry than if you find you are filling up on fries and chocolate. If you are eating well but still piling on the pounds, then it's time to see a dietician who has experience of working with pregnant women. She will help you to find out how to make the best of your nutrient intake without loading up on calories.

Your best strategy is to eat healthily and incorporate regular exercise into your daily life. Evidence has shown that exercise in addition to a healthy diet during pregnancy results in less weight gain than eating a healthy diet alone. The researchers also found that the women who exercised reduced their risk of giving birth to a large baby.

If you're a relative newcomer to exercise, though, you should start with low-impact exercise such as walking, swimming, or low-impact aerobics (see p.57). And never begin a new exercise regimen without first discussing with your doctor what you can do safely.

"Keeping a food diary **will show** if your diet is **well balanced**."

Getting ready for pregnancy

Staying safe and healthy

Your pregnancy diary

Birth and beyond

FIRST TRIMESTER	SECOND TRIMESTER	THIRD TRIMESTER

▼ Your body at **22** Weeks

22 Weeks

❋ At this point, you'll probably notice a steady gain in weight—about ½ pound each week.

❋ You may notice increased vaginal discharge. It's due to increased blood flow in that part of the body.

Have you found yourself longing for hotdogs with ice cream,

or salivating over cheese and chocolate? Don't worry—lots of women have weird and wonderful food cravings in pregnancy.

Cravings in pregnancy

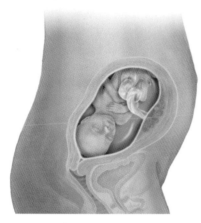

▼ Your baby at **22** Weeks

Now the baby inside you is beginning to look like a miniature newborn.

❋ This is a very exciting time because your baby is now looking recognizably like a baby. His lips are becoming more distinct and his eyes have developed; though the irises don't have their color yet, his eyebrows and eyelids are in place. His pancreas, which is essential for hormone production, is developing steadily and the first signs of teeth are there now, showing beneath his gum line. If you could see inside your uterus, you would be able to spot the fine hair (lanugo) now covering his body.

Don't be surprised if you find you have a craving to eat something particular during pregnancy. This kind of yearning is an undeniable part of carrying a baby for many women, and not all of these cravings can be neatly catalogued—or stomached. You may find yourself yearning for pickles wrapped in cheese, or mayonnaise spooned straight from the jar—or even seeking out a good helping of pure steak fat!

Some pregnant women develop strong cravings for non-food items such as dirt, ashes, clay, chalk, coal, ice, laundry starch, baking soda, soap, toothpaste, paint chips, plaster, wax, hair, coffee grounds, and even cigarette butts. This phenomenon is called pica, which is Latin for magpie—a bird that will eat almost anything.

The causes

No one knows what causes these cravings, but a combination of biochemical, psychological, and cultural factors may be at work. In some studies, these bizarre cravings have been linked to an iron deficiency—even though none of the craved items contain a significant amount of iron. Some women who have iron-deficiency anemia crave ice until the deficiency is cured. And pica is sometimes listed as a symptom of iron-deficiency anemia.

If you crave non-food items, it doesn't necessarily mean you have any sort of deficiency, and it definitely doesn't mean you should consume them! In fact, eating non-food substances can interfere with your body's ability to absorb nutrients and may even cause a deficiency. And while eating ice is not likely to be harmful (except possibly to your teeth!), eating dirt and most of the other items mentioned can lead to illness, such as lead poisoning or bowel blockage, which could have very serious consequences.

Get some advice

If you're having strong cravings for any non-food items, it's a good idea to talk to your doctor. While this kind of craving does occur in healthy pregnant women, it's worth getting yourself checked for any underlying physical or psychological problem. You may also be able to curb unhealthy cravings by eating breakfast every day (just some fruit would do), getting plenty of exercise, and ensuring that you have a wide ranging and healthy diet.

Planning ahead for working parenthood

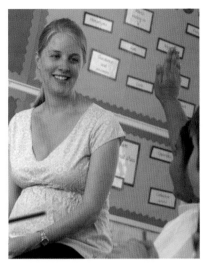

If you have a job you enjoy, finding dependable child care means you can return to work after the birth.

All parents work, of course, and staying at home with a demanding baby or toddler is equally, if not more, taxing than going back to your old job. There are new skills to be learned, but there is no one around to train you. Added to that, there is no recognition of the hard work done and no pay check at the end of the month. It's not all about money, of course, but losing one person's income is something that many couples find difficult to afford.

Deciding to return to work means balancing your time between work and family, and you will need to develop a raft of new skills. One of the most valuable is the ability to plan and juggle your time so that you meet different demands. You will also need to develop strong organizational skills.

Solid and dependable child-care arrangements are a must if you want to enjoy your new life fully. Be prepared to devote plenty of time to choosing the right option for you, since you are handing over a huge responsibility to someone when you employ them to care for your baby. You have to be confident that you are leaving your little one in the hands of a skilled and caring professional. You don't want to be worrying about your baby's well-being while you're trying to work.

If you have a job that you find satisfying and your child is entrusted to capable hands, you can have a very rewarding life as a working parent. Work can give you a challenge, an income, and the pleasure of adult company during part of the day. Then, you can return home and really enjoy spending time with your child.

Working mom

It can be hard to know when—and how—to tell your work colleagues you're pregnant.

"It's so much easier now that my work colleagues know I'm pregnant. I don't need to hold in my stomach any more! I was really nervous before I told them, so I told the colleagues I work with most closely first. It didn't take long for the news to travel after that. I've had lots of congratulations—everyone seems to be really happy for me. It created a bit of a buzz in the office for the morning. A couple of my co-workers even said that they suspected I might be pregnant—I guess I wasn't that good at hiding my nausea and fatigue after all!"

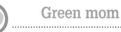
Green mom

Urinary tract infections (UTIs) are common in pregnancy, but there are ways of avoiding them.

"Over the years, since I had my last baby, I've learned quite a few natural methods for warding off UTIs. I think they're better than taking pills and medicines and they seem to have worked, since I haven't had a UTI during my pregnancy so far. By this stage last time around, I'd already had a couple and I was really over it.

Firstly, when I go to the bathroom, I always make sure to wipe myself front to back and empty my bladder completely. And I always make sure I go to the bathroom soon after having sex.

Then, whenever I have a shower, I wash carefully between my legs with an organic body wash. And of course it helps to always wear cotton panties and change my underwear and hose every day. And I also drink two glasses of low-sugar cranberry juice a day. In addition to being full of antioxidants and vitamin C, it's said to help flush out the bacteria which cause UTIs."

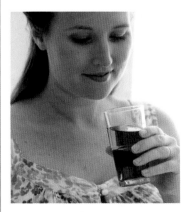

Many women find that drinking a glass or two of low-sugar cranberry juice daily helps treat UTIs.

Getting ready for pregnancy

Staying safe and healthy

Your pregnancy diary

Birth and beyond

▼ Your body at **23** Weeks

23 Weeks

✳ You may notice some bleeding when you brush your teeth—it's a common pregnancy complaint.

✳ Your belly button, once an "innie," may now stick out. Don't worry. It'll revert soon after you give birth.

Are you a blossoming mom-to-be, or just feeling awful? Remind yourself why pregnancy makes you beautiful. And if you're still struggling to choose a name for your baby, we have a few tips.

You're blossoming!

Even though you're probably overjoyed by the new life that's been growing inside you for the last 23 weeks, there may be days when you can't wait for the whole thing to be over. As your breasts grow, your abdomen swells, and your waistline disappears, you may long to have your old shape back—or even to remember what it was! While you're reveling in being pregnant, you may not be reveling in looking pregnant.

The second trimester of pregnancy is usually when women are looking—as well as feeling—at their best. Read on for a reminder of some of the beauty bonuses of pregnancy.

● **You will probably have that celebrated "glow"** You may notice that your skin looks brighter than usual. Hormones are partly responsible, but an increase in blood volume brings more blood to the skin, which helps to give it that radiant look.

● **Fast-growing fingernails** Around the fourth month, your nails may start to grow faster than usual. Pregnancy hormones get the credit, but also the blame, since fingernails may also become softer or more brittle.

● **A fabulous head of hair** Many women find that pregnancy brings out the best in their hair. You might start to notice your hair has more volume.

● **Bigger breasts** It's common to go up a cup size or two during your pregnancy, so by now you may have new cleavage to show off!

● **A very happy mate** Believe it or not, your partner may be crazy about your new physique. Men tend to see the sensuality in blossoming breasts and soft curves. The sight of your pregnant form is a constant reminder of his virility too, and we all know how important that is to him!

Whether or not you're blossoming and blooming, it is worth trying out these two look-good strategies:

● **Emphasise the positive** If your legs are gorgeous, flaunt them by wearing a short dress. Upper arms like a supermodel's? Show them off with a sleeveless top. Proud of your new, improved cleavage? Don't be shy—highlight it with a scoop- or V-neck top.

● **Spoil yourself occasionally** Treat yourself to a pedicure, a manicure, a new lipstick, or some lacy underwear.

▼ Your baby at **23** Weeks

Her hearing's well established now so she's getting used to all kinds of sounds.

✳ She can make out a distorted version of your voice, the beating of your heart and your stomach rumblings. Loud noises that she has often heard in the uterus—a dog's bark, the vacuum cleaner—probably won't bother her when she is born. She now weighs a little more than one pound and measures about 11½ inches.

Anything you do that's just for you will make you feel more glam. Meanwhile, don't forget to exercise. It'll make you feel better about the way you look, keep your energy levels up and help you bounce back after the birth.

And here's a little perk that no one told you about: pregnant women often bring out the kindness in people. People fall over themselves to hold doors open for you. They give up seats on trains and buses. Enjoy it while it lasts!

45–50% more blood will be running through your veins and arteries

by the time you get to the end of your pregnancy. This is all part of the way your body adapts during pregnancy to meet the demands of your baby.

Dad's **Diary**

Coming to terms with being a stay-at-home dad

"Our child-care plans were turned upside-down when I was laid off. My wife was just three months pregnant, and our little girl was almost three. After months of job hunting (and our baby's birth just weeks away) we started to think seriously about me staying at home with the children. Laura earns more than I did anyway, and had planned to go back part-time after the birth. Her company has happily agreed to her returning full time, so she'll be the main breadwinner. Now that we've made the decision, I'm not worried about staying at home—I'm not hugely career minded and I don't have a problem with not being the primary earner. I'm happy at the thought of being able to spend more time with my children."

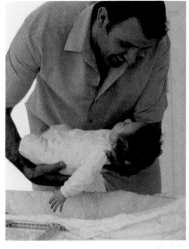

Many fathers relish the thought of being a stay-at-home dad.

Choosing a name

If you've already started thinking about baby names, you'll know that naming your baby is one of the best parts about being pregnant. But it's a big responsibility too. After all, your baby

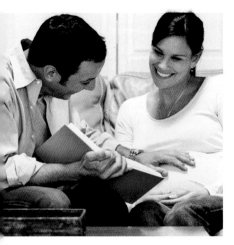

will have the name you choose for life. Here are a few things to consider before you make your choice:

● **Sound and compatibility** How your baby's name sounds when it is said aloud is one of the most essential things to think about. Is it melodious? Harsh? Does it go well with your last name? Often, longer first names work better with shorter last names, and vice versa.

● **Uniqueness** An unusual name has the advantage of making the bearer stand out from the crowd. On the other hand, a name that no one has heard of and can't pronounce can draw unwanted attention.

Choose what you will name your baby with careful consideration. Remember, she'll be stuck with your choice for life.

● **Relatives and friends** Many parents choose to name their babies after a grandparent, other relative, or close friend. This option can provide you with a good pool of names to consider.

● **Ancestry and heritage** Your child's heritage is an essential part of who she is, and you may want her name to reflect that heritage.

● **Meaning** No one is likely to treat your daughter Ingrid differently because her name means "hero's daughter," but the derivation of your baby's name is something you may want to think about.

● **Initials and nicknames** People, especially children, can be cruel when it comes to nicknames, so try to anticipate any potentially embarrassing ones that your little one may be given if you choose something unfortunate.

Getting ready for pregnancy

Staying safe and healthy

Your pregnancy diary

Birth and beyond

| FIRST TRIMESTER | SECOND TRIMESTER | THIRD TRIMESTER |

Your body at **24** Weeks

24 Weeks

❉ By now, you probably have a definite "pregnant" shape and the linea nigra down your abdomen.

❉ You may notice faint red streaks—striae or stretch marks—on your belly, hips, buttocks, and breasts.

If you're feeling hot, heavy, and over it, it's time to spoil yourself with a few treats. Don't feel guilty if you have the urge to splash out on a bit of pampering and de-stressing now and again.

Go on, treat yourself

You're a few weeks past the halfway point in your pregnancy but the end probably still feels a long way off. You can be excused if you sometimes feel a little down, but if ever there was a time to pamper yourself, then pregnancy is it. Banish the blues by trying some of our indulgent ideas.

● **Give yourself a home spa** Make your bathroom a tranquil space: dim the lights and add scented candles and a relaxing CD. Have some fluffy bath towels handy—keep them on a warm radiator or heated towel rail for added comfort. Then get the facemasks, bubbles, and nail polish out and enjoy.

● **Get a great haircut** Make an appointment for a consultation and cut with a really good stylist. He'll be able to help you find a lower-maintenance style that will see you right through pregnancy and into those first few weeks of living with a baby. While you're there, ask about nourishing salon products. Pregnant women often find their hair is much glossier, so now is the time to make the most of that shine.

● **Go out on a date** Spend a romantic evening with your partner this week,

at the theater, movies, a favorite restaurant, or somewhere else where you can appreciate each other's company. If you already have children, ask a favorite grandparent or friend to do the babysitting.

● **Ditch the lenses** The shape of your eyeballs can change during pregnancy due to fluid retention, or you may even be suffering from dry eyes. If you wear contact lenses and they're becoming uncomfortable, think about investing in a chic pair of glasses instead. Some designer frames can look very stylish and sexy. Glasses could be a good investment for your early days of motherhood too, when you might not have time to fiddle around with your contact lenses—especially in the early hours of the morning.

● **Buy even more shoes!** If your feet are swollen, it might be wise to invest in a pair of shoes in a size bigger than you normally wear. Opting for shoes that are practical and comfortable doesn't mean that you need to sacrifice style—flat shoes can be just as pretty as their high-heeled counterparts and they look great with the right outfits.

▼ Your baby at **24** Weeks

If your baby arrives from now onward, he may survive, with special care.

❉ If your baby is born this week, it is still possible that he could survive with a lot of special care in the neonatal intensive care unit (NICU). His skin is thin and fragile but his body is filling out and taking up more room in your uterus. His taste buds are now forming and, believe it or not, your baby may already have a sweet tooth.

Looking at child-care options

It is important to start thinking about child care early on, and certainly once you're into your second trimester of pregnancy, because the best child-care choices are often snapped up very quickly. The first thing to do is to look at all the options that are available in your area. You can do this by talking to other parents and parents-to-be or by contacting the Childcare Aware hotline (800/424-2246), which can give you the number of your local child-care resource and referral agency for referring you to licensed centers and home day cares.

If you are looking for a nanny, it may be hard to find someone who is prepared to commit themselves to a job before handing in their notice to their current employer (usually a month beforehand). However, you can start a general search for nanny agencies, begin to see people, and build up a picture of quality and availability.

If you are looking at child-care providers you may find that the same principles apply. Many child-care providers are unwilling to commit themselves too far in advance. You may be asked to pay a fee to keep a place.

When you start looking, don't expect to find someone immediately—in fact, it's best to see a number of different people and places so you get an idea of the variety in quality, price, and style.

If your first choice is oversubscribed or out of your reach financially, don't despair, but be prepared to compromise. and consider alternatives. The only thing you should not compromise on is your certainty that your child will be taken care of by caring, qualified people.

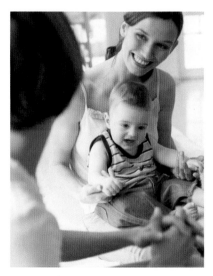

Finding good child care takes time. Make sure you start researching your options as early as possible.

Premature labor

A premature birth is when a baby arrives before 37 complete weeks of pregnancy. It's difficult for doctors to predict which women will go into labor prematurely, but there is evidence that certain bacteria in your urine make premature labor more likely. It is now recommended that all women have their urine tested for bacteria early in pregnancy.

Other risk factors include smoking, using recreational drugs, expecting twins or more, and previous premature births. If your water breaks or you start contractions before 37 weeks, you should contact your doctor or hospital immediately.

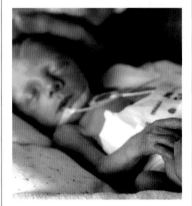

Many premature babies do well nowadays, but you can minimize your risk of having a premature labor.

Parents**Talk...**

"I'm about halfway through my pregnancy and my skin is really itchy. It's especially bad on my belly, and my doctor says that's because the skin is stretching there as my belly grows, which I guess makes sense. Apparently general itchiness of the skin is pretty normal. Fingers crossed it stops once my baby has arrived. Scratching in public is not a good look!"
Jen, 24, pregnant for the first time

"I was diagnosed with obstetric cholestasis (see pp.230–31) at 27 weeks and I'm 32 weeks now. The itching is really bad on the soles of my feet, but it's actually everywhere and I've made myself bleed by scratching. It drives me crazy. Long, cool baths and calamine lotion help to ease the itching. There's no cure for it, but I'm having extra prenatal checkups to monitor my baby."
Shola, 27, pregnant for the first time

Getting ready for pregnancy

Staying safe and healthy

Your pregnancy diary

Birth and beyond

FIRST TRIMESTER	SECOND TRIMESTER	THIRD TRIMESTER

Your body at **25** Weeks

25 Weeks

❋ Hormone surges and the extra weight you're carrying can make you ache all over.

❋ Your growing belly may make it hard to get into a comfortable position to sleep.

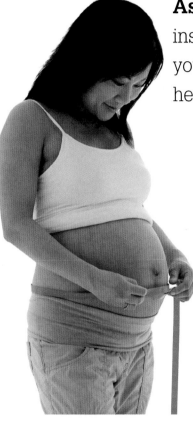

As your baby grows and takes up lots of room inside you, indigestion, gas, and heartburn can make you really uncomfortable in later pregnancy. Eating a healthy, high-fiber diet will help ease the symptoms.

Digestive matters

Pregnancy has a way of making you feel more relaxed about your bodily functions. Which is probably just as well, given what may be happening to your digestive system these days.

There's the gas for starters. The pregnancy hormone progesterone slows your digestive processes, which can cause more gas and bloating, especially after a big meal. To help ease matters, try not to eat big, heavy meals and take your time eating. Reducing your intake of common culprits like beans and broccoli may help too.

Heartburn and indigestion

You may experience heartburn and indigestion during your pregnancy. Heartburn causes a burning sensation in your upper chest. It happens because progesterone relaxes the valve that separates your esophagus from your stomach, allowing stomach acid to seep up the esophagus. Also, as your growing baby crowds the abdominal cavity, it can push acid up into your esophagus.

The same process that causes you such discomfort may actually be of some benefit to your baby because the nutrients that linger in your bloodstream can be absorbed more fully into your baby's system.

To prevent heartburn, avoid rich or spicy dishes, eat little and often, and chew your food slowly and thoroughly. Give yourself two or three hours to digest any meals before going to bed. It may even help to sleep propped up in bed to give gravity a chance to keep the stomach acids down. You can also talk to your doctor about finding an over-the-counter antacid that is safe to use during pregnancy.

Constipation

Constipation is another common problem in pregnancy: about 30 to 40 percent of pregnant women get constipated at some point. The culprits

Fact: In later pregnancy, your growing baby crowds your abdominal cavity. This can slow down your digestion and pushes on your stomach, making you feel even more bloated when you've eaten.

▼ Your baby at **25** Weeks

Your baby now weighs nearly 23¼ ounces and is about 13½ inches long.

❋ There's no air in her lungs yet—just amniotic fluid—but she's making movements that look like breathing. She's getting some baby fat, too. As this happens, her wrinkled skin will begin to smooth out. She's also growing more hair—if you could see it, you would be able to discern its color and texture.

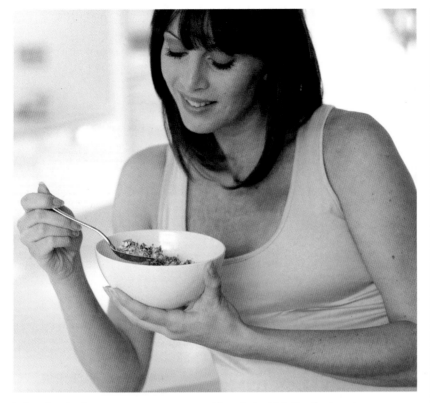

Constipation is a common pregnancy problem. Eating high-fiber foods such as whole-grain breakfast cereals, whole-grain bread, and plenty of fresh fruit and vegetables can help prevent it.

are the pressure of your growing uterus on your rectum, along with pregnancy hormones, which slow the transit of food through your digestive tract. Some iron pills can make constipation worse, so be aware of this side effect.

If constipation persists, mention it to your doctor. If changes to your diet and lifestyle don't make a difference then your doctor can prescribe a laxative that is safe to use in pregnancy. Sometimes, constipation can lead to hemorrhoids

"**High-fiber** foods and gentle **exercise** can ease **constipation**."

Eating high-fiber foods, such as whole-grain cereals, whole-grain bread, fresh fruit, and vegetables every day, and drinking plenty of fluids, should help. Gentle exercise such as walking, swimming, and cycling can ease constipation, too.

(see p.236). These varicose veins in the bottom can be painful, itchy, and uncomfortable but they can be treated with a range of creams and ointments to ease the symptoms. Hemorrhoids usually resolve themselves fairly soon after your baby is born.

Working mom

Office work brings special challenges for you and your ever-increasing belly.

"My belly and my desk appear to be having a fight at work—and I think the belly may be winning! I've really noticed it moving higher this week and now it's got to the point that the baby is really pushing against me and the desk. It's a bit uncomfortable to say the least. I wish there was a desk pillow that I could use as a buffer. Or even a special ergonomic desk for pregnant women with a belly-shaped cut-out!

I've already asked HR for a footrest. I'm starting to get swollen ankles, too, so I'm hoping having something to raise my feet up will help. I try to get away from my desk every hour or so to stretch my legs, and I go out for a walk and some fresh air every lunch time. But the bigger I get, the more I look forward to maternity leave."

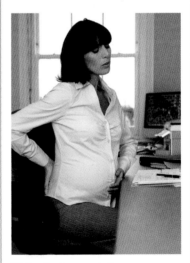

Sitting for long periods can cause a backache, but more so if you're pregnant. You need plenty of breaks.

Getting ready for pregnancy

Staying safe and healthy

Your pregnancy diary

Birth and beyond

| FIRST TRIMESTER | SECOND TRIMESTER | THIRD TRIMESTER |

▼ Your body at **26** Weeks

26 Weeks

✲ You may see a slight increase in your blood pressure. Don't worry: it's normal.

✲ Fend off constipation with fiber-rich foods like whole-grain breads and cereals, lentils, and brown rice.

A birth plan is a useful part of your baby preparations. It gives you a chance to decide how you want your baby's birth to be managed. Having a written record will also give you confidence during labor.

Preparing your birth plan

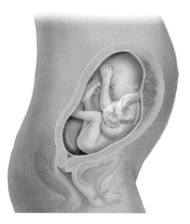

Your baby at **26** Weeks

His eyes begin to open around now and his response to sound is more consistent.

✲ Toward the end of the seventh month, the network of nerves to your baby's ear is complete, which makes his response to sound better. He now measures about 14 inches from crown to heel and weighs a little more than 1½ pounds. He is still continuing to take small breaths and, although he's only breathing in water and not air, it's still good practice for when he's born. If you are having a boy, his testicles are beginning to descend into his scrotum—a trip that will take about two to three days.

A birth plan is a way of communicating with the nurses and doctors who will care for you in labor. It will tell them about the kind of labor you would like to have, what you ideally want to happen, and anything you definitely would want to avoid.

The best birth plans acknowledge that events may not go as expected. You need to write yours in such a way that your doctor's hands aren't tied. She may need to recommend a course of action that isn't what you had hoped for, but which is in your baby's best interests.

Doing your research

Before you start writing get as much information as you can.

● **Go to childbirth classes** A good childbirth teacher will help you make the best choices for you.

● **Talk to other women** Women who have given birth at the hospital or birth center you're going to or who've had a home birth, if that's what you'd like, can tell you how easy or difficult it was to get the kind of care they wanted.

● **Talk to your partner or birth companion** What kind of labor and birth would they like for you? Ask how they see their role. Then jot your "birth

wishes" down just as they come to mind. You can figure them out later.

Here is a list of headings that you might want to use in your birth plan. Take a look in your medical records and see whether there are any suggestions for birth plans in there as well.

● **Birth partner** Write down who you want to be with you in labor and whether this person should stay the whole time. There may be certain procedures or stages when you'd prefer him or her to leave.

● **Positions for labor and birth** Mention which positions you would like to use during labor and for the birth. For some useful positions, see pp.266–7. Also say how active you would like to be: would you like to remain upright and mobile for as long as possible, maybe using a birth ball, or would you prefer to be in bed?

● **Pain relief** Say what kinds of pain relief you want to use, if any, and in what order (for example, you might prefer to try Demerol before an epidural). If you'd like to try for a natural birth (no pain-relieving drugs at all), make this clear.

● **Monitoring baby's heart rate** Say how you want your baby to be monitored during labor—whether you

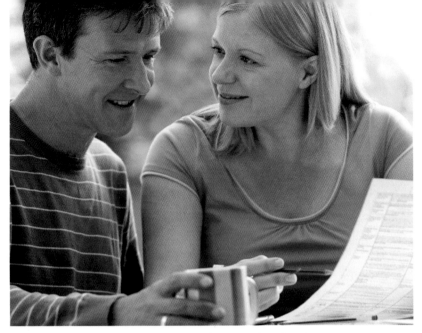

Discuss your birth plan with your partner but remember, when the time comes, you will both need to be flexible in case anything unexpected happens.

would like your doctor to listen to your baby's heart intermittently using a handheld device (Doppler) or whether you prefer to have electronic monitoring using a belt strapped around your waist.

● **Speeding up labor** If your labor slows down, you might want your doctor and nurses to use interventions to speed it up again, such as breaking your waters, or you may prefer to wait and see what happens naturally.

● **Birth pool** If your maternity unit has a birth pool, or if you are renting one to use at home, make a note of whether you want to use it for pain relief as well as or instead of to give birth in.

● **Assisted birth** You might want to express a preference for forceps or vacuum if you need some help to deliver your baby.

● **Third stage (delivery of placenta)** You can choose to have an injection to speed up the delivery of the placenta, or you might prefer to have a natural third stage without drugs.

● **Feeding your baby** Be clear about whether you want to breast-feed or bottle-feed. Also be clear about whether

your breast-fed baby may have any formula. If you definitely don't want her to have bottles, say so.

● **Unexpected situations** Some women write down in their birth plan what they want to happen if their baby has to go to the NICU. They might want to care for him as much as possible themselves and be transferred with him to another hospital if that's needed. They might ask for their partner to stay with them at the hospital.

Special needs

You may have special requirements to mention in your birth plan. If you have a disability, write about the help you will need in labor. Say whether there is any special equipment you need.

If you have religious needs, be sure to include these. It might be important for certain rituals to be performed when your baby is born. Or you might require a special diet during your hospital stay. Write all of these things down. Hospitals and health professionals are committed nowadays to being culturally sensitive and treating people as individuals.

Organized mom
....

Make your birth plan as demanding as you like but prepare to be flexible, too.

"I've included as much detail as I possibly can in my birth plan. I want my doctor to be clear on what I would like to happen and what I want to avoid if possible. I'd like to have my husband and best friend in the delivery room with me, but I want Sophie to leave when it's time for me to actually push. I've also made it clear that I want to try for as little pain relief as possible and would like to use the birth pool for pain relief and relaxation. I want to breast-feed my baby as soon as I can and prefer him not to have any bottles of formula. I know I sound demanding, but I just want to have the best experience for me."

Laid-back mom
....

Your birth plan doesn't have to be long. You may prefer to go with the flow and see how things develop.

"I've just written my birth plan and to be honest it's really short! I've pretty much only said who I want my birth partner to be and stated that if it's possible, I'd like to try for a water birth. When it comes to pain relief, I really don't know how high my pain threshold will be. If I can do it with as few drugs as possible then that would be great, but if I'm suffering, I want them to hit me with everything they've got. I'm happy to be flexible about positions for labor. I'll just see what's comfortable at the time."

Your body at **27** Weeks

27 Weeks

✳ If you're unlucky you may discover the delights of leg cramps, hemorrhoids, or varicose veins.

✳ If you're experiencing an odd rhythmic sensation, it may be that your baby is hiccupping.

Laboring and giving birth in water can be a very good experience. Being in water is relaxing and reduces the need for pain relief. Some believe it's completely safe for mom and baby.

Planning a water birth

If you would like a water birth, the first thing to do is to talk to your doctor at one of your prenatal appointments. She can tell you if the hospital you are going to has a pool available. More maternity units have facilities for water births than before, but some may be less encouraging about them than others. These days all maternity units should have doctors and nurses who are trained to care for women who want to labor or give birth in water. You can get an idea of how much experience your hospital has of water birth by asking the following questions:

● How many women each year use the birthing pool for pain relief during labor?
● How many women give birth in the pool each year?
● How many nurses are trained in the use of the birth pool?
● Are there any times when the pool is not available?

If you are very enthusiastic on the idea of a birthing pool and your local hospital doesn't have one, or doesn't have the staff to cover it on a 24-hour basis, you might consider transferring to another hospital. Another possibility is a home water birth. Your doctor or midwife should be able to tell you about local companies that rent birthing pools. Otherwise, try contacting Waterbirth International, or look for an independent birthing center that supports water births.

Researching water birth

There are several ways to find out more:
● **Learn about other people's experiences** Talking to women who have labored and given birth in water is best. Talk to some who have used a birthing pool just for pain relief and to some who have given birth in water. Ask them when they got into the pool, when they got out, what they found helpful about being in water, and what they didn't like.

Fact: 1803 is the date of the first recorded water birth in Europe.

It happened in France when a mother whose labor had been extremely long and difficult was finally helped to give birth in a tub of warm water.

▼ Your baby at **27** Weeks

This week sees activity in your baby's brain as more of her brain tissue develops.

✳ At the same time, the characteristic grooves start to appear on the brain's surface. She now weighs nearly 2 pounds and measures 14½ inches from head to toe. Her eyes open and close, and she sleeps and wakes at regular intervals. Some experts believe that babies begin to dream by the 28th week.

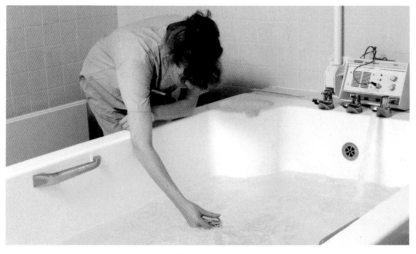

Some maternity units have a birthing pool, but not all encourage their use. You should ask probing questions to gauge how much they're used.

● **Childbirth classes** These are a good source of information about what happens during a water birth. When you book your classes, remember to ask whether they will include information about laboring in water. At the beginning of the course, your teacher will probably ask what topics to cover, so that's your opportunity to ask for water birth. Others in the group will almost certainly be interested as well!

● **Books** Most up-to-date books about pregnancy and childbirth will include a section on water birth.

Dads and family leave

If your partner is having a baby, you may be entitled to family leave. If not, you can probably use sick days or vacation time to support your baby's mother in the tiring first week and learn the basics of baby care.

A few employers formally offer paternity leave, and a few states offer paid family leave. Many employers are required by federal law to allow their employees (both men and women) 12 weeks of unpaid family leave after the birth or adoption of a child under the Family and Medical Leave Act (FMLA). Talk to a human resources representative at your company to find out what options are available to you.

Parents who plan to take leave under the FMLA must request their leave 30 days before they plan to take it, but you may want to give your boss earlier notice. You could take your leave all at once, or spread it out in smaller chunks over the first 12 months after your baby's birth.

If you aren't eligible for any paid leave, you may want to try to negotiate a leave of absence anyway.

Fathers who can't get time off work can still take steps to make the most of their time at home. Or you might consider working overtime before your baby arrives and exchange it for time off after the birth.

Getting ready for pregnancy

Staying safe and healthy

Your pregnancy diary

Birth and beyond

Braxton Hicks contractions

Some time toward the middle of your pregnancy, you may notice the muscles of your uterus tightening for anywhere from 30 to 60 seconds. Not all of us feel these random, usually painless contractions, which get their name from John Braxton Hicks, the English doctor who first described them in 1872.

There are a variety of different opinions about these contractions and about what purpose they serve. Some experts think they play a part in getting your cervix ready for labor (also called "ripening"). Others believe that Braxton Hicks contractions do not lead to changes to the cervix and that ripening doesn't happen until the pre-labor stage, when the first real contractions of labor start, or until labor itself.

Dad's **Diary**

Timing paternity leave

"I've decided to take two weeks' paternity leave after our baby is born. It'll mean a bit of a financial sacrifice but I think we'll be able to manage. The only thing I haven't yet decided is when to take the time off.

Jenny's mom is coming to stay for a week or so after the baby's born, so, although I'd really like to be at home right after the birth, it might be better for me to take the time off when she's gone back home. Otherwise, Jenny will be bombarded with support for the first two weeks and then left all alone soon afterward. And I'm also thinking that it will give us the chance to spend time together as a new family, just the three of us. I can't wait."

The third trimester

The home stretch

You are probably becoming impatient to meet the baby whose squirms and kicks you've become so familiar with over the weeks. Indulge yourself by buying some little undershirts and diapers and daydreaming about the sleepless but happy time after your baby is born.

What to expect

At this stage you're probably veering from feeling "I've been pregnant for ever" one minute and "Help, I'm not ready for this!" the next. You're not alone. Swapping experiences with other women in your childbirth class can be reassuring.

Oh, the joys of pregnancy!

Sleep gets more difficult as your belly grows. Backache is a common problem, while some women also develop pelvic pain. Braxton Hicks contractions may become more intense or frequent. As early as 33 weeks your baby's head may engage (dip into the pelvic cavity in preparation for birth), making you feel like you need to urinate all the time. By 35 weeks your uterus is 1,000 times its original volume and has expanded up under your ribs. Together with hormonal changes, this causes heartburn in around 70 percent of women in late pregnancy. Your feet, hands, face, and ankles can become swollen too.

Your growing baby

At the beginning of the third trimester your baby can open his eyes and turn his head toward the source of any continuous bright light. His brain is growing rapidly and his lungs and digestive tract are maturing. From 32 weeks your baby gains around a third to a half of his birth weight, getting fattened up so he's ready for survival outside the uterus. With six weeks to go, he could measure as much as 17¼ inches long from top to toe. He's getting so big and snug in your uterus that you may notice he isn't moving around so much. By the end of week 36 your pregnancy will have come full term but it's best for your baby to stay in the uterus for 40 weeks.

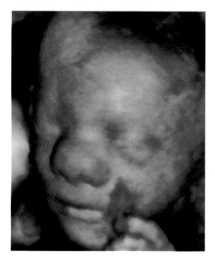

The facial features of this baby are all well developed and his tiny fingers can be seen near his mouth.

> ### Organized mom
>
> *Now that you're in the final stretch, it's time to make sure you're on top of all the details.*
>
> "I've now gone completely list crazy. I'm so worried that I've forgotten to buy something vital that I've been carrying a notepad and pen around with me so I can jot things down as I remember them.
>
> I've also got the contact details of all our close friends and family pinned to the note board above the phone, and I'm planning to pack my hospital bag a couple of weeks before my due date."

Make life easier

Now is the time to make sure you're organized for the home stretch. Stock up on shopping to save time and effort later. Make a list of important numbers—your doctor and the hospital—and keep it by the phone or stored on your cell. It's a good idea to have your hospital bag packed from 36 weeks onward, so that you're not rushing around in early labor trying to get everything done.

Getting ready for pregnancy

Staying safe and healthy

Your pregnancy diary

Birth and beyond

Your body at **28** Weeks ▼

28 Weeks

❉ Your breasts may start producing colostrum—the concentrated early milk. They may leak a little.

❉ Most women will gain an average of 11 pounds during the last trimester, which starts this week.

As you count down the days to your due date,

your doctor will keep a close eye on your baby's growth and activity. You, meanwhile, may be getting curious about how big your baby will be.

Prenatal appointments from now onward

During this trimester, you'll probably have a checkup every two weeks from 28 to 36 weeks, then once-a-week visits. Here's what to expect:

Physical exam

As in the second trimester, you'll be weighed and your blood pressure will be taken. Your urine will be tested for signs of preeclampsia (see p.233), UTIs (see p.228), and other problems. Your ankles, hands, and face will be checked for swelling (see p.238).

Your doctor will check your baby's heartbeat and feel and measure your belly (see p.147) to estimate his size. If he seems either too big or too small, you'll get an ultrasound to evaluate his growth and to check your amniotic fluid levels. You may be asked to start counting your baby's movements for a set period of time each day.

At 36 weeks or so, if she suspects he's breech (see pp.286–7), she'll order an ultrasound—and you'll probably be offered an external cephalic version (ECV; see p.287) to try to turn the baby.

Tests

If you're Rh-negative, you may need a blood test at 28 weeks to check for antibodies, followed by an Rh-immune globulin injection (see p.233). Between 35 and 37 weeks, your practitioner will swab your vagina and rectum to check for a group B strep (see pp.226–7). If your test is positive, you'll be given antibiotics during labor.

If your blood glucose level was high and you haven't yet had a glucose tolerance test to ascertain if you have gestational diabetes (see p.229), the test will be done early in this trimester.

Your blood may be checked again for anemia and if you're at risk for sexually transmitted infections (STIs), you'll be tested again. If you were found to have placenta previa or a low-lying placenta, you'll have another ultrasound to check the location of your placenta.

Near your due date

Your doctor will discuss the signs of labor and when you should get in touch with her. This is the time for you to

---

▼ Your baby at **28** Weeks

This week your baby can blink his eyes. They now sport lashes.

❉ He'll also turn in the direction of light if he notices bright light shining through the wall of your uterus. He now weighs a little over 2½ pounds and measures about 15 inches. His fat layers are starting to form as he gets ready for life outside the uterus. His bones are nearly developed, too, but they're still soft and pliable.

resolve any lingering concerns you may have about the way your labor and delivery will be handled.

If you go past your due date, your doctor will check your cervix to see if it's softening, effacing (thinning out), and dilating (opening) because this may help her decide if and when labor should be induced.

Between 40 and 41 weeks, you may get a full biophysical profile or a modified one, which includes a nonstress test to assess your baby's heart rate and an ultrasound to check your amniotic fluid level. These tests are usually performed twice a week.

Even if everything looks normal, your doctor will induce labor if you haven't had your baby by 42 weeks. (If your cervix is ripe, you may be induced even sooner.)

How big will your baby be?

How big your baby will be depends on a number of factors. Probably the most influential factors are genetic. Big parents often have bigger babies.

Even your baby's sex can play a part, since boys are often bigger than girls. If your baby is overdue, he'll probably be bigger since he's had more time to grow.

Thankfully, you usually grow a baby to fit you. So even if your partner is much taller or heavier than you, your baby is likely to fit through your pelvis. It's not just size that matters—the position your baby is in influences labor, so you can have a big baby in a good position and an easy birth, or a small baby who has managed to get into a difficult position that can make things more complicated.

Some medical conditions are linked to an increased risk of a big baby. These include obesity and gaining a lot of weight during pregnancy. Unmanaged high blood sugar levels from gestational diabetes (see p.229) or diabetes mellitus (the chronic form of the condition) can lead to a bigger baby, as the baby uses the extra sugar to grow.

Factors that affect baby's birth weight

Many moms-to-be wonder how big their baby will be at birth. These factors affect baby's birth weight:

- your height
- the baby's father's height
- your weight before pregnancy
- the weight you have gained during your pregnancy
- the sex of the baby
- uncontrolled gestational diabetes
- whether you smoke while pregnant
- whether the baby is overdue (comes late) or premature (early)

Parents**Talk...**

"I loved my childbirth classes. It was so nice to be able to talk to women who were going through exactly the same as me. I could share my worries and concerns because they were all so supportive. One of the women I met there is my best friend now. We have such a strong bond because we're raising our children together."
Louise, 29, mom to two-year-old Tom

"What I learned in my childbirth classes was invaluable. The relaxation techniques helped keep me calm and feel more in control during labor. Rather than panicking I could focus on getting my breathing right and telling my husband what kind of massage I needed and when."
Anna, 35, mom to six-month-old Joel

"Being informed about my pain relief choices helped me feel like I had some say in how my labor was going to go. I have a really low pain threshold, so just assumed that an epidural was the only way for me to get through it. But my childbirth teacher took the time to explain to me that this wasn't the case and that breathing exercises might be enough. It turns out she was right!"
Paula, 27, pregnant for a second time

You can easily strike up new friendships at your childbirth classes. It's good to share your worries with other pregnant women.

Getting ready for pregnancy

Staying safe and healthy

Your pregnancy diary

Birth and beyond

Diet in late pregnancy

As your pregnancy progresses you might be finding that, no matter how much or how often you eat, you still feel ravenous at all hours of the day and night. That's not surprising, because the rapidly growing baby inside you needs extra calories of his own.

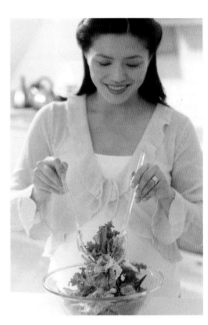

Keep a supply of salad fixings and fresh fruit and vegetables at home, and you'll be less likely to snack on unhealthy foods.

Keep the calories in check

You may feel permanently starving these days but that doesn't mean it's a good idea to eat anything and everything. Remember, you're eating for yourself and a baby, not another adult!

Quality not quantity

In addition to avoiding overeating, you should watch the quality of what you eat. When you have a craving for junk food, try to opt for a healthier choice. Help yourself to do this by keeping your fridge and cupboards well stocked with quick, healthy snacks, such as cottage cheese, hard-boiled eggs, whole-wheat bread, and fresh fruit and vegetables.

When you're going out and about, don't leave home without putting a bag of nuts and raisins or a piece of fresh fruit into your bag. You never know when you'll need a quick energy boost, and by tucking into something wholesome you'll hopefully be able to avoid the temptations of the nearest fast-food restaurant.

You will of course already be following our useful advice on eating in pregnancy (see pp.48–51 and 120–21) but it bears repeating during this last trimester that you should also try to eat natural foods that have been processed as little as possible. For example, choose whole-wheat bread or brown rice rather than white bread or white rice, and stick to fresh fruit as opposed to canned fruit in syrup. We should all keep fatty foods and sweets to a minimum but the occasional treat won't hurt.

Special needs of the last trimester

As your pregnancy progresses, heartburn becomes all too common. This is due to hormonal and physical changes in your body. Although you may not be able get rid of the heartburn completely, you can minimize it. Try cutting out rich or spicy dishes, citrus fruits, chocolate, alcohol, and coffee. Eat small, frequent meals, take small mouthfuls, and chew your food well.

Top eating tips for the last trimester

During these last weeks, focus on not overeating and on eating healthily.
- Stock up on healthy snacks—for example, hard-boiled eggs and fresh fruit.
- Be prepared—carry healthy snacks when you are out and about.
- Avoid heartburn—eat small, frequent meals and chew your food well.
- Drink plenty of water.

- Get your vitamin K—from green beans, leafy green vegetables, and cauliflower.
- Don't overeat—you only need about 300 extra calories a day at this stage. That's about the equivalent of a glass of milk and a banana.
- Don't forget your antioxidants—a diet that's rich in vitamins C and E may help prevent preeclampsia.

You need vitamin K in your last trimester because it helps blood to clot. If you have low levels of vitamin K you may bleed more at birth, and babies with low levels can also bleed internally. This is why babies are given vitamin K when they are born. Good sources include green leafy vegetables, cantaloupe, cauliflower, green beans, and whole-wheat bread, and pasta.

You may also be suffering now from swollen ankles and feet (edema; see p.238). You can help relieve it by drinking more water during the day and by cutting down on salty foods, such as olives and salted nuts.

Some experts believe that a diet that is high in antioxidants can help to prevent preeclampsia (see p.233).

Vitamins C and E are two important antioxidant vitamins. For vitamin C, eat citrus fruits, green and red peppers, melon, potatoes, tomatoes, strawberries, cabbage, and broccoli. Foods rich in vitamin E include vegetable oils (especially corn, soy and wheatgerm oil), sunflower seeds, wheatgerm, corn, cashews, almonds, corn oil, margarine, and peanuts. Taking a general pregnancy multivitamin supplement may also help you to lower your risk of getting preeclampsia.

Make sure you spend the last few weeks eating well and getting plenty of rest. You can make life easier for yourself if you spend some time now making simple recipes that you can freeze and enjoy after your baby is born.

Active mom

Drinking plenty of water is essential, especially when you're exercising and pregnant.

"I've always found it difficult to drink plenty of water. When I got pregnant I knew I had to, not only for my sake—it can help prevent water retention—but for my baby's too. Whenever I have a glass, I add a wedge of lemon or a little fruit juice to make it more interesting. If I have a day at home, I fill a big jug with water and try to finish it by the end of the day. When I'm out, I always take a bottle of water to sip regularly throughout the day."

Getting ready for pregnancy

Staying safe and healthy

Your pregnancy diary

Birth and beyond

Healthy main meals

In your last trimester, you're allowed an extra 300 calories a day to match your baby's growth spurt. But try to resist eating too many cakes, candy, and fast food snacks. Three hundred calories is less than you think—it's the equivalent of only two and a half cups of low-fat milk. Try these healthy main meals to fill you up when you're hungry.

Ragu sauce

Serves four to six ● 1 lb 2 oz lean ground beef ● 1 medium onion, finely chopped ● 1 clove garlic, crushed ● 3½ oz bacon, cut into small pieces ● 4 sundried tomatoes in oil, drained ● 14 oz can chopped tomatoes ● 4¼ fl oz red wine (optional) ● 1 tsp oregano

Gently heat the beef in a nonstick pan, stirring and breaking it up. Add the onion, garlic, and bacon and increase the heat to sautee gently. Cook for 5–10 minutes, stirring frequently, until the onion is softened. Chop the sundried tomatoes and add to the pan with the canned tomatoes, oregano, and wine (if using). Bring to a boil, stir and reduce the heat. Cover and let simmer gently for 35–40 minutes, stirring frequently. Serve with any pasta.

Salmon with pine nuts and lime

Serves two ● cooking oil spray ● 2 salmon fillets ● juice and grated zest of 1 lime ● a little finely chopped lemon grass (optional) ● 1 tsp chopped parsley ● black pepper ● 2 tbsp pine nuts

Preheat the oven to 350° F. Lightly spray two pieces of foil with oil. Place a piece of salmon on each piece of foil. Squeeze over half the lime juice. Sprinkle on the grated zest and lemon grass (if using). Sprinkle with parsley and season with pepper. Close the foil, place in the oven and cook for 15 minutes. Remove, open the parcel, sprinkle with the pine nuts, and return to the oven to brown the pine nuts and finish cooking the fish (5 minutes). Pour the cooking liquid from the parcel over the salmon. Serve with new potatoes and steamed broccoli or green beans.

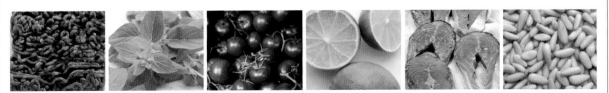

FIRST TRIMESTER   SECOND TRIMESTER   THIRD TRIMESTER

Your body at **29** Weeks ▼

29 Weeks

❋ Be sure to get enough iron to help your baby make red blood cells. Eat meat and leafy greens.

❋ Are you feeling less pressure in your lower abdomen? If so, your baby has probably shifted position.

You don't need to give up your workouts just because you're getting bigger; exercise prepares you for the hard work of labor ahead. But do make sure that you're not exercising too hard.

Exercise for the last weeks

Exercise does wonders for you during the last few weeks of pregnancy. It makes perfect sense: the better shape you're in, the stronger you'll be to cope with labor and the birth. Keeping physically active during pregnancy is also good preparation for the hard work of labor that lies ahead.

It also makes getting your body back in shape once the baby's born much easier. If you've managed to maintain your strength and muscle tone all through your pregnancy by staying fit, your body will have an easier time bouncing back after you give birth.

What's more, any type of aerobic exercise helps increase the body's ability to process and use oxygen, which is important for you and your baby.

Importantly, exercise at this stage will help you sleep better, too. When you're carrying all that extra weight in front of you, you'll quickly see that finding a comfortable position to sleep in at night can be a real challenge (see p.198). Exercise will help you work off any excess energy, and will tire you enough to lull you into a deeper, more restful slumber.

Don't go for the burn

Staying active doesn't necessarily mean going for the burn. Your body releases a hormone called relaxin during pregnancy which loosens your joints in preparation for delivery, so you need to be careful with the choice of exercise and pay attention to technique. It's important to find exercises that won't injure you or harm the baby.

As you grow bigger, you'll be better off avoiding activities that could put you at risk of slips and falls, such as cycling, rollerblading, horseriding, and skiing, although people who take part in these sports competitively often continue well into their pregnancies.

However, most pregnant women should stick to low-impact, gentle exercise such as walking, yoga (see p.59), and Pilates (see p.57). Swimming is great, too. It improves circulation, increases muscle tone and strength, and builds endurance—while the water supports your weight (see p.57). Whatever exercise you choose, you should always start slowly, stretch well before and after, warm up and cool down gradually, and don't overexert yourself.

▮ Your baby at **29** Weeks

This week your boy baby's undergoing some changes to his sex organs.

❋ His testicles now descend from near the kidneys through the groin en route to the scrotum. In girls, the clitoris is rather prominent because it's not yet covered by the still-small labia. These will grow to cover it in the last few weeks before birth. Your baby now weighs around 2½ pounds and measures about 15 inches.

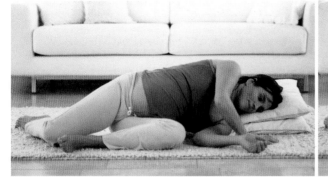

Getting up from lying down is harder the bigger you get. Start by rolling onto one side, with one or both knees bent.

Push down on your arms to come up fully, then unbend your knees. You can reverse the process when you want to lie down.

Help me get up!

Getting out of bed won't be a problem until your belly starts to bulge in your second or third trimester. Then you need a safe, comfortable way to get up, especially if you have back pain.

● **Getting out of bed** Roll onto your side with your knees bent up, drop your feet over the edge of the bed, and push yourself up sideways with your arms. Reverse the process when you lie down. If rolling onto your side is too painful, try the following technique: lying on your back, bend both knees up as far as they will go and separate them to clear your belly. You may need to use your hands to help pull your legs up. Put your chin on your chest, and use your arms to pull yourself directly up, keeping your knees bent up as high as you can. This may work for you but you may find that your belly is too big or your stomach muscles too weak to perform this maneuver.

● **Getting out of the bath** Roll onto your side in a sitting position and move onto your hands and knees. Lean on the sides of the bath to stand, and perch on the edge. Holding firmly onto the sides of the bath behind you, arch your back and lift one leg at a time over the bath sides. Use a bath mat to prevent slipping.

Cord blood banking

Umbilical cord blood is a source of lifesaving blood stem cells. Cord blood banking involves collecting blood left in the umbilical cord and placenta and storing it for future medical use. Stem cells can develop into other types of cells, so they can help repair tissues, organs, and blood vessels, as well as treat a host of diseases. For instance, stem cells may be used to create a new blood and immune system in patients with conditions such as leukemia. If you want your baby's cord blood to be saved, you can donate it to a public bank for use by anyone who is a match, or pay to store it in a private bank for your own use. If you'd like to donate or privately bank your cord blood, talk to your doctor. You'll need to prepare and sign up for these options well before delivery.

Parents**Talk...**

"I had backache when I was pregnant; it was really painful in the third trimester. I found the gentle exercises and stretching I learned at prenatal yoga very helpful, though. Swimming worked wonders, too— just gentle walking in the pool helped to relax the muscles."
Fran, 26, first-time mom

"I joined a pregnancy yoga class when I was 20 weeks pregnant and I love the way it makes me feel afterward. It also made realize how stiff I am in certain places. I'm sure the exercises will help me prepare for labor, too."
Mica, 24, seven months pregnant

"I love nothing better than a soak in a warm bath, but getting out has become a bit of a challenge now that I'm bigger. I have to get onto all fours and hold on to the sides. My partner is usually there to help me, too. I even bought a bath mat to make sure I don't slip."
Magdalena, 31, first-time mom

FIRST TRIMESTER	SECOND TRIMESTER	THIRD TRIMESTER

Your body at **30** Weeks ▼

30 Weeks

❋ Do you misplace your car keys and forget your appointments? Don't worry—pregnancy is to blame.

❋ Don't be alarmed if you feel breathless. It's just your uterus pressing against your diaphragm.

By this stage you may have come to love your increasing size, but not the clumsiness it causes. Remember, though, that annoying symptoms like this will disappear after your baby is born.

Clumsy and forgetful?

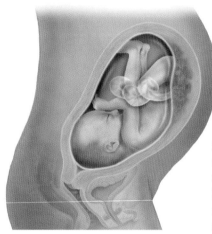

Your baby at **30** Weeks

At this stage it is believed that your baby can probably distinguish light from dark.

❋ This week he will continue to open and shut his eyes, and if you shine a light on your stomach, he may well reach out to try and touch it. While he may soon slow up growing in length (by now he measures about 15¾ inches from crown to toe), he will continue to gain weight steadily until the time he's born. Right now there's about two pints of amniotic fluid surrounding your baby, but that volume will decrease as he gets steadily bigger.

Feeling graceful and dextrous isn't part of the pregnancy package and you may be a little clumsy from now on. You may find that your memory isn't what it was, either. It's all perfectly normal.

Clumsiness should come as no surprise if you consider what your body's going through: you're carrying more weight, your center of gravity has changed, and many of your joints are loosening up. You may even experience numbness and weakness in your arms as your posture changes.

Be reassured that, if you were to take a tumble, your baby would be well protected by your pelvis and the fluid he floats around in. Even so, try not to get into situations where you have a high risk of falling, like climbing steep steps or walking on wet, icy, or uneven surfaces. And don't carry anything that you can't safely drop. If you do fall, you should contact your doctor just to make sure everything is all right.

If your clumsiness is accompanied by sudden swelling of the hands or feet, headaches, blurred vision, vomiting, or upper abdominal pain, contact your doctor immediately. These can be signs of preeclampsia (see p.233).

Are you forgetting things?

Becoming forgetful in pregnancy is pretty common, too. If you get forgetful, it's not something you need to worry about and isn't a medical problem, although it may well have a physical cause. Several small-scale studies have suggested that the size of women's brain can alter during pregnancy.

Forgetfulness may also stem from feeling a little overwhelmed by the huge life changes you are about to experience. And expectant mothers often have a lot going on, what with planning for birth and life with a baby, and maybe moving house as well.

Forgetfulness may be your cue to simplify your life but meanwhile, devise strategies to help you remember what's important and so reduce frustration:
● Carry a small notebook in which you can jot down reminders.
● Keep a detailed daily calendar.
● Assign items you use often, such as keys, to one place.

You don't absolutely have to wallpaper that room right now or clean out your cupboards just because a new baby is arriving. This kind of self-imposed stress can lead you to forget things, so cut yourself a little slack.

Specialized prenatal monitoring

If you've got special problems, such as a preexisting medical condition like diabetes or epilepsy, or if you develop a problem during your pregnancy, you'll need to talk to your obstetrician. You may need to go for more regular checkups than other mothers-to-be.

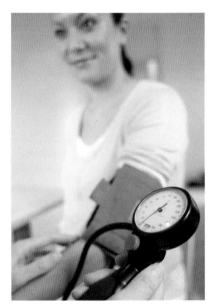

If you have a preexisting condition or develop a problem in pregnancy, you'll have extra prenatal checkups.

If your blood pressure starts to rise toward the end of pregnancy, the results of your regular urine test will be crucial to what happens next. If your urine has protein in it, you may be in the early stages of preeclampsia (see p.233), which means that you'll need more frequent prenatal checkups.

If your doctor discovers that your baby is too small or too large for dates, she may want to refer you for an extra ultrasound scan just to make sure. This is a much more accurate way of measuring your baby's growth than using a tape measure.

If you do have a problem during late pregnancy, such as a rise in blood pressure or your water breaks but labor hasn't started, you may find that you have to be hospitalized. This is so that you can be monitored. You may also need to be induced.

Fact: Smoking in pregnancy greatly increases the risk of SIDS.

Statistics suggest that the risk of sudden infant death syndrome is four times higher if you smoke between one and nine cigarettes a day during pregnancy, rising to eight times higher if you smoke 20 cigarettes or more daily.

Parents**Talk...**

"I was really struggling to give up the cigarettes until I had my scan picture. I uploaded it onto my computer and used Photoshop to put a cigarette in my baby's mouth. It was such a disturbing image that something in my brain finally clicked into place."
Tina, smoker from the age of 20

"It took a few months into my pregnancy but I did eventually stop. Patches work, good thoughts about your baby's health work, support from your husband or partner works, too."
Agnes, smoker from the age of 16

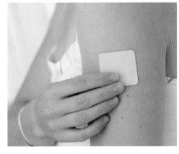

Determined to stop smoking now you're pregnant? Nicotine patches help.

Parents**Ask...**

My last baby was premature. Will the same thing happen in this pregnancy?

If you have already had one premature birth, you do have a greater chance of having another, but you should try not to let this worry you. Most women whose first baby was premature go on to have their next baby after they are 37 weeks pregnant, or at full term.

There is about a one in five chance that your next baby will be premature, so you have a four in five chance that you will not have another premature baby.

The earliness of your last birth seems to influence your chances of having another premature birth. If you gave birth very early, when you were between 20 and 31 weeks pregnant, you'd have a much higher chance of having another premature birth than if you'd given birth when you were between 32 and 36 weeks pregnant.

Knowing that you are at increased risk of having another premature birth can be a frightening thought. However, the fact that you have already been through it means you'll be well-placed to monitor your pregnancy.

Getting ready for pregnancy

Staying safe and healthy

Your pregnancy diary

Birth and beyond

Your body at **31** Weeks ▼

31 Weeks

✶ Is your belly giving you a backache? Switch to low-heeled shoes and avoid heavy lifting.

✶ Gaining one pound a week is normal during the last trimester as your baby has a final growth spurt.

It could be your partner, your mom, or your friend. Whoever you choose to be with you, having a trusted companion by your side during labor will help you feel calmer and more relaxed throughout.

Birth partners

As your pregnancy progresses, you may start to feel worried about how you'll cope during labor and childbirth. A birth partner, who stays with you throughout it all, will help to make the experience less scary and bolster your confidence. He or she can also provide practical help and can communicate on your behalf with hospital staff.

Since the 1970s, fathers have tended to attend births but they don't have to. If your partner doesn't want to be there, decide what's right for both of you. If he isn't going to be there, you may want to enlist the services of a close friend, your sister, your mother, or a paid birth companion called a doula (pronounced "doola"; see p.194).

Going to childbirth classes with you is a good way for your labor partner to prepare. So, too, is talking through together what you're hoping for at the birth. If you write a birth plan (see pp.174–5), your birth partner should be aware of its contents. It's also a good idea for your birth partner to meet the doctor or doctors who may be with you during the labor and birth.

Your labor partner's job is to encourage, reassure, and assist you in

---

▼ Your baby at **31** Weeks

If your baby isn't moving so much now, don't worry. She's running out of space!

✶ Her arms, legs and body are continuing to fill out—and at last they are proportional in size to her head. In fact, she is looking more like a newborn. She's now weighing in at about 3¼ pounds and measures about 16 inches from crown to toe. It's no wonder that she's running out of space in your uterus.

Dad's **Diary**

Military route planning
Our route to the hospital has been planned with almost military precision. I have two routes planned: one for a rush-hour hospital dash—that's my newly found back streets and traffic-light-free roads, and one for an off-peak, middle of the night run. I'm pushing (excuse the pun) for the latter—although when the time comes, I don't think I'll have a lot of say in the matter.

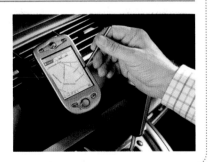

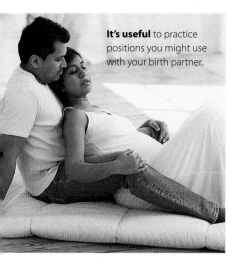

It's useful to practice positions you might use with your birth partner.

any way you find comforting and useful. You can practice some of the ways your partner can help—massaging your lower back, for example, and coaching you with your breathing—but you both need to keep an open mind about what needs to be done, because you won't really know what you want until you finally go into labor.

Another useful role for a labor partner is that of prompter—for example, you may forget about how important it can be to keep moving around in labor and your partner can remind you if necessary. If a medical intervention is suggested, your partner can help to ensure that you are as aware as possible about what is going on.

Flexibility is key during labor and birth and it's essential that your partner is as aware of this as you are. It's important for him to remember that things can change quickly and that you may have to change your mind or make a new decision about some aspect of your care or treatment. So it's important that he doesn't cling to something you said before the event, not realizing that your views have now changed. He must be aware that you have the final word; although he might want to help you in making a decision, or in communicating that decision to your caregivers, your views are what count.

Top tips for labor partners

Preparing yourself to be a birth partner? Follow these succinct tips to be sure of being the best.

- Ask questions.
- Bring a few things for yourself, such as a clean T-shirt and some food.
- Know what to expect—labor isn't the right time to be flipping through a birth manual.
- Be flexible.
- Find useful distractions for your partner, such as rhythmic breathing.
- Be a one-person support team— you are her main emotional and physical support.
- Be ready to take charge of the situation if necessary.
- Be aware of what you're ready to do and what to leave to the professionals.
- Be there—just showing up is the most important thing of all.

Backaches in late pregnancy

Back pain can be divided into two categories. True back pain happens when ligaments, muscles, discs, and joints are placed under strain from poor posture, bad lifting technique, weak or tight muscles, or injury. It often gets worse toward the end of the day or if you have spent a long time on your feet.

The second type of pain is posterior pelvic pain. Most women who seek help because of back pain in pregnancy have this type of pain.

Research shows that you can reduce your chances of developing back pain in pregnancy by getting weekly exercise, having a good upright posture and avoiding heavy lifting (see p.150).

Below are a range of other measures that may also help:
- Massage to the lower back can often help tired, aching muscles. Try leaning forward over the back of a chair or lying on your side.
- A warm bath, a heating pad, or a warm jet of water from a shower head can all help with back pain.
- A physical therapist may recommend a special back support to take some of the weight of your baby off your belly muscles and back.
- Sleeping on your side with a wedge-shaped pillow tucked underneath your belly can help to reduce back pain.

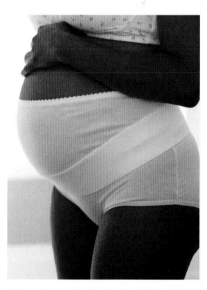

If you have a backache it might be helpful to use a special pregnancy support to take the weight of your baby off your back.

Getting ready for pregnancy

Staying safe and healthy

Your pregnancy diary

Birth and beyond

32 Weeks

❊ Pressure on your bladder may mean frequent bathroom trips, making a good night's sleep difficult.

❊ Constipation, increased blood circulation, and the pressure of your uterus may give you hemorrhoids.

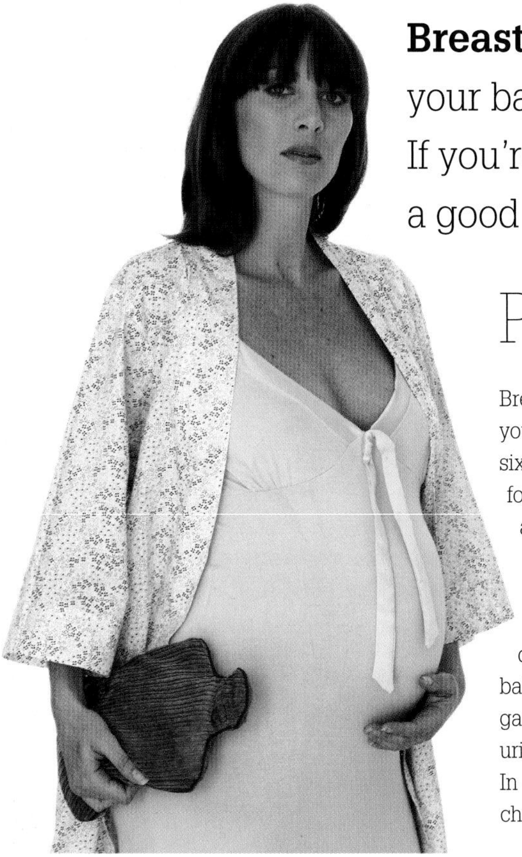

Breast-feeding is the most natural way to feed your baby, but it doesn't always come naturally. If you're planning to breast-feed your baby, now is a good time to find out as much as you can about it.

Preparing for breast-feeding

Breast-feeding gives all the nutrients your baby needs to thrive for the first six months of life, and alongside other foods after this time, it's an important and healthy part of the diet.

The health benefits

Research shows that breast milk contains antibodies that protect your baby against infection—including gastroenteritis, respiratory illness, urinary infections, and ear infections. In addition, it reduces the risk of childhood diabetes and leukemia.

As well as the anti-infective properties that are always in breast milk, the breast-feeding mother makes specific antibodies when she comes into contact with an infection. These transfer to her milk, ready for the baby to receive as soon as he next comes to the breast.

Breast-feeding is the healthiest choice for mothers, too. It gives them a reduced risk of premenopausal breast cancer, ovarian cancer, and of fractures caused by osteoporosis.

As long as you're healthy, there's not much more you can do to prepare your body for breast-feeding. But you can prepare your mind. Learn as much as you can about breast-feeding before your baby is born. Talk to other breast-feeding mothers, read books to familiarize yourself, and contact local breast-feeding support organizations.

Try to go to a breast-feeding class or a preparation for breast-feeding session (offered by many hospitals, and La Leche League International also has support groups in communities across the country) some time during your last few months of pregnancy. The more you know about breast-feeding, the more likely you are to succeed at it.

Whether you think about it or not, your pregnant body is busy preparing itself for breast-feeding. That's one reason why your breasts get so much bigger during pregnancy—your milk ducts and milk-producing cells are developing, and more blood goes to your breasts than before.

But don't worry. Breast size has nothing to do with the ability to breast-feed successfully—even if you stay small-breasted, that will not reduce your chances of being able to feed your baby yourself.

Your baby at **32** Weeks

By now your baby may have a full head of hair—or perhaps just a few wisps.

❊ He now weighs approximately 3¾ pounds and measures about 16½ inches long from head to toe. Although his lungs won't be fully developed until just before birth, your little one is busy inhaling amniotic fluid. This is to exercise his lungs and practice breathing for after he's born.

Escape routes

If you're starting to feel a little, well, bored of being pregnant, you're not alone. What was exciting and new during the first few weeks and months of pregnancy can become pretty tedious by the sixth or seventh month.

Sometimes you need a break from all things baby-related. So, take on tasks and dabble in activities that a new mom couldn't possibly squeeze into her busy schedule. Below are some ideas:

- **Make dates with friends** Take time to enjoy a good leisurely talk with your pals over a lunch or coffee.
- **Streamline your space** Clean out your files, sift through the kitchen drawers, or put those boxed-up photos in the attic into photo albums.
- **Connect with your partner** Enjoy some romantic dinners together and focus on each other while you can.
- **Set up time-savers** Make an appointment for a new, easy-to-manage haircut, collect takeaway menus from restaurants near your home, set up an online bank account so that you can manage your finances easily, hire a house cleaner if you can afford to and don't have one already, and learn to master online grocery shopping.
- **Pamper yourself** If you can possibly afford it, a pregnancy massage at a spa is well worth the money.
- **Indulge in some retail therapy** Treat yourself to a pretty new maternity bra or some elegant ballet flats to wear in late pregnancy.
- **Do some exercise** Go for a gentle swim at your local pool and enjoy the sensation of weightlessness! If swimming isn't your thing, go for a stroll in the fresh air instead.
- **Escape to another world** Tuck into a nice big novel or rent a few DVDs that sweep you off to another place for a little while.

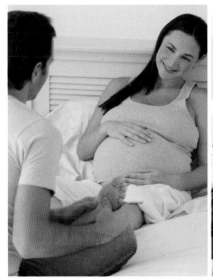

Ask your partner for a massage. It will help him feel involved, will help you relax, and will give you extra time together.

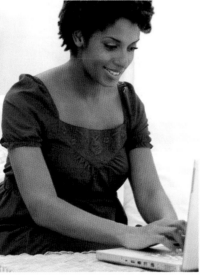

An online bank account is a real time saver for new moms. Setting up one will give you a break from thinking about your pregnancy.

ParentsAsk...

My hips are sore at night. How can I relieve the pain?

Hip pain is common in pregnancy and is often a problem in bed at night. Try sleeping on your side with legs bent and a pillow between your knees supporting the whole length of your leg. A pillow under your belly is also helpful to stop you from rolling forward. An extra layer of padding, such as a sleeping bag or quilt, under your bottom sheet can improve matters. You may also find gentle heat on your hips—a hot water bottle—helpful. Avoid activities that seem to aggravate the pain, too.

You will probably find that your pain is worse if you have had a busy day. Try to spend time resting on an exercise or birthing ball or on your hands and knees. This takes the weight off your hips and gives them a rest.

Do I need to toughen my nipples or do anything else before I can breast-feed?

The hormonal changes pregnancy brings to the breasts are sufficient preparation for most women. You don't need to use creams to soften your skin beforehand or express colostrum either. In particular, don't rub or scrub your nipples—this will only hurt you and make breast-feeding difficult. The best preparation for breast-feeding is getting your partner to support you in your decision to breast-feed, so that you and your baby can get off to a good start. Research shows that you are more likely to breast-feed longer if your partner is well informed.

The other thing you can do to help breast-feeding is to make sure that the doctor who attends you during your baby's birth knows that you would like plenty of skin-to-skin contact with your baby when he or she is born. This early skin-to-skin contact has been shown to increase the length of time that women breast-feed for.

Getting ready for pregnancy

Staying safe and healthy

Your pregnancy diary

Birth and beyond

Your body at **33** Weeks ▼

33 Weeks

✳ Mild, irregular contractions, known as Braxton Hicks, may become more noticeable around now.

✳ You may notice that your feet, hands, face, and ankles have become a bit swollen.

It's hard to imagine how life will be once your baby's born. One thing is sure, though—it's going to be busy. Making preparations now will make life easier in those sleepless early days.

Stocking up

As you head into the final weeks of pregnancy, it's time to make life easier for yourself. In the first weeks after your baby's birth, it may not be so easy to pop out to the supermarket, so it's worthwhile stocking up on basics— everything from cereal to toilet paper— before shopping becomes a real chore.

Buying in bulk is good advice—the prices really are better, so you'll save yourself some money, too. But if you're not careful, you can also spend a lot on items you don't need or that will go bad before you can eat them. Below are a few bulk-buying tips:

● Make a list of things you use a lot, such as laundry detergent or bottled water. These are perfect to buy in bulk.

● Concentrate on nonperishable and long-life items, such as canned soups and vegetables, grains and dried pasta, and tea and coffee.

● When you get home, repackage perishables into smaller quantities. Big packages of steaks or chicken breasts,

for example, can be divided into daily portions and frozen until needed.

● Don't forget to stock up on non-food products too—you won't want to run out of dish washing liquid or tissues.

Feed the freezer

It's also a great idea to start cooking extra portions to freeze as easy meals for the early weeks. This will prove to be a godsend when you're getting used to

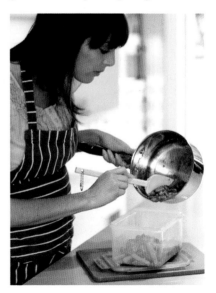

Cooking extra meals and freezing them for later use will be a lifesaver once you're in the throes of new motherhood.

▼ Your baby at **33** Weeks

She might be positioning herself for birth now—upside down and head down.

✳ Your doctor will be paying careful attention to your baby's position during the coming weeks. Although she may be perfectly positioned now, some babies do decide to turn around again. She now weighs in at about 4½ pounds and measures approximately 17½ inches from head to toe.

caring for your new baby. So, for example, the next time you make a lasagne, a stew, or casserole, make double the batch, then freeze half of it. It won't just save you time when the baby's born; homemade meals are also much healthier and more nutritious than fast-food and ready meals that you buy from the supermarket.

Nutritious homemade soups are also freezable, and get into the habit of putting leftovers into the freezer rather than the fridge. Milk and bread can be frozen, too, so keep a couple of cartons of milk and a few loaves in the freezer. And remember, frozen vegetables are just as nutritious as fresh, and will be more convenient once the baby is born.

Still commuting?

The trip to and from work can be the most stressful and tiring part of your day, especially if you have to stand for long periods. While traveling as part of your job can be assessed for possible risks to you or your baby (see p.62), unfortunately the commuting part can't. But there are strategies that you could try to improve matters. For example, you could suggest to your employer that you change your working hours so that you are traveling outside rush hours. It wouldn't affect the number of hours you work, but it might mean you get a seat on the bus or train. Or would your employer consider letting you work from home one or two days a week to help reduce the strain on you?

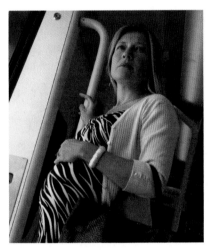

Ask your employer if you can change your working hours to avoid commuting in rush hour so you might get a seat.

"Try changing **your working hours** to avoid **rush hour**."

You could also talk to your doctor, who might suggest you take a period of sick leave if the commuting is affecting the well-being of you or your baby. If you're eligible for short-term disability leave through state or employer benefits, you may be able to take four to six weeks. Some plans also cover bedrest before birth. And if you're eligible for leave

under the FMLA, you can start taking unpaid leave anytime during your pregnancy—or anytime thereafter — as long as you conclude your leave within the first twelve months after your child's arrival. Check with your human resources department to find out if any limitations apply under your company's leave policies.

Active mom

Bored by the last few weeks of pregnancy? Most moms are, especially if they're usually active.

"I'm in my third trimester and can categorically say that the novelty of being pregnant has well and truly worn off! I'm used to being fit and active so I hate having to roll out of bed sideways just to get up.

I've worked hard in the gym to get a body that I'm happy with, so to have people constantly commenting on my size, not to mention touching my stomach, is getting really tedious.

And I'm bored by the fact that everyone assumes that all I want to talk about is the baby and my pregnancy. I am open to other topics! I don't think there's been a single non-work related conversation with any of my co-workers that hasn't been centered around children for months!"

Green mom

Cloth diapers plus flushable disposables are eco-friendly and kind to your baby's skin.

"I'm happy to say I've bought some shaped one-size cloth diapers. In addition to being economical and made from organic cotton, they'll be soft and gentle on my baby's skin. I'll wash them carefully, too, to protect the environment. For vacations and day trips I'm getting some flushable disposables. They're a little bit more expensive than ordinary disposables, but I can sleep well at night knowing I'm not contributing to the mass of diapers on landfill sites."

Getting ready for pregnancy

Staying safe and healthy

Your pregnancy diary

Birth and beyond

Your body at **34** Weeks ▼

34 Weeks

✳ If you notice a tingling sensation or numbness in your pelvis, it's the pressure of the baby on the nerves.

✳ Try the relaxation, positions and massage learned at childbirth classes to help relieve any discomfort.

The big day is only a few weeks away. If you're one of the many women whose mother has offered to come and help, you can start to make plans now. Otherwise, a doula may be for you.

Moms and doulas

Most women need someone they can count on for support, strength and guidance during childbirth, in addition to their midwife or doctor. Usually this special person is their partner, but for others it will be a close friend or their own mother. Although lots of moms want to support their daughters during labor, only you can decide if having your mother in the delivery room with you will be a help or a hindrance. You may feel you can't give birth without her, or you may prefer to keep it as a special time for just you and your partner. Don't rush or be pushed into a decision and, if you don't want mom there, let her down gently.

Another alternative is to employ a doula. She is an experienced woman who offers emotional and practical support before, during and after childbirth. The idea is to "mother the mother," nurturing her during pregnancy, birth, and the early days as a new mom.

A doula is trained in childbirth and has a good knowledge of female physiology, but she isn't a replacement for the medical staff. You can find out if

there is a doula in your area and details of costs from the website for Doulas of North America (www.dona.org).

In many cultures, women rest for up to 40 days after giving birth. In the West, however, social pressures mean that moms are rushed back into normal day-to-day activities much sooner. If your partner has taken time off, he is likely to return to work when your baby is still only one or two weeks old. It can feel overwhelming to take care of a newborn on your own, particularly if you've had stitches or a cesarean. With the help of your mom, close friend, or postpartum doula, you can enjoy some of the benefits of a prolonged "lying in" period, giving you the chance to bond with your new baby and spend extra time with your other children.

66% of new moms think that their parenting style is more like their own mother's than they thought it would be—even though they were sure they'd do things differently!

▼ Your baby at **34** Weeks

Now your baby's building his fat layers to help keep him at the correct temperature.

✳ These fat layers show in the way he's gradually filling out and getting rounder. The fat helps him to regulate his body temperature after birth. He now weighs more than 5 pounds and is around 17¾ inches long. If you don't already talk to your baby, this is a good time to start— by 35 weeks his hearing's fully developed.

In addition to doing the everyday chores that you haven't had the time or energy for—shopping, cooking, and cleaning—moms can help hugely by preparing some homemade meals and putting them in the freezer for you to enjoy when you need them. As all moms know, good nutrition is vital to a speedy recovery after the physical demands of pregnancy and labor. A little forward planning goes a long way!

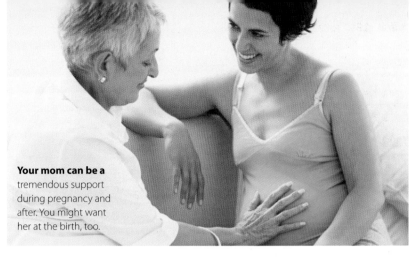

Your mom can be a tremendous support during pregnancy and after. You might want her at the birth, too.

Go shopping: nursing bras

When you are breast-feeding your breasts expand enormously, but that doesn't mean you have to settle for a bra that would look better on a granny. You can look good as well as be comfortable.

A good nursing bra needs to be flexible, allowing extra room for when the milk comes in and when your breasts reduce in size (usually after 12 weeks or so). It almost goes without saying that the cups should open and close easily, preferably using only one hand. The opening should allow plenty of room for your baby to feed and never constrict or squeeze your breast since this can lead to blocked ducts or mastitis. When it comes to comfort, the same tips apply as to maternity bras (see p.92). Make sure you get a professional fitting. When trying on, be sure that the cups fit snugly and cover most of the breast. The center seam should lie comfortably against your breastbone. Also make sure your maternity bra has:

- four hook and eye fastenings
- wide nonslip shoulder straps for extra support
- broad side and back for extra support
- deep center at the front for extra support
- drop-cup feature

ParentsAsk...

I'm 34 weeks pregnant and my breasts are leaking. Is it normal?
Leaking breasts late in pregnancy are perfectly normal, so don't worry. What they are leaking is called colostrum (see p.93). Some women leak quite a lot before their babies are born and others don't leak at all. There doesn't seem to be any link between how much you leak before the baby's birth and how much milk you produce afterward.

This leaking can be embarrassing for you or your partner if you leak when you are making love. But you should both be assured that this is quite normal.

When you are out and about, wearing breast pads inside your bra will help prevent wet patches on your shirts. You should change the pads at regular intervals during the day to keep you feeling fresh and comfortable. This will also help to prevent any smell of stale colostrum.

Organized mom

There's no doubt that your life and your partner's is about to change. It pays to prepare well.

"My husband Dan and I have been talking about how our lives will change after our baby is born. It's hard for us to imagine now how different things will be after the birth, but I've been speaking to friends and trying to plan as much as I can.

Dan thinks that our lives will continue as they were before, but I know that it will be hard for us to travel and go out as much as we do now, especially in the early days when I'm sore and we're feeling exhausted.

I've been reading lots of books about baby care and I'm going to try and get my baby in a gentle routine as soon as possible, so that hopefully she'll sleep better and we'll be able to get our lives back on track. I really want to breast-feed too, so I've been reading up on how to do it and going to some breast-feeding preparation classes. I think I'm quite prepared now (Dan jokes that I have a degree in parenting!) but I fear my darling husband is going to have more of a shock in store."

| FIRST TRIMESTER | SECOND TRIMESTER | THIRD TRIMESTER |

Your body at **35** Weeks ▼

35 Weeks

❋ You may feel that you've run out of room—your uterus has expanded to 1,000 times its original volume.

❋ Don't be surprised, but you'll gain little or no more weight from now until your due date.

As you head toward your baby's birthday, now is a good time to try to encourage your baby into a good position for birth. Here are a few techniques you can try.

Positioning baby for birth

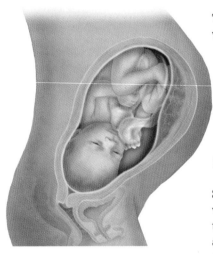

▼ Your baby at **35** Weeks

Do you see the occasional protrusion from your belly? That might be baby's foot.

❋ When she stretches and squirms around, your baby's elbow, foot, or head may now protrude from your stomach. She weighs about 5¼ pounds and measures around 17¾ inches. Soon, as the wall of your uterus and your abdomen stretch thinner and let in more light, she will develop daily cycles of sleeping and waking. Your little one is now sporting full-length fingernails and toenails, and has a fully developed pair of kidneys.

The best position for your baby to be in when you start to go into labor is head down, with the back of her head slightly toward the front of your abdomen. In this position, it's simple for her to move gently downward during labor, so labor is nearly always shorter and easier. Your doctor describes a baby in this position as being in an anterior position.

But nature isn't always so helpful. Some babies go down into the pelvis with the back of their heads toward their mothers' spines. This is called a posterior position and it can lead to several things happening:

- Your water is more likely to break at the beginning of labor.
- You have a lot of backache during and in between contractions.
- Labor is slower.
- You may need forceps or a vacuum to help you give birth to your baby.

There are some techniques that people say get the baby to enter the pelvis in an anterior, rather than a posterior, position. This is called "optimal fetal positioning" and should be done from about 35 weeks of pregnancy. It's all about making sure that your knees are always lower than your hips:

- Sit on a cushion in your car to lift your bottom up.
- Check that your favorite chair doesn't make your bottom go down and your knees come up.
- Take regular breaks and move around, especially if your job or leisure activities involve you in a lot of sitting.
- Watch television kneeling on all fours for 10 minutes every day.
- Scrub all your floors and baseboards— our grandmas used to say that washing the kitchen floor was a good way of preparing for labor. And they were certainly right! When you are kneeling on all fours, the back of your baby's head can't help but swing around to the front of your abdomen.

Sometimes women have a lot of minor pains for several days before labor really starts. These pains might well be due to the fact that your baby is trying to turn from a posterior position into an anterior one. If this happens to you, get as much rest as possible during the night, and during the day try to remain upright and active, leaning forward while you are having the pains. Don't despair. This is nature's way of getting your baby into the best position, so she is ready for birth.

Presentation positions

By around eight months, there's not much room in the uterus. Most babies settle in head down—known as a cephalic presentation. At full-term, nearly 97 percent come out head first. Most of the rest are breech, but there are several other positions.

Anterior position The best position for labor, with the back of baby's head slightly toward the front of your abdomen.

Posterior position Also known as "sunnyside up"; your baby has the back of her head toward your spine. You are likely to have a slow backache labor.

Breech position Your baby is bottom-down. Vaginal delivery is usually attempted, but you may need a cesarean.

Brow presentation Your baby's head is extended slightly. Unless it flexes, it is very unlikely you'll have a vaginal delivery.

Transverse Your baby is lying horizontally across your uterus. In this position your belly will feel tight and firm.

Oblique Your baby is lying diagonally across your uterus. In this position you're likely to have a cesarean.

Anterior position   **Posterior position**   **Breech position**

Brow presentation   **Transverse**   **Oblique**

Baby car seats

A car seat is one piece of equipment you really need before your baby is born. If you are having your baby in the hospital and are going home by car, you are legally obliged to put her in a car seat.

Choosing the right car seat for your baby's age and weight is very important. You must also make sure that the seat is properly installed. Some seats work better in some models of cars than others, so try before you buy. If a car seat doesn't seem to fit your car perfectly, or if it seems difficult to fasten in place, do not buy it. The seat should

be held tightly by the seatbelt with very little sideways movement. Practice putting the empty seat in and tightening the seatbelt. If the seat moves around, it's not safe.

Rear-facing car seats should never be used on a front seat if there are airbags in the car. To make sure that your car seat is safe, have it checked by a professional. The National Highway Traffic Safety Administration's website lists child safety seat inspection stations, or ask at car dealerships, since some are happy to do a free check.

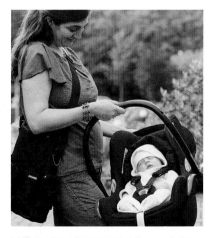

When choosing a car seat for your baby, make sure it's right for your baby's age and weight, and that it's correctly installed.

Sleep in late pregnancy

Is a good night's sleep nothing but a distant memory now?
Lots of women have trouble sleeping as the birth gets closer, and maybe some rather strange dreams, too. Find out here what to expect sleep-wise during your third trimester, and why it's happening.

Meeting the challenge

Most women have trouble sleeping at some stage of their pregnancy and often remember a good night's sleep as a distant memory as the birth gets closer.

During your third trimester, just lying down comfortably might be a challenge.

Your belly is now simply too big. If sleeping on your left side with pillows wedged between your legs and behind your back doesn't help, try settling in a comfy chair instead. In the final four to six weeks, you may find that you get

your best rests by sleeping sitting up.

And if that weren't enough, remember during your early pregnancy days when it seemed as though you spent more time in the bathroom than out of it? Well here we are again. This

---

Comfortable sleep positions

Finding it impossible to get comfy in bed? Try curling up or stretching out on your left side with a pillow between your legs. (And keep returning to that position if you wake up at night on your stomach or back.) You can buy a number of different maternity pillows, although you may find that your usual pillows work just as well. Arrange them between your legs, under your belly, and behind your back for extra comfort and support.

You might find that wearing a sleeping bra and a maternity belt gives you extra support and aids sleep.

Finally, if lying on your side puts too much pressure on your hips, sleep on a piece of soft foam. The foam layer goes on top of your mattress and under the sheet for added comfort and air circulation. You should be able to buy soft foam in a range of sizes at most large department stores.

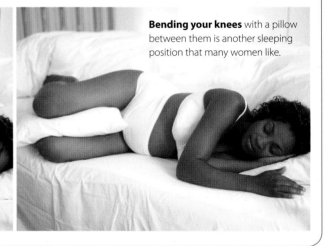

Lying stretched out on your left side with a soft pillow between your legs can be comfortable at this late stage.

Bending your knees with a pillow between them is another sleeping position that many women like.

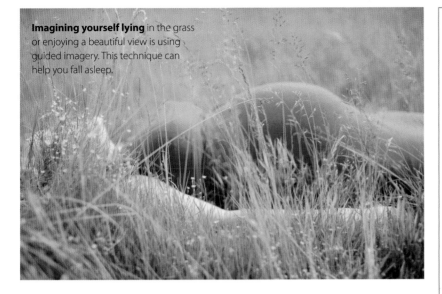

Imagining yourself lying in the grass or enjoying a beautiful view is using guided imagery. This technique can help you fall asleep.

time it's thanks to your growing baby, who's putting pressure on your bladder. You can try to reduce the number of trips to the bathroom by cutting back on fluids in the late afternoon and completely emptying your bladder on every trip to the bathroom by leaning forward when you urinate. Another technique is to rock back and forth while you are urinating, or to stop, wait for 30 seconds, then squeeze again to get out any last drops.

Heartburn and other sleep stealers

Don't be surprised if heartburn, leg cramps, restless leg syndrome, and snoring, not to mention your baby's kicking and squirming, keep you awake at night during your third trimester. Studies show that pregnant women in their third trimester have fewer periods of deep sleep and wake up more often during the night. In short, the quality of your sleep is heading toward an all-time low.

Try to catch up during the day if the opportunity arises. Otherwise you can become really run down and exhausted. This can become a bit of a vicious circle

though, since cat naps during the day will reduce your requirement for sleep during the night. Nevertheless, this pattern of needing less sleep at night will continue when you are dealing with night feedings so it may be some time before you will need to get back to a normal diurnal (asleep at night and awake during the day) rhythm.

Bizarre dreams

Are you having strange dreams now that you're in the third trimester? Many moms-to-be find that during pregnancy, their dreams become more bizarre than ever before. It's all because of the changes taking place with your hormones, perhaps combined with mixed feelings about your changing shape—and maybe the added ingredients of anxiety and excitement about the prospect of becoming a mother.

A taste of things to come

Although you can ease or avoid some of these sleep disturbances, it's likely that you will have to endure some sleepless nights. Think of this time as a dress rehearsal for life after your baby is born!

Nighttime survival tips

Add to the bedtime ritual tips we gave you on p.130 with the extra ideas below for the third trimester:

● **Massage** A foot, hand, or neck massage from your partner is a perfect way to wind down before bed.
● **Deep breathing** Breathing deeply and rhythmically can ease muscle tension, lower your heart rate, and help you get off to sleep.
● **Progressive muscle relaxation** Lying in bed, start by tensing and releasing your hand and forearm muscles, followed by your biceps and triceps, and so on until you reach your feet. The concentration you need for this, together with the relaxation it gives, can help get you off to sleep.
● **Guided imagery** Picture yourself in a quiet, relaxing scene—lying on a warm sandy beach, walking in fields full of beautiful-smelling wild flowers, or sitting on a secluded hilltop.
● **Drinking** Drink plenty of fluids during the day but less in the evening. You will be less likely to need to get up for the bathroom at night.

Dad's **Diary**

Neither of us can sleep now!
Sleep is a real problem for Karen as she nears her due date. She struggles to get into a comfortable position and then, when she does, she finds that she's too hot and the stretch marks on her belly start itching like crazy. I wake up in the middle of the night shivering to find that she's opened the window to let in the freezing fall air. Of course, I can't complain, so I just find the nearest blanket and try to go back to sleep.

Your body at **36** Weeks ▼

36 Weeks

✳ More pressure in your lower abdomen? Your baby is dropping as his head engages ready for birth.

✳ By now, you may feel as if you need to urinate all the time as your baby presses on your bladder.

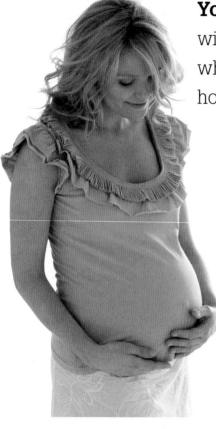

Your baby could arrive any day, so fill the car with gas and make sure you know where to park when you get to the hospital. If you're planning a home birth, other children will need to be cared for.

Be prepared

As your due date approaches, make sure you've got the practical preparations in place for the day (or night) you go into labor. Make sure your partner (or whoever will be driving you) memorizes the route to the hospital. If you're in the throes of labor in the passenger seat, your partner may not be in a fit state to navigate. So do a dry run and make sure you know the route as well. It's also a

else lined up to take you to the hospital; maybe one of your parents, or a friend, or relative. You probably won't need their help but it'll give you peace of mind that you're prepared for any last-minute changes to your plans.

If you have a child already, arrange alternative care for her for when you go into labor. A trusted friend or relative will need to be able take care of her at

"Your partner **has to be ready** for that **'drop-everything' call**."

▼ Your baby at **36** Weeks

Although many babies born at 36 weeks do just fine, some babies will develop respiratory distress syndrome and also have problems with eating properly.

✳ Barring medical reasons, doctors discourage any elective delivery before 36 weeks. A typical 36-week-old weighs 6 pounds. You may now be feeling increased pressure in your lower abdomen as your baby engages in your pelvis, ready for birth.

good idea to plan a few alternative routes in case there are obstacles when the big day arrives. Keep the car filled with enough gas to get you there. A last-minute stop at the gas station is the last thing you need when you're battling through contractions.

Make sure that you can contact your partner no matter where he is when you need him. He has to be ready for that "drop-everything" call. In the unlikely event that your partner isn't around when you go into labor, have someone

the drop of a hat. Even if you have a home birth, you'll need someone to come and take care of her, or to take her to their home. If the caregiver is someone who has never spent the night with your child, it might be helpful to have a practice run first—especially if you'll be sending her to stay at the caregiver's house. Arrange a sleepover sometime before the birth with games or other simple, fun activities so that she'll have happy memories of spending the night with this person.

Parents**Talk...**

"When my due date was a week away, the reality of what was about to happen set in. I felt like I was going to run a marathon and hadn't done enough training."
Bella, 34, mom of six-month old Anna

"I'm most scared about the pain. I'm not planning on having pain relief, but I'm worried that it'll be so agonizing I'll ask for it anyway."
Rani, 33, first-time mom

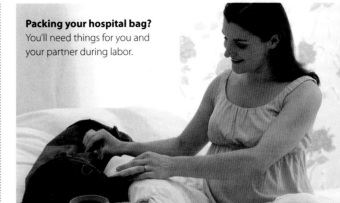

Packing your hospital bag?
You'll need things for you and your partner during labor.

Getting ready for pregnancy

Staying safe and healthy

Your pregnancy diary

Birth and beyond

Packing for hospital in preparation for labor

This is the final stretch, with only a few weeks to go before your due date. Now's the time to pack a bag for all the essentials you'll need during labor and after your baby is born. Find out what the hospital provides and what you can bring yourself, but be aware that hospitals can be short on space—there may be only a small cabinet by your bed for your things.

What to pack for labor
- Picture ID, your insurance card, and any necessary hospital paperwork.
- Your birth plan.
- Robe, slippers, and socks.
- An old nightgown or a T-shirt to wear in labor.
- Massage oil or lotion.
- Lip balm.
- Toothbrush and toothpaste.
- Snacks and drinks for while you are in labor, or some glucose tablets.
- Watch with a second hand—to time contractions.
- Digital camera or camcorder (not all hospitals allow camcorders during delivery so check beforehand).
- Relaxation materials—books, magazines, portable DVD player, handheld games console, and games.
- Toiletries.
- Water spray—or a handheld fan.
- Music to listen to—on a CD or MP3 player, but check with the hospital in case they won't let you plug anything in to re-charge it, in which case you'll need to take a battery-operated machine.

For your birth partner
- A change of clothes.
- Toothbrush and toothpaste.
- Snacks and drinks.
- Book or games console.

For after the birth
- Going-home outfit and loose, comfortable clothes to wear while you're in the hospital.
- Nursing bras and breast pads.
- Maternity pads—a couple of packs.
- Nightshirt or T-shirt—front-opening shirts are useful for breast-feeding.
- Toiletries.
- Towels, hairbrush, toothbrush, and toothpaste.
- Old panties/cheap panties/disposable panties—don't bring your best ones since they will get messy.
- Arnica tablets which may help with bruising after the birth.
- Ear plugs, in case you end up on a noisy ward!
- Address book—unless all your numbers are stored on your cell phone.
- Fully charged cell phone and charger (if allowed in hospital).
- Coins/card for using hospital phone.

For your baby
- Towel.
- Infant car seat.
- One outfit for the trip home.
- Baby blanket (a warm one if the weather is cold).
- Diapers.
- One pair of socks or booties and a hat.
- Jacket or snowsuit if you are having a winter baby.
- Burp cloths.

| FIRST TRIMESTER | SECOND TRIMESTER | THIRD TRIMESTER |

Your body at **37** Weeks ▼

37 Weeks

❊ If you need help to conquer the late pregnancy blues, read up on what your newborn will be like (see pp.302–309).

❊ It may be harder than ever to get to sleep at night. Take it easy during the day if you can.

The next couple of weeks are a waiting game. Try to enjoy this time before your baby arrives—eat well and get plenty of rest. And if you already have a little one, make the most of this special time together.

Dealing with a toddler

Your toddler may become anxious in the month or so before you give birth. As you get bigger, less energetic, and more focused on the labor, he may become clingy, develop new fears, and even regress slightly. This is normal. Acting like a baby may be just his way of exploring how babies behave and what it felt like to be your baby. Lots of love and affection during this time will help him regain his confidence.

Try to avoid any other major changes that might unsettle your toddler, such as moving or starting a new preschool. Now isn't the best time to pressure him to complete potty training or ask him to give up security items such as his pacifier, either. Keeping to his regular routine as much as possible is key in helping him feel secure.

Spend as much time with your child as possible in the last few weeks of your pregnancy. It's likely that you're going to be pretty busy with the baby when she arrives, so make the most of your time together. He will really appreciate it and remember this special time when he had you all to himself.

How will we manage in the early days and weeks?

It will be hard at times, but it won't be impossible. Below are our top tips on how you can cope.

● Make your toddler aware from the very start that the baby is interested in him, is watching him, and loves him. Say things like, "She's following your game with her eyes" and "She's very interested in what you're doing."

● Involve him in games with the baby from the earliest days, and always tell your toddler how much you value his help and assistance at bathtime, or getting a clean diaper, and so on.

● Buy a few small presents for him, wrap them up and leave them by the door so that visitors with gifts for your newborn can also give him something.

60% of moms think that 18 months to three years is the best age gap to have between siblings. Just 10 percent think that 18 months or less is ideal, while eight percent think the age gap doesn't matter.

Your baby at **37** Weeks

With baby's head now in your pelvis, she has more room for her growing legs.

❊ If your baby's head has engaged (see pp.204–5) and is cradled in your pelvis, she will now have a bit more room for her 6¼-pound body and her 19½-inch length. Many babies now have a full head of hair, which may be around one inch long. But don't be surprised if her hair isn't the same color as yours.

Your last prenatal appointments

You will be seeing your doctor weekly at this point. She will continue to check your blood pressure and urine, and measure your belly. She'll examine your abdomen to determine your baby's position and growth, and she'll listen to your baby's heartbeat.

If you haven't had your baby by 41 weeks, your doctor may offer to strip the membranes to try and kickstart labor. If you choose not to have this done, or if it doesn't make you go into labor, you'll be offered an induction. Your doctor will also review with you the signs of labor and when you should contact her.

Before your appointments, make a note of any questions you'd like to ask your doctor. It's an ideal time to raise any last-minute worries or fears you have about the labor, or about taking care of your baby after she's born. Your doctor will able to reassure you and offer you help and advice during these last few days. Be sure to talk about care for you and your baby after delivery. If you haven't found a pediatrician yet for your baby, ask your doctor for some names.

Finally, remember that due dates aren't always accurate. Though you think you're overdue and may start worrying, you may not be overdue at all.

"Your doctor will **reassure you** during these **last few days**."

Organized mom

The last few weeks may bring some new symptoms. If you're at all worried, tell your doctor.

"Now that I'm officially in the home stretch I've been feeling really tired again, and I've even been feeling a bit breathless from time to time, especially when I'm climbing the stairs or rushing around. I'm sure it's normal to feel like this, but I'm definitely going to mention it to my doctor when I see her again, just in case. I've also been having the odd painless 'tightening', and I'm not sure if these are Braxton Hicks contractions or not, so I'm definitely going to mention them.

I can't believe it's my last prenatal appointment next week. I'm writing down a list of any important symptoms so I don't forget to ask my doctor—it may be a while before I see her again!"

ParentsTalk...

"When my breech baby simply refused to turn, I was booked for a cesarean. I was okay about it until I got into the operating room. All of a sudden, after a day of just relaxing, watching TV and talking with my husband, the reality of what was about to happen just hit me. I was trying hard not to cry, but as they gave me the epidural I burst into tears! It wasn't until my doctor reassured me that everything would be fine that I started to calm down and enjoy the whole experience."
Maggie, 30, first-time mom

"During my cesarean I asked for the curtain to be lowered so I could see my twins being born. It was a weird experience but totally incredible. It's something I'll always remember and will tell the twins about when they're older."
Jenna, 37, mom to Rosie and Harriet

"Having a cesarean doesn't make you any less of a mom or woman. Remember that how you give birth isn't the measure of being a good mother—it's what you do afterward that really counts."
Sheena, 24, mom to two-year-old Josh

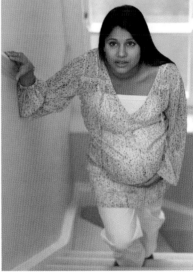

During these last weeks even climbing the stairs can be an effort. Tell your doctor if you develop any worrying symptoms.

Getting ready for pregnancy

Staying safe and healthy

Your pregnancy diary

Birth and beyond

FIRST TRIMESTER	SECOND TRIMESTER	THIRD TRIMESTER

Your body at **38** Weeks ▼

38 Weeks

❄ Your due date is right around the corner and your baby's just waiting for the right time to be born.

❄ Take it easy during the final week or so—this may be your last opportunity to relax for a while.

You may now feel more pressure in your lower abdomen and notice that your baby is gradually dropping. This is called lightening, or engagement. Your lungs and stomach now get a chance to expand.

Rules of engagement

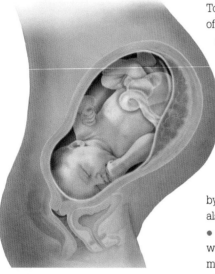

▼ Your baby at **38** Weeks

Baby is still growing and laying down the fat reserves that regulate body temperature.

❄ Although your baby is still growing, boys tend to have a slightly heavier birth weight than girls. The average baby at 38 weeks weighs about 6½ to 7 pounds. Your little one's organ systems are now fully developed, but his lungs will be last to mature, which is why premature babies need help breathing.

Toward the end of pregnancy, the shape of your uterus, your liver, and intestines encourage your baby's presenting part (usually his head, but sometimes his bottom) to dip down into your pelvis. This can occur as early as 33 or 34 weeks of pregnancy, but may not happen until labor starts.

If your baby engages in the pelvis early this does not mean that you will give birth early.

Usually he will engage in the pelvis by 37 to 38 weeks, but this process can also be affected by lots of other things:

● If you are very athletic and have well-toned abdominal muscles, this may mean that your belly is held in tighter, which changes the angle of the baby's body and presenting part to the pelvic brim. In this position it is harder for him to engage in the pelvis. To encourage his head to engage you need to relax your abdominal muscles and "dangle your belly" out at the front.

● There is some data to suggest that if you spend a lot of time sitting down at work, in a car, or in soft easy chairs or on a squishy sofa to watch TV, your baby is more likely to be lying in a posterior position—that is with his back to your back. In this position it is harder

for him to enter your pelvis. This is not the best position for an efficient labor, partly because the presenting part of the baby remains high for so long. Make sure to sit leaning forward whenever you sit down, with your knees below your hips. This will help your baby to turn his back toward your front and move down. A kneeling chair is ideal for you to adopt this position.

● If you have had several babies before, your abdominal muscles may be loose, which makes it easy for your baby to move and change position frequently. Sometimes he may lie across your abdomen (transverse) or at an angle (oblique). If he gets into one of these positions (see p.197), it is less likely that he will manage to engage in your pelvis before the start of labor.

● Your baby may be a large one. If this is the case, he may not be able to descend into your pelvis until your contractions start.

● Sometimes the entrance to your pelvis is narrow. If that is the case, it may take a long time for your baby's presenting part to enter your pelvis but, once he is in position, birth is generally rapid because the pelvic outlet usually tends to be roomy.

Enjoying the last weeks together

If you're expecting your first baby, your relationship is facing one of its toughest tests. Going from being partners to parents is a steep (some would say perpendicular!) learning curve. No one can predict how you will manage, but one thing is for sure: nothing will be the same again. That's why you and your partner should make the most of your last few weeks alone together.

First there were two

With the excitement of your imminent new arrival, it's easy to lose track of where it all began: your relationship with your husband or partner. Take time out to remind yourself of your shared history and how you've dealt with life's ups and downs so far. Taking stock like this gives you confidence that you will manage whatever life throws at you. It's also an opportunity to discuss your plans for the future.

A kiss and cuddle

Research shows that sharing affection every day boosts the chances of a partnership lasting. Like children, adults who do not get hugged, praised, or supported start to feel cut off and out of touch with others. Regular shows of affection deepen the bonds between you and set you up for the challenges of parenthood that lie ahead.

You can show that you love and care for each other in little ways every day. Cuddle up on the sofa together, or hold hands as you walk along. Try a peck on the cheek when you make them a cup of coffee, put a loving note on the fridge or in their pocket, or buy a small surprise gift to show that you've been thinking about them during the day. Remember, too, that sex is not a replacement for affection, and that when it comes to lovemaking, it's quality, not quantity, that's important.

Invest in your relationship

Investing in your relationship as a couple will be just as important once your baby is born. The demands of parenthood, work, and social life can often mean that partners start to take their relationship for granted. If that happens, you may begin to lose sight of what you both want and need from each other. So you should always make sure to find regular time for just the two of you throughout the coming weeks, months, and years.

60% of new moms say that having a baby has strengthened their relationship with their partner. It takes time for a couple to adjust to their roles as parents but for many it strengthens the bond they share.

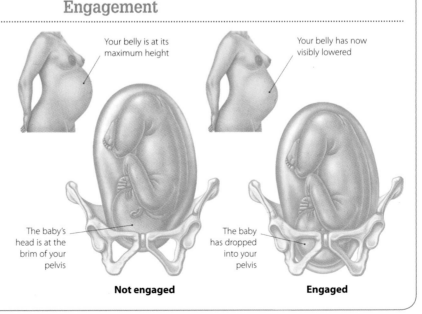

Engagement

During these last few weeks of pregnancy, your baby's head will drop down into your pelvis, ready for the birth.

A sense of relief

As your baby's head engages, you will find that eating and breathing become easier as your baby frees up space for your lungs and stomach. However, walking may become increasingly uncomfortable—some women even say it feels as if the baby is going to fall out. (But don't worry, it can't happen.)

You may also feel as if you need to go to the bathroom more as your baby squashes on your bladder. Practicing your Kegel exercises (see p.135) can help.

Your belly is at its maximum height

Your belly has now visibly lowered

The baby's head is at the brim of your pelvis

The baby has dropped into your pelvis

Not engaged

Engaged

Getting ready for pregnancy

Staying safe and healthy

Your pregnancy diary

Birth and beyond

Your body at **39** Weeks ▼

39 Weeks

✳ These last few days will probably drag as you wait impatiently for the arrival of your baby.

✳ You and your partner might try relieving the tension with a little love-making. It might get labor started.

With your baby about to arrive any day, it's an exciting time, but you're probably a bit apprehensive too. How will you know when you've started labor? What will happen if the baby comes suddenly?

Last-minute fears

It's perfectly normal to feel anxious as the big day draws near. You may have heard some childbirth horror stories, or believe that all labors start a certain way and progress at a certain rate. The truth is, every single birth is different.

Feeling in control

Some of the most common fears women have about childbirth are worrying about being able to deal with the pain, losing control during labor, and any problems arising that might require medical intervention. That's why it's a good opportunity to use these last few days to review your birth plan in case you've missed anything. Make sure it's clear in your head and talk to your birth partner about it, too, so he's sure about his role during the birth.

If you still have any last-minute worries about the forthcoming birth, speak to your doctor—she is the most qualified to put your mind at rest.

The countdown continues…

You're probably as big as you're going to get now, and likely to be feeling tired and uncomfortable with it. Your uterus fills your entire pelvis and abdomen and, with all the excitement of baby's imminent arrival, you may be finding it increasingly difficult to sleep at night. Try to make up for it during the day, and put your feet up whenever you can.

Remember, too, that the days leading up to the birth can be a confusing time for any other children you may have. Involve them as much as possible in the preparations and excitement to help manage their natural feelings of jealousy (see p.219).

Finally, don't worry if by the end of this week you're still waiting—only a tiny proportion of babies are born on their due date, many are born later. You and your partner might try relieving the tension with a little lovemaking—sex has been known to get labor started. It is thought to stimulate the uterus during orgasm into triggering the release of oxytocin, the "contraction" hormone. Semen also contains a high concentration of prostaglandins which help to prepare the neck of the uterus for labor. But if passion is the last thing on your mind, don't worry—your baby will be born in her own sweet time.

▼ Your baby at **39** Weeks

Your baby's about to greet the world! But don't worry if you're still waiting.

✳ Only 5 percent of babies are born on their due date and a whopping 75 percent are born later. She's still building a layer of fat and is shedding the greasy, white substance which has been protecting her skin. It's likely she already measures about 20 inches and weighs a bit over 7 pounds—a mini watermelon.

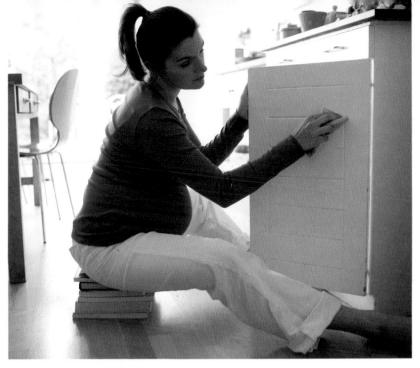

Suddenly feeling the urge to clean every surface in sight could mean that your baby's birth is just around the corner.

Signs of labor

Pregnant first-time moms often worry they won't know when they're in labor. Here are the signs you should watch out for:

● Persistent lower back or abdominal pain, often accompanied by a crampy premenstrual feeling.

● A bloody show (a brownish or blood-tinged mucus discharge).

● Painful contractions that occur at regular and increasingly shorter intervals and become longer and stronger in intensity.

● Broken water, but you're actually in labor only if it's accompanied by contractions that are making your cervix dilate.

The nesting instinct

As well as the physical signs, of labor (see Signs of labor, above right) a very common clue that labor is just around the corner is the sudden emergence of the "nesting instinct." If you're close to your due date and find yourself frantically cleaning out drawers, organizing cupboards, and dusting like crazy, it may be that you'll soon be welcoming your baby into the world.

Nesting is probably prompted by your pregnancy hormones and the instinctive desire to prepare the "nest" for the new arrival. In the animal kingdom female animals and birds have similar patterns of cleaning and preparation before they give birth. By having the house spotlessly clean, your baby's room ready, and all her clothes organized, you are ensuring that she will have the best chance for growth and survival once she is born.

Don't worry if you haven't had a nesting instinct—many women are simply too tired and worn out by now! But if you do find yourself packing and repacking your hospital bag, cleaning every room, or rearranging your kitchen cupboards, don't push yourself too hard. Rest frequently and eat regular, healthy meals. Remember, you'll need your energy for labor and the wakeful nights that lie ahead…

Meanwhile, plan something good to do each day so you have something (else!) to look forward to.

ParentsAsk...

I've heard about stripping the membranes. What is it?

Stripping or sweeping the membranes can be a way of bringing on labor. While not exactly controversial, not all doctors or midwives will do it. If your doctor feels it is needed, she can strip the membranes while she examines you internally. She simply "sweeps" a finger around your cervix. The aim is to separate the membranes around your baby from your cervix. This releases hormones called prostaglandins, which may help to kick-start your labor.

Membrane stripping is usually offered only if your cervix is already a bit dilated and there's no urgent reason to induce. It is typically done during an office visit.

Membrane stripping can be uncomfortable because the cervix is often hard to reach. It doesn't increase the risk of infection to you or your baby.

| FIRST TRIMESTER | SECOND TRIMESTER | THIRD TRIMESTER |

Your body at **40** Weeks ▼

40 Weeks

❋ After months of anticipation, your due date rolls around, and… you're still pregnant.

❋ You still have a couple of weeks before you're considered to be having a "prolonged pregnancy."

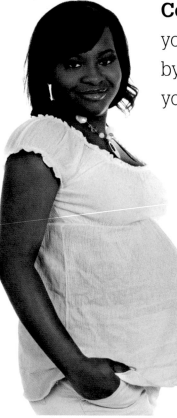

Congratulations! You've made it to the end of your pregnancy. If the last nine months have flown by, be prepared for time to slow down drastically as you count down the days to your baby's birth.

Your due date's arrived

So you've made it to your due date but there's no sign that your baby is on his way. You may not only be just plain fed up with the whole, long, drawn-out process, but also worried in case there is anything wrong. Well, first of all, calculating the due date isn't an exact science, so although you may think you're now overdue, you may not be yet.

But if you want to get labor going, there are a few old-fashioned remedies that you could try to kick-start your contractions. Unfortunately there is no research to show that any of these is effective, but there's probably no harm in trying a spicy food, a long walk, or making love (see p.206). If nothing else, they might well help you to relax.

▇ Your baby at **40** Weeks

His skull bones won't fuse until after he's born to help him through the birth canal.

❋ Mother Nature thinks of everything. Those unfused skull bones will be able to overlap a bit when he's going through the birth canal. This is the reason your baby's head may look a little cone-shaped after birth. Rest assured, it's normal and only temporary. The average newborn weighs 7½ pounds and is 20 inches long.

Parents**Talk...**

"As my due date came and went without so much as a hint my baby was on its way, I used the time to prepare for the chaotic weeks after the birth. I stocked up the freezer with dinners, spent lots of time with my feet up, went to the hair salon (since there was no way I'd have time for the next couple of months!) and enjoyed one or two last romantic evenings out with my husband before we were transformed into fatigued and disheveled versions of ourselves."
Chris, 34, mom to six-month old Ben

"When I got to 39 weeks I got obsessive about trying to bring on labor. I had as much sex as I could manage, ate fresh pineapple and spicy food, drank raspberry leaf tea, and walked and swam. And by 41 weeks it happened—a few days before I was due to be induced!"
Katie, 32, first-time mom

"I ended up being induced at 42 weeks. If you're overdue, don't worry—just take it easy and make the most of some time to yourself."
Frances, 28, mom to one-year old Alex

Still going strong

If you're still pregnant by 41 weeks, you'll have an prenatal appointment with your doctor. She will examine your belly to check the position and size of your baby and will do an internal examination to see if your cervix feels ready for labor. If you haven't had one already, she may offer to strip your membranes (see p.207) to see if this triggers labor. She'll discuss with you whether or not you want to be induced if stripping the membranes doesn't work. As an alternative to induction she may offer that you have your pregnancy monitored on a regular basis (see p.250).

By 42 weeks obstetricians usually recommend that you have an induction.

5%

of babies are actually born on their expected due date, while a whopping 75 percent are born later. So if you've gone beyond 40 weeks, don't worry. You're in the majority.

The reason for this is that the very small number of babies who die unexpectedly while they are still in the uterus increases after 42 weeks of pregnancy, and again after 43 weeks. However, do not be alarmed since the numbers are still extremely small.

Take your mind off things

For the time being, it's a good idea to try to have something planned for every day. Don't stay at home wondering whether you can feel anything happening. Get out of the house—but don't go too far! Make an appointment with the hairdresser and ask for a nice long head massage, or make an appointment for a pedicure. If you haven't already stocked up the freezer, do so now. Tell friends and relatives not to call every day to find out what's happening—say you'll call them when the big event has taken place.

A visit to the hairdresser will help take your mind off the fact that you've been pregnant for weeks and weeks and weeks!

If you can manage it, go for a few walks; it might get things started. Enlist the help of friends and family to keep you entertained—meet up for lunch, or invite them over for coffee.

But above all, rest, rest, rest. Labor requires a great deal of energy and stamina, so make the most of your last few days by putting your feet up whenever you can.

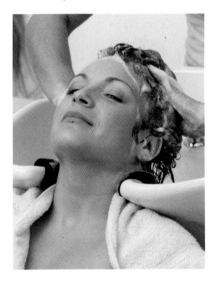

Your full-term baby

The average baby measures about 20 inches long from head to toe and weighs approximately 7½ pounds at birth, but anywhere between 5½ and 8½ pounds is a healthy range for newborns. Your amniotic fluid, once clear, is now becoming pale and milky as your baby sheds the vernix caseosa (the waxy coating that was protecting his skin). The outer layers of his skin are still continuing to slough off as new skin forms underneath.

In TV soaps, labor always begins with the water breaking—in the middle of a crowded room, of course—just

before contractions start. If you've been worrying that this scenario will happen to you, then stop.

Membranes rupture in less than 15 percent of pregnancies and, when they do, the baby's head tends to act as a cork at the opening of the uterus. You should stay calm—it may be hours before you feel your first contraction—and call your doctor right away. Your body will produce more amniotic fluid until the baby is born, so your caregivers may suggest you wait at home until contractions are under way or they may suggest an induction.

ParentsAsk...

What is a biophysical profile?

A biophysical profile (BPP) is an ultrasound that looks at your baby's overall movements, his breathing, and muscle tone, and the amount of amniotic fluid (important since it shows how well the placenta is supporting your baby).

After 40 weeks, fetal heart rate monitoring (called a nonstress test or NST) is usually also done. Or, you may have a modified BPP—an NST and an ultrasound to assess the amount of amniotic fluid.

If the fetal testing isn't reassuring, you'll be induced. If there's a serious, urgent problem, you may need to have an immediate cesarean.

Getting ready for pregnancy

Staying safe and healthy

Your pregnancy diary

Birth and beyond

Common concerns in pregnancy

Getting ready for pregnancy

Staying safe and healthy

Your pregnancy diary

Birth and beyond

It's natural to worry

Worrying is a way of coping with major life changes. Share your concerns with your partner, midwife, or doctor. Talk with other mothers at the same stage of pregnancy as you. They will understand how you feel.

Reassurance needed

Many pregnant women worry about how they'll deal with labor and whether their baby will be born healthy. It's normal to spend a few nights tossing and turning as you ponder best and worst-case scenarios. Your worries may continue during the day, too.

But if your anxiety starts to become all-consuming and regularly disrupts your sleep, then it's time for you to find a better way to deal with it. Share your fears with your partner—he's probably harboring similar concerns. Turn to friends or family for support. And of course, talk to your doctor, who should be able to reassure you.

If you're feeling extremely anxious or have a particular reason to be concerned about your baby's health, you may be able to arrange to have an ultrasound scan. Although this can't detect every potential problem, you may find it comforting to see even a fuzzy outline of your growing baby.

"Remember that **most babies** are born **completely healthy**."

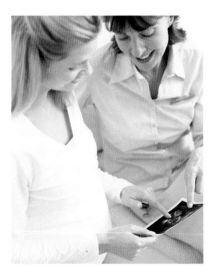

Of course, if your scan suggests that there is a problem, you will naturally be very worried. Rest assured that a range of specialists, from pediatricians to physical therapists, will be on hand to support and guide you through the options available. You can also be put in touch with community and nonprofit organizations that can help.

But remember—most babies are born completely healthy, so relax and enjoy your pregnancy!

Having an ultrasound scan can help allay any particular fears you may have. It's reassuring to see how your baby's growing.

ParentsAsk...

If I have a high-risk pregnancy do I have to stay in the hospital or stop work early?
Not necessarily. A high-risk pregnancy is one in which you or your baby are at higher than average risk of experiencing complications. For example, this might be if you have a preexisting medical condition such as a heart problem, previous pregnancy-related complications (such as cervical weakness), or a history of pregnancy loss.

Your pregnancy will be more closely monitored than usual and extra tests may be recommended. If complications do arise—or seem likely to arise—you may be advised to avoid strenuous activity and to rest as often as possible.

Dad's **Diary**

Is it "sympathetic pregnancy"?
"I've been feeling easily exhausted and sick to my stomach on and off for weeks. Friends say I should stop eating in fast-food restaurants, but could this be a sign of couvade syndrome or 'sympathetic pregnancy'? I've heard it's a controversial topic, since there hasn't been much scientific research on it. Of course, I don't want the doctor to scrutinize my body as well as Karen's, but maybe, on some level, I would like to be involved as much as possible in her pregnancy."

Baby-safety worries

Some drugs can be harmful to you and your unborn baby, but try not to worry if you took a headache or cold remedy before you knew you were pregnant. Chances are your baby will be absolutely fine—just exercise a little caution from now on.

Could I have harmed my baby?

It always pays to think twice before you take any medication while you're pregnant, but you may worry about medicines you took before you actually knew you were pregnant. These might include the pill.

Active mom

It's great to stay in shape but you should always listen to your body and don't overdo it.

"I've always been a bit of a fitness fanatic. Looking good and feeling healthy are both so important to me. Before I became pregnant, I went to the gym at least five times a week for an hour and a half. I'd feel guilty if I missed a session. When I found out I was expecting, I dropped down to four workouts a week but still really went for it. That's until my ninth week of pregnancy, when I woke up one morning to find I'd bled a little at night. My doctor asked me if I'd been overdoing it and I realized that I had. I spent the next three days in bed and, thankfully, the bleeding stopped and baby is well. I've since substituted the gym for the much more relaxing yoga."

In the past, when doses of hormones in the pill were higher, there used to be worries that getting pregnant while taking the pill, or just after stopping, would be harmful to the developing embryo. But more recent research has found no evidence of an increased risk of abnormalities.

Aspirin and ibuprofen aren't usually recommended in pregnancy, but if you have taken them—or cold remedies containing them—without knowing that you were pregnant, they are unlikely to

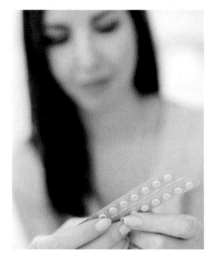

If you took the pill before you knew you were pregnant, don't worry. There's no evidence that it will cause any problems.

have harmed your baby. Acetaminophen is considered safe to use throughout pregnancy, as long as you stick to the recommended dosage and only use it occasionally.

Likewise, doctors advise against taking some of the ingredients in cough remedies, such as codeine, ephedrine, and phenylephrine, while you are pregnant. But they are unlikely to have harmed your baby if you have taken them unknowingly. From now on, though, just stick to a simple hot drink of honey and lemon.

Treatments to avoid

However, there are some treatments that are known to be potentially harmful to unborn babies. These include:
- Isotretinoin and accutone which are used to treat acne.
- Psoriasis drugs, such as acitretin and methotrexate.
- Mebendazole and other drugs used to eliminate pinworms.

If you have taken any of these while unaware that you were pregnant, or if you are taking medication for an ongoing condition, such as epilepsy or diabetes, talk to your doctor. The chances are that your baby is fine, but she can reassure you and order extra tests if necessary.

Has my baby stopped growing?

Sadly, just over one in 115 pregnancies ends in stillbirth in the United States. One of the first signs that something might be wrong is if you notice that your baby is moving significantly less than he was previously or has stopped moving completely. You may also have

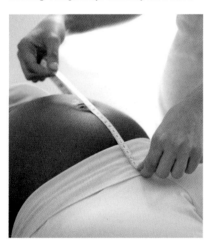

Measuring the height of the fundus (the top of the uterus) is one of the methods used for checking that your baby's growing.

vaginal bleeding. In some cases, the first sign that there is a problem is going into premature labor. If any of these things happens, you should contact your doctor immediately.

More than half of stillbirths are classified as "unexplained," which means that doctors are unable to identify the exact cause of death. However, some of the things that are known to cause stillbirths include a genetic or physical defect in the baby, placental abruption (when the placenta begins to separate from the uterus; see p.232), preeclampsia (see p.233), and infections, such as listeriosis, salmonella, or toxoplasmosis. When a baby dies before birth and premature labor doesn't

occur, labor may have to be induced. Some parents decide that they want to have the induction as soon as possible; others prefer to wait for a few days so that they have time to take in what has happened and to see if the labor starts naturally. Depending on the circumstances of your loss, you may be asked if you would like to see, touch, or hold your baby. Many parents find this extremely helpful.

Note: If you've had an unexplained stillbirth, it may be comforting to know that there is no increased risk of it happening again. However, if your baby was affected by a genetic abnormality, you may be referred for genetic counseling to assess the risks and discuss future options.

After a stillbirth

It may seem cruel that, at this time of shock and grief, there is paperwork to be done. However, some parents appreciate the formal recognition of their baby's existence and treasure the certificates that they receive.

- **Certificate** States typically issue a death certificate, but no birth certificate, for stillborn babies. In recent years, however, several states have begun to offer stillbirth certificates as well.
- **Burial or cremation** Hospital staff and your doctor will be able to put you in touch with counselors and others who can advise you as you make necessary decisions after a stillbirth. One decision will be whether to have a stillborn baby buried or cremated. Parents may also

want to place a notice in the births or deaths column of the local newspaper.
- **Take your time** Don't feel pressured to make decisions too quickly. Your baby's body will be kept safely by the hospital until you have decided what arrangements you wish to make. Many parents take photographs or videotape their baby.
- **Saying goodbye** There is no obligation to hold a service before burial or cremation. You can say goodbye to your baby in almost any way you choose. This could mean letting the hospital make all the arrangements for you, or holding a religious or non-religious, traditional, or personally designed ceremony.

Dad's **Diary**

Anxious times

"There's nothing worse than suddenly thinking there might be something wrong with your baby. We had a worrying time at around 22 weeks when Laura hadn't felt the baby move for a couple of days.

She tried lying down on her side in a quiet room—nothing. She tried drinking a very cold drink—still nothing. We called the doctor and she reassured us that the baby might have shifted to a position where his movements wouldn't be felt. But to be on the safe side, she also made an appointment for the next day so that she could listen to the baby's heartbeat. Everything was absolutely fine—but it was an anxious wait before the appointment."

Getting ready for pregnancy

Staying safe and healthy

Your pregnancy diary

Birth and beyond

Worries about birth defects

Discovering that your unborn baby has a birth defect is devastating, but it does give you and your doctors the chance to plan her care before she's born. Some defects may be corrected soon after birth, but others have lifelong implications for your baby and your family.

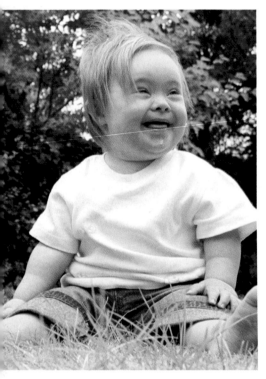

It's a shock to have a baby with Down syndrome but support groups offer help and put you in touch with other parents.

Fact: Spina bifida is becoming an increasingly rare condition— mainly because pregnant women are now advised to take folic acid supplements (see p.49) to prevent neural tube defects.

Will my baby be normal?

Every parent-to-be worries at some point about whether or not their baby is going to be born normal. Luckily, serious birth defects are rare and prenatal care is so good now that problems often get picked up well in advance of your baby's birth. But, although serious defects are rare, it's wise to be aware of the kind of problems that can affect babies. Below are some of the more common ones.

Heart defects
Some heart problems are detected during a prenatal ultrasound scan. Others are picked up during your baby's newborn examination when the doctor hears a heart murmur—unusual sounds that blood makes as it passes through the valves and blood vessels of the heart.

Most heart murmurs are completely normal or "innocent" and cause no symptoms. However, some are a sign of a heart defect. Serious heart defects may need surgery. Many children make a complete recovery and can lead a normal life afterward. Others may need more surgery when they are older.

Cleft lip and palate
A cleft lip is a split in the upper lip between the mouth and nose caused because separate areas of the face did not join properly during pregnancy. A cleft palate happens when the roof of the mouth has not joined completely. Clefts sometimes run in families.

A cleft lip is usually repaired by surgery by the time a baby is two to three months old. A cleft palate is usually repaired by the time a baby is a year old. Like the lip repair, the surgery is performed under general anesthetic.

Babies born with clefts can have problems with latching on to the breast or sucking on a nipple, which can make feeding difficult. However, a feeding specialist should be able to help you feed your baby successfully.

Down syndrome
Down syndrome is a genetic condition that affects just over one in every 1,000 babies born in the United States. We don't know what causes Down syndrome, but there is a definite link with older mothers.

Children born with Down syndrome all have a degree of learning disability, but this will vary from child to child. They also have certain physical characteristics. For example, your baby may have looser muscles and joints than other babies and she may possibly have a lower than average birth weight. Babies with Down syndrome often have

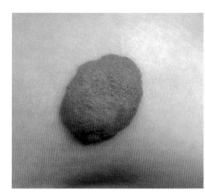

Strawberry marks are thought to be caused by abnormalities in the way blood vessels have developed. They are harmless.

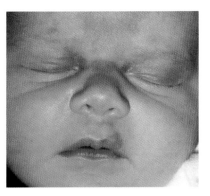

Many babies are born with "stork marks" or "angel kisses." They're nothing to worry about and will eventually disappear.

eyes that slant upward and outward. Their eyelids may have an extra fold of skin that appears to exaggerate the slant. Many babies with Down syndrome also have a single crease on their hands, which runs right across the palm.

Spina bifida

Spina bifida is when the spinal cord doesn't fully close, leaving a gap. There are three types: spina bifida occulta (hidden) is the most common and mildest form, myelomeningocele is the most serious, while spina bifida meningocele is less serious than meningomyelocele and is the most rare form.

It is estimated that approximately 5 to 10 percent of people may have spina bifida occulta without realizing it. Around one in 800 babies is born with myelomeningocele, the most serious form of spina bifida.

Spina bifida can be picked up either during a routine ultrasound scan or following a blood test. Babies with severe spina bifida will need surgery during the first two days after birth to repair the gap in the spinal cord. Some doctors do not use surgery but let the area heal on its own.

Birthmarks

Birthmarks are markings on your baby's skin that may be permanent or may fade away over time. The most common are caused by tiny blood vessels just beneath the skin. These small red, mottled spots are sometimes called "stork marks" or, when they're on the forehead or eyelids, "angel kisses." They are harmless and usually disappear in a few months but, sometimes, over years. Other birthmarks can be caused by abnormalities in the blood vessels.

The most common birthmarks are strawberry marks—raised, crimson marks that develop on about five percent of babies—and port-wine stains—flat red or purple marks ranging in size from a few millimeters to several centimeters in diameter. About three in 1,000 babies are born with this type of birthmark, often on one side of the face. Port-wine stains can be lighter with laser therapy.

Congenital moles are another type of birthmark. These can be brown colored in fair-skinned babies, to almost black in dark-skinned babies. Some are raised or hairy.

Most birthmarks don't cause any physical problems, but it's worth showing the birthmark to your doctor to monitor it.

Organized mom

Finding out your baby has a heart defect is a shock, but there is lots of help available.

"We discovered that our baby had a heart defect at our 20-week anatomy scan. The sonographer told us that he suspected she had a ventrical septal defect—a hole in the heart. We were referred to a cardiac specialist, who confirmed the diagnosis. Fortunately, we were told that the hole was quite a small one, which might heal by itself once our baby was born. But she'll need regular checkups to make sure the hole is getting smaller and there's also a chance that she might need heart surgery to correct the problem when she's a little older.

It's really frightening to be told that your baby has something wrong with her heart. I found it much easier to deal with it once I knew all the facts. Our doctor gave us some information to take home with us and there are lots of websites and support groups for parents of children with heart defects. It also helped to talk online to other parents in a similar situation."

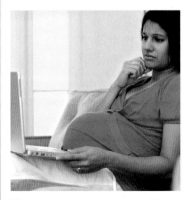

Most parent support groups will have a website and a helpline to give you information and advice.

Getting ready for pregnancy

Staying safe and healthy

Your pregnancy diary

Birth and beyond

Worries about labor day and after

Whatever stage of your pregnancy you're at—but especially in those last weeks—your head is bound to be full of worries about what exactly will happen on labor day and how you'll cope. This is all perfectly normal. The key is always to be well prepared.

ParentsTalk...

"I got very excited a week before my due date when I started to have contractions. These felt different and stronger than the Braxton Hicks contractions. After five hours, they were about five minutes apart and becoming more painful. I phoned my husband at work and told him to come home immediately. An hour later I was at the hospital. And that's when the contractions stopped! My cervix hadn't dilated at all. The nurse said it was just my body getting ready to have my baby. I gave birth two weeks later."

Kim, 28, mom to two-month-old Ryan

"I'd been having very strong contractions for about two hours when Ken and I got in the taxi. Then I suddenly had the most overwhelming urge to push. Even the panic in the driver's eyes wasn't going to stop me! He pulled over and he and Ken made me as comfortable on the back seat as they could while they called an ambulance. I gave birth before the paramedics arrived, though."

Helena, 32, second-time mom

Worries about the day

If you're having a hospital birth, you may well be wondering whether or not you'll reach the hospital or birthing center in time. Providing that you've prepared well, you'll have nothing to fear. Those preparations include making sure that your hospital bag is packed (see p.201) and that your car has a full tank of gas. Also check that your partner or friend has figured out the best route to the hospital, and if you're planning on taking a cab, make sure you've set your phone to speed dial the taxi company number. The last thing you want to do is to have to rummage around trying to find the number between contractions.

And if you're planning a home birth, rest assured that your baby is unlikely to arrive before the midwife does! That only happens in very few cases. To be

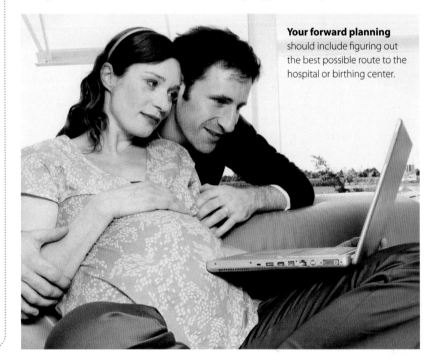

Your forward planning should include figuring out the best possible route to the hospital or birthing center.

on the safe side though, all moms-to-be should read pp.292–3 for tips on how to manage if your baby decides he's in a hurry to make an appearance.

Labor and after

You may also have worries about the labor itself. Will you be able to deal with the pain? Will you make a fool of yourself in labor? How will your partner manage? Will they follow your birth plan? What happens if you have complications and need a cesarean? How long will you stay in the hospital?

When these worries trouble you, take a few deep breaths and just visualize yourself holding your new baby. If you find that hard, take a look at those tiny baby clothes you have ready. That will remind you why you are on this journey.

Will my breasts do the job?

If you're not generously endowed in the breast department, don't worry about your ability to breast-feed. Most differences in breast size are about the different amounts of fat in the breasts. You need milk-producing and storing tissue to make milk, and this is laid down in pregnancy. Most women find this means their breasts do get bigger, especially toward the end of their pregnancy. Even with this extra growth, some women still have smallish breasts at the end. They are just as likely as anyone else to breast-feed effectively.

Flat or inverted nipples shouldn't cause difficulties with breast-feeding, either, though you may find you are a little sore in the early stages. Preparing your breasts before birth with breast shells or nipple-rolling exercises seems to make little difference. In any case, you often find that flat nipples stand out when your baby nurses because of the drawing-out action of his jaws.

Like all new moms, you'll need help latching your baby onto the breast for the first few feedings. He has to learn how to open his mouth wide so that he draws in a deep mouthful of breast. Discuss this with your doctor or the La Leche League before you deliver, to be sure you get the right help once he is born.

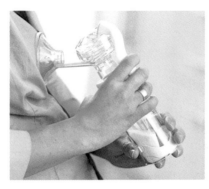

Flat or inverted nipples can sometimes be drawn out if you use a breast pump before feedings.

If you do experience problems, using a breast pump before feedings may help to draw out inverted nipples. And avoid engorgement as much as possible so that your baby can "practice" while your breasts are soft. Speak to your doctor or breast-feeding consultant if you need help with this.

10%
of women have flat or inverted nipples but this won't prevent you from breast-feeding. If one nipple is flatter than the other, your baby may prefer the more accessible side, but persevere.

ParentsAsk...

What's my risk of getting an infection at the hospital?

The risk of contracting an infection in a maternity unit is very low. Hospital-acquired infections, such as MRSA—or methicillin-resistant Staphylococcus aureus—are more likely to occur in patients who are elderly or very ill, or who have an open wound from an operation. Maternity ward patients tend to be young and healthy.

You can minimize your chances of infection. Anyone attending you or your baby, or simply visiting, should wash their hands thoroughly or use alcohol-based hand sanitizer before touching or examining you.

If you get an IV or catheter, be sure it's inserted under sterile conditions. Your skin should be sterilized at the site of insertion, and the person performing the procedure should wear clean gloves.

If you're concerned about germs on surfaces in your room, such as the telephone, table, or TV remote, ask the hospital staff to wipe them down.

Your temperature will be taken frequently to monitor for fever, which can be a sign of infection. If you have a cesarean, be sure to ask your doctor about caring for your postsurgical incision and about signs of infection.

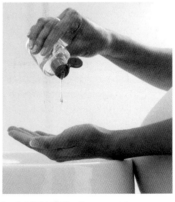

In the hospital, take precautions to reduce the risk of infection.

Getting ready for pregnancy

Staying safe and healthy

Your pregnancy diary

Birth and beyond

Different moms, different worries

Becoming a parent isn't always easy. And if you are a young parent, you may find that the changes ahead are even more challenging. Make sure you build a strong support network around you and take any offers of help (including financial) that you are given.

Concerns of very young moms

If you're still only in your teens, one of the most difficult aspects of pregnancy is the sense of isolation. Your parents' first reaction to the news may have been shock or rejection, rather than delight. You may also be the first in your group of friends to be pregnant and feel as if you have little in common with them any more, which can make you feel very lonely. Pregnancy can be scary and confusing at the best of times. But having no one to confide in and share the experience with can make dealing with the big physical and hormonal changes doubly difficult.

Not only that, but expecting a baby in your teens can disrupt your school or college studies. It could even force you to postpone or abandon your career dreams. If you have a partner, you might also worry that having a baby on the way will put too much pressure on your relationship, and that your partner may leave you to bring up the baby alone.

But with the right support you can overcome many of these challenges. Often, after the initial shock, parents come around to the idea of their own "baby" being pregnant. A supportive mom or dad helps to ensure you get the right prenatal care. Teachers, too, can push for special provisions to help you continue your studies if possible.

Financial help for young moms

One of your concerns if you're very young and pregnant may well be money. Don't despair. Financial help is available if you know where to look for it. Each state has its own welfare program, so eligibility requirements and benefits vary according to where you live. Here are some of the programs you might be eligible for:

● **Temporary Assistance for Needy Families (TANF)** This supports very low-income families by providing monthly cash assistance.

● **Food** If you need food for you and your baby, you can apply for aid through the Women, Infants, and Children program, or WIC. Local food banks can also help you put nutritious food on your table.

● **Medicaid and the Children's Health Insurance Program** These can help ensure you have access to medical care.

● **Early Head Start programs** These aim to promote prenatal care for pregnant women, development of very young children, and healthy family functioning. Look for programs operating in your area.

● **Child Care Assistance** To find out if you qualify for this, visit the National Child Care Information Center website to contact your state agency.

For more help, get in touch with your state child welfare agency, public health department, and education department to find information and programs.

 ### Single mom

If you're single and pregnant, you may feel lonely and worried. Try turning to a best friend.

"Being single and pregnant is really scary. I always imagined I'd be sharing this experience with someone I loved, and who loved me. I've been feeling very lonely and have been panicking about money as well. I have some savings and a job that'll provide good maternity pay, but I'm still concerned I'll struggle while I'm on leave. Above all, I'm terrified of being alone when I go into labor. Luckily, my best friend has offered to move in with me for the last couple of weeks of my pregnancy."

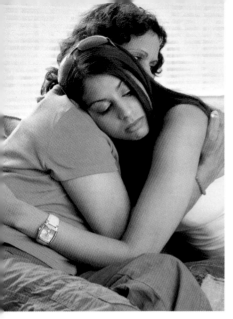

Parents may be shocked at first, but most will eventually offer the support you need.

And your friends and partner can help by just listening and being there for you through your emotional ups and downs.

Remember—all new moms struggle. But with youth on your side, you probably have more energy than most to deal with the physical demands of pregnancy and having a child!

ParentsTalk...

"I dreaded telling my mom and dad I was pregnant. Having a baby at 15 certainly hadn't been part of my life plan. I couldn't believe my parents' reaction, though, when they found out. They just hugged me and told me not to feel anxious because they were going to support me every step of the way."
Meg, 17, mom to two-year-old Ben

"My mom and dad weren't pleased when I told them I was pregnant at just 16. When they'd had time to take it all in and realize how scared I was, though, they became much more supportive. They were with me at every scan and my mom was my birth partner. I just know that I could never have got through it without their help."
Bella, 17, mom to three-month-old Dee

"I became pregnant at 18 and was so worried I was going to lose my friends because all our nights out revolved around drinking and clubbing. They were amazing, though, and organized more DVD nights and lunches, specially for me. Now that my son is here, one of my friends will often offer to babysit so I can have a night off and go out with the others."
Sophie, 19, mom to four-month-old Josh

"I was absolutely terrified since I was expected to take my SATs the week my baby was due. My English teacher was amazing, though, and arranged it so I could take them a year later. I'm happy to say that my SAT scores were good, and thanks to my mom's help with my lovely baby, I'm planning to go to college!"
Amy, 18, continuing in education

Concerns of second-time moms

If you're already mom to a toddler, you may wonder how he's going to take to being an older sibling. It can be hard for him but you can ward off upsets by telling him about the coming birth.

Four or five weeks before is a good time to talk to your toddler. Explain what will happen once the baby arrives, and get him involved in the preparations. For example, invite him to help you make simple decisions, such as whether he thinks the baby would prefer bunnies or ducks on the nursery curtains.

Once your baby comes home, try to involve your toddler in taking care of her. He can help you hold towels or get

diapers. When she cries, he can sing or talk gently to her. Ask him for advice and help, too: "Do you think the baby would like to wear her red hat or her white one?" And set aside some time each day to do something just with him, even if it's only a few minutes of drawing or building with blocks.

Your toddler will sometimes feel jealous. Don't be surprised if he hits or throws something at his new sibling. Make sure you prevent him from hurting the baby, and encourage him to talk about how he feels. Tell him that it's natural to feel this way, but make it clear that trying to hurt the baby is not okay.

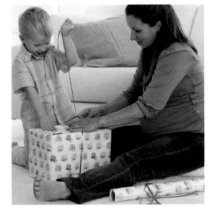

Inviting your toddler to get involved in preparing for your new baby's arrival can help him get used to the idea.

Getting ready for pregnancy

Staying safe and healthy

Your pregnancy diary

Birth and beyond

Recurring pregnancy problems

It's very normal to feel anxious at certain points in your pregnancy, particularly if you experienced problems last time around. Keep in mind that every pregnancy is different and you and your baby will almost certainly be fine. If you do feel concerned, talk to your doctor.

I've had a problem pregnancy before

If you had difficulties with your last pregnancy or birth, it's natural that you might feel a little anxious this time around. Try to remember that this experience is different. Also, try to stay positive and look forward to your future with this baby.

Miscarriage

Most women who have had a miscarriage (see pp.42–3) go on to have healthy pregnancies. Even women who have had unexplained recurrent miscarriages (three or more in a row) have about a 75-percent chance of having a healthy pregnancy next time.

When you have had a miscarriage, it's normal to worry that you might lose this baby, too. It may be particularly stressful up to the stage where you lost your baby last time. You will probably feel more sad and anxious as the date approaches, and that's perfectly normal and understandable. Don't be too hard on yourself for not feeling happy all the time, especially during the first weeks. Allow yourself to vent your feelings; a good cry now and then will help to relieve a lot of tension.

Stillbirth

If you've had an unexplained stillbirth, it may be comforting to know that there is no increased risk of it happening again. But of course you will want to take every precaution to make sure this baby is healthy. Eating well (see pp.48–51, 120–21, 148–9, and 182–3), quitting smoking, drugs, and alcohol (see pp.118–19) and taking care of yourself are the best ways of protecting your baby. You may have extra prenatal appointments and tests as well, partly to reassure you and partly to pick up any problems early. And your doctor will understand if you need to check out any twinges or spotting immediately.

Cesarean

If you had a cesarean section (see pp.288–91) last time, you may wonder about a vaginal birth this time. Occasionally there is a recurring problem (such as having a very small pelvis), which means you have to have another cesarean.

Parents**Talk...**

"I had a miscarriage six months ago when I was nine weeks pregnant with my first child. I was so scared when the bleeding started and, as the hours ticked by, it gradually became heavier and heavier. I called my doctor and a scan revealed that I had lost my baby. I never even knew if I was having a boy or a girl, although for some reason I feel strongly that it was a boy. I'm now in the early stages of my second pregnancy and I feel so nervous that I'm going to lose this one, too."
Renée, 28, pregnant for a second time

"I had high blood pressure when I was pregnant and, at 30 weeks, they found protein in my urine. I had to have an emergency cesarean and Aiden was whisked off to the Neonatal Intensive Care Unit. I found it hard to bond because it was ages before I could hold him. I'm scared it'll end up the same this time. I got plenty of exercise and got my diet on track before I became pregnant this time, though, and, so far, thank heavens, my blood pressure has been fine. Fingers crossed!"
Joanna, 31, mom to Aiden

About 75 percent of women who choose to have a vaginal birth after a first baby by cesarean (VBAC) go on to have a successful vaginal birth. If you have had a previous vaginal birth, you will have an even higher success rate—it can be up to 90 percent.

You also have a better chance of a vaginal birth if you previously had a cesarean for one of these reasons since they are unlikely to reoccur:

- Your baby was in the breech position (see pp.286–7).
- Your baby was becoming tired and distressed during labor.
- Your labor happened very slowly.
- Your induction failed.
- You requested a cesarean.

Doctors do tend to be a bit more cautious during labor if you have previously had a caesarean section. This is because there is a very small risk (one in 200) of the scar from your last cesarean tearing during your contractions. This is called uterine rupture. It will probably mean that you and your next baby will be monitored closely during labor.

Premature baby

If you have had a premature baby (see pp.280–81) before, you are slightly more at risk of having another premature

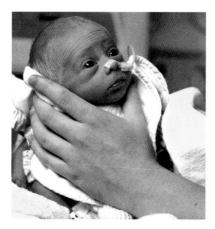

baby. That can be a worrying thought, but the risk only increases a little. The general rate of premature births for all women is about 10 percent, but if you have had a premature baby before, it rises to about 20 percent. But, of course, you may be one of the lucky 80 percent of women who do not go on to have another premature birth.

Having had a premature birth already means your awareness of what might happen will play an important role in monitoring your new pregnancy, particularly when you get to the same stage in pregnancy when your last premature labor started. That increased awareness also means you can be extra careful with your diet, can stop smoking and other risky activities, and make sure you get to all your prenatal appointments.

If you've had a premature birth, there is a slight risk that you will have another one. You'll be better prepared the second time.

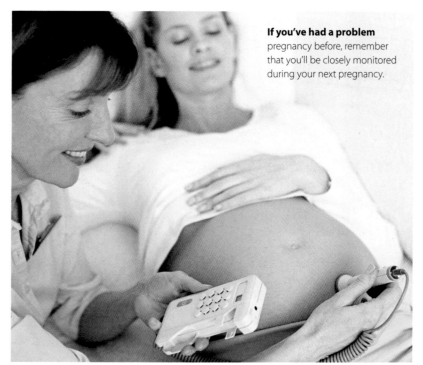

If you've had a problem pregnancy before, remember that you'll be closely monitored during your next pregnancy.

Dad's **Diary**

Fourth time lucky?

"After having three miscarriages (two in the second trimester) in the past two years, my wife and I can't help but worry that this pregnancy might end the same way. Leandra had a vaginal scan early in this pregnancy and it revealed that she may have a weakened cervix. The doctor advised us to have a cervical stitch inserted as a precautionary measure after 14 weeks. We know it doesn't work for everyone, and that there are risks involved, but it has made us feel more positive that we'll carry this baby to full term.

We're still extremely cautious, though. It's hard for Leandra—and me!—not to worry about every twinge or if she gets any vaginal discharge. We're regularly in touch with our doctor. She's given us a lot of support, and we're not afraid to call her if we're at all worried."

Genetic disorders

Having a genetic disorder may mean that you need extra care during pregnancy. It could also mean that your baby is affected by the same disorder as you, so you and your partner will have some serious thinking to do. Your doctor will support you with this.

I've got a genetic disorder

If you have a genetic disorder, you may feel anxious about whether or not your baby will be affected. You are probably already an expert on your condition. Talk with your specialist or doctor to see if it may affect your baby.

Thalassemia

Thalassemia is a genetic blood disorder that causes the body to make fewer healthy red blood cells and less hemoglobin (the iron-rich protein in red blood cells). If you have thalassemia during pregnancy, you might be more prone to iron-deficiency anemia (see p.229). Certain kinds of thalassemia can affect blood test results, causing them to indicate that your iron reserves are low when they are not. As a result, you should have additional blood tests to confirm that you are iron-deficient before you take iron supplements. If you have thalassemia, you will also benefit from taking 5 milligrams (mg) of folic acid a day.

Your baby can be tested for thalassemia during pregnancy using a diagnostic test, such as chorionic villus sampling (CVS; see p.136) or amniocentesis (see p.147). If you or your

---

ParentsAsk...

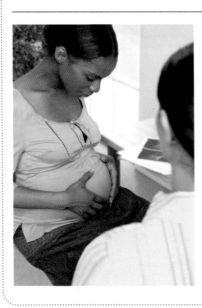

Should I seek genetic counseling?
You may want to talk to a genetic counselor before you try to become pregnant if you, your partner, your children, or any other family member has an inherited condition, such as cystic fibrosis or sickle-cell anemia.

A genetic counselor is a medical professional who can help you sort through complex information about your chances of having a child with a genetic disorder or birth defect and about the testing, treatment, and other options available. The counselor's role is to explain the technical and scientific information you need to understand to make informed choices.

If you are already pregnant and your baby has been diagnosed with a genetic disorder through prenatal testing such as CVS (see p.136) or amniocentesis (see p.147), there will

be a counselor available to offer you support and guidance. Genetic counselors have been trained to work with you and your family to help you absorb, digest, and understand information. They can put the risks in perspective by giving you information and helping you articulate your feelings.

Genetic counselors won't make any decisions for you, nor will they suggest that you follow any particular course of action. A good counselor will explain to you the outlook for a child with an abnormality and will describe the treatments that might be necessary, both immediately after birth and throughout the child's life. Once you have understood all the facts, it will be up to you to decide what to do.

Carrier screening

Carrier screening is a special type of testing that's done to find out whether you or your partner carry a genetic mutation that could cause a serious inherited disorder in your baby. Some of the more common disorders that are screened for include cystic fibrosis, sickle-cell disease, and thalassemia.

These disorders are recessive, which means that a person must inherit a defective gene from each parent to have the disease. If you're a carrier of a defective gene for a recessive disorder, that means you have one normal copy of the gene from one of your parents and one defective copy from the other. (Carriers don't usually have any symptoms of the disease.)

If both you and your partner are carriers of a disorder such as sickle-cell disease or cystic fibrosis, your child will have a one in four chance of inheriting one defective gene from each of you and of having the disease. This is why some people choose to find out if they are carriers for certain diseases.

Risk factors include having a family member with the inherited disorder (or a family member who's a known carrier) or being part of an ethnic group at increased risk for the disease.

If you opt for this kind of screening, you'll probably be asked to give a blood or saliva sample first. Then, if you're found to be a carrier, your partner will be screened also. (Both partners may be screened at the same time to get the results faster.)

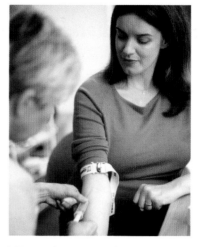

You can have a screening test to see if you are a carrier of a genetic mutation that might be passed on to your baby.

---

baby is tested for thalassemia you will be offered some counseling so you can make informed medical and personal decisions.

Cystic fibrosis

Cystic fibrosis (CF) is an inherited condition that affects the internal organs, especially the lungs and digestive system, by clogging them with thick, sticky mucus. This makes it hard to breathe and digest food.

If you have CF, pregnancy shouldn't adversely affect your health provided your CF is mild to moderate. If it is severe, you are more likely to develop pregnancy complications. It is important to continue your treatment for CF throughout your pregnancy to get the best outcome for both you and your baby. Sign up for prenatal care as soon as possible so an appointment with an obstetric team that has experience in CF can be made for you early on. They will monitor the growth and

development of your baby, and will review and adjust your medication if necessary. If both you and your partner are known to be carriers or affected by CF, you will usually be offered a diagnostic test, such as CVS (see p.136), during pregnancy, to see if your baby is also affected.

Sickle-cell anemia

Sickle-cell anemia is an inherited condition. People affected by it have abnormal hemoglobin, which causes their red blood cells to become misshapen or "sickled." These sickled cells then get stuck in the tiny blood vessels, blocking the flow of blood and producing pain.

For sickle-cell anemia to affect your child, both parents must carry the gene responsible for sickle cell, and are usually Asian, African, Caribbean, Mediterranean, or from the Middle East.

It is possible to test an unborn child for sickle cell from as early as 11 weeks

50%

is the chance that a baby who has one parent

with thalassemia minor has of inheriting the gene defect from the parent and of also being a carrier. Babies who inherit the gene disorder from both parents have a double dose of the gene and can sometimes have thalassemia major.

of pregnancy by using tests such as amniocentesis (see p.147) and CVS (see p.136). Fetal blood sampling may be carried out after amniocentesis if results suggest further testing may be needed. Your doctor will be able to give you more information.

If your baby has sickle cell, he may need to take penicillin every day to prevent infections. Children with sickle-cell disorder also need folic acid to help them make blood and prevent them from becoming run down.

Getting ready for pregnancy

Staying safe and healthy

Your pregnancy diary

Birth and beyond

Medical problems in pregnancy

Some women bloom during pregnancy, feeling better than ever, but for others it can be a time of discomfort and worry. You and your baby are vulnerable to common infections, and your body may no longer feel your own, as you adapt to the physical changes of pregnancy.

There are many physical conditions that are linked with pregnancy that are neither serious nor lasting, but which can make life when you're pregnant a bit of a drag. During pregnancy your body has to adapt to the changes in your hormone levels, your circulation, and the increasing weight that you're carrying. These changes are great for taking care of your baby, and preparing for labor, but some of them may not feel quite so great for you.

Physical changes

Inside your abdomen, everything shifts to make room for your growing baby. Your organs and bowels are squashed up or pushed to one side, and you'll feel extra pressure on your bladder or stomach depending on your baby's position. It's amazing how your body adapts but it can be an uncomfortable experience, causing pain, indigestion, and incontinence.

The blood volume in your circulation increases during pregnancy and the tissues in your muscles and joints also take on more fluid. You may notice some swelling in your ankles and other parts of your body.

The hormone relaxin (see p.74) makes your ligaments and joints more mobile and flexible, so there is room for your baby to move through your pelvis during labor. The down side to this is that it can make some parts of your body too loose, resulting in pain, and problems with your pelvis and other joints. Pregnancy hormones also have an effect on the walls of your veins and arteries, which is why varicose veins and hemorrhoids are another common complaint of pregnancy. All these physical changes can be uncomfortable, painful, and embarrassing, but most of them will clear up in the hours, days or weeks following your baby's birth.

Infections in pregnancy

Infections can be much more significant during pregnancy. First, your immune system doesn't work so well so you're more vulnerable to them. Second, you may find it harder to get rid of an illness. Third, you're more likely to develop complications with some infections, which you'd have sailed through if you weren't pregnant. Finally, an infection that is fairly harmless to you may be dangerous for your growing baby.

Some infections only cause a problem if you catch them at a certain stage of pregnancy. For some infections, there are treatments that can reduce the risk of harm to your baby while, for others, you just have to wait and see if your baby is going to be okay. In many cases, there are things that you can do to prevent you getting an infection in the first place, such as avoiding certain foods (see pp.52–3) and following good personal hygiene. You may also already be immune to some infections, so your baby will be protected by the antibodies in your blood.

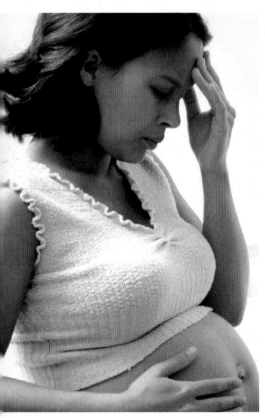

The changes in your body during pregnancy help your developing baby, but may make you feel unwell.

Infections

Chicken pox

Chicken pox is a mild but highly infectious disease that usually affects children. If you had it as a child, you probably have no reason to worry. Your body will have developed antibodies to the virus, making you immune to further infection. However, if you think that you've never had the virus before, you should avoid contact with people with chicken pox. This is because the virus can lead to serious complications for you and your baby. You also need to be aware that you can catch chicken pox from someone who has shingles, which is a related condition caused by the same virus as chicken pox.

Causes Chicken pox is an illness caused by the varicella-zoster virus (VZV). It usually spreads via sneezes and coughs from an infected person.

Symptoms The most common symptom of chicken pox is a red rash. Other symptoms may include nausea, fever, and aching, painful muscles. Chicken pox can be more severe if you catch it while pregnant, and you are more likely to develop dangerous complications, such as pneumonia.

There are other potential problems if the virus affects your baby during pregnancy or as a newborn. These may include eye problems and shortened limbs. Possible neurological problems may also mean your baby is slow to reach his developmental milestones.

Treatment Your doctor may offer you hyper immune globulin, a concentrated antibody that reduces the severity and duration of chicken pox. Alternatively, if it's been no more than 72 to 96 hours since you were exposed to chicken pox, you may get a shot of varicella zoster immune globulin.

Amniocentesis can show whether there are signs of the virus in your amniotic fluid, but this does not necessarily mean that your baby was infected. Your doctor may arrange for you to have a detailed ultrasound scan to check that your baby's vital organs look healthy.

Cytomegalovirus (CMV)

At least 50 percent of women already have antibodies to CMV before they get pregnant, meaning they were previously infected. Most people with CMV don't develop any symptoms, so you probably wouldn't know if you'd ever been infected.

Causes CMV is a common virus that is part of the herpes family of viruses. It's spread through bodily fluids such as saliva and urine, and can be transmitted from person to person through close bodily contact.

Symptoms Most people don't know when they have a CMV infection. Those who do know tend to have symptoms such as fever, swollen glands, and a sore throat. You may also feel tired and achy.

CMV is the virus most frequently passed to babies during pregnancy. About 1 to 4 percent of previously uninfected women have a first (or primary) CMV infection during pregnancy. Among these women there's about a 30 to 50 percent chance that the baby will become infected in the uterus.

Most babies won't have any symptoms at birth or develop any CMV-related problems later on. However, some babies born with CMV are very sick at birth and may end up with a number of long-term problems. Others may seem fine initially but develop hearing loss or other complications months or sometimes even years later.

Treatment There are blood tests to check for CMV, but you would only have one in certain circumstances, for example, if you suspect you've recently been exposed to CMV. If the blood tests show that you've had a recent infection, you'll get a thorough ultrasound to look for CMV-related abnormalities in your developing baby or the placenta. You may also have amniocentesis to see if your baby has CMV, but this test won't tell you whether your baby will develop health problems from the infection.

Fifth disease

The chances are that you've already had fifth disease, since most people are exposed to the virus in childhood some time between the ages of three and five. Fifth disease is also called slapped cheeks disease.

Causes Fifth disease is passed from person to person in saliva, through close contact or via the air, such as through coughing and sneezing. It is highly contagious and can spread quickly through schools or day-care centers.

Symptoms In children, fifth disease may cause mild respiratory symptoms, which are sometimes accompanied by a temperature. A distinctive blotchy red rash may begin to appear on the face, which gives the appearance of "slapped cheeks." Once the facial rash has appeared, the disease is no longer contagious.

Adults may have no symptoms at all, or they might experience a sore throat, headache, itching, or fever. Very occasionally, slapped cheek disease causes painful joints.

It's rare but, if caught between nine and 20 weeks of pregnancy, the virus can cause a condition called hydrops fetalis in unborn babies. This is when

Getting ready for pregnancy

Staying safe and healthy

Your pregnancy diary

Birth and beyond

an unusual amount of fluid builds up in a developing baby's tissues and organs, and it can be picked up by an ultrasound scan. Sometimes a baby can recover from this condition on her own and is born healthy but, occasionally, she may need a blood transfusion to improve her chances of survival.

Treatment A blood test will be able to determine if you're immune, but can't tell whether you have been exposed to the disease during your pregnancy or many years ago.

If you think you've been exposed, you will be offered extra ultrasounds because your risk of miscarriage and other complications is higher. If your baby develops hydrops fetalis, a blood transfusion in the uterus may help.

Flu

The flu (or influenza) is a viral disease of the lungs and upper airways. The symptoms of the flu—fever, headaches, chills, achiness, fatigue, and loss of appetite—can really lay you low when pregnant. This is your body's way of telling you that you need to take it easy.

Causes The flu virus is usually spread in the small droplets of saliva coughed or sneezed into the air by an infected person. Direct contact can also spread infection. It takes an average of two days to go from being infected to having the full symptoms.

Symptoms The main symptoms are a high temperature that comes on quickly, and general aches and pains. You may also experience a loss of appetite, nausea, and a harsh dry cough. Your symptoms will usually peak after two to three days and you should begin to feel much better within five to eight days.

Treatment If you develop flulike symptoms, speak to your doctor. It's important to keep your temperature as normal as possible while you are

pregnant, so avoid the temptation to sweat it out snuggled under a comforter. Acetaminophen helps to lower fever and is safe to take at the recommended dose. Make sure you drink plenty of water and juice, get plenty of rest, and give yourself time to recover completely before picking up your daily routine again. Always ask your pharmacist's advice before buying over-the-counter cold and flu remedies since some are not appropriate for pregnant women.

The flu vaccine used in the United States is prepared from an inactivated virus and there is no evidence that it's harmful to unborn babies. The US Centers for Disease Control recommend that all pregnant women receive a seasonal flu shot.

Genital herpes in pregnancy

If you suffer from genital herpes there is a very small risk that your baby will catch the infection and, if she does, the results can be serious. That's why it is important to tell your doctor if you or your partner have ever had genital herpes. Extra care can then be taken of you and your baby.

Causes Genital herpes is usually caused by herpes simplex virus type 2 (HSV-2). It's usually spread during sexual activity.

Symptoms Most people with the herpes simplex virus (HSV) do not experience any symptoms when they are first infected. If you do get symptoms, they may include:
● Painful sores over your genitals and buttocks.
● Itching, burning, painful, or tingling sensation in the groin area.
● Stinging when passing urine.
● Vaginal discharge.
● Swollen glands in the groin area.
● Flulike symptoms including fever, headache, and aching muscles.

With a second or later infection you may get no symptoms at all, or just a small area of irritation.

Treatment If you catch genital herpes for the first time in the first or second trimester of your pregnancy, there is a slight risk of complications such as miscarriage, intrauterine growth retardation (IUGR), and premature labor. Your doctor will probably give you a five-day course of an antiviral medicine, usually acyclovir. This is safe to use during pregnancy.

Your baby is at greater risk if you catch genital herpes for the first time in late pregnancy. She can catch the virus through direct contact with an active sore during birth. If you suspect you have an active genital herpes infection in the last trimester of pregnancy it is vital that you tell your doctor. You may be advised to have a planned cesarean section to minimize the risk of transmitting the virus to your baby. If you caught herpes early in your pregnancy, and it has been successfully treated, you will still be able to have a vaginal birth.

Group B streptococcus

Group B streptococcus, also known as group B strep or GBS, is one of the many bacteria that normally live in our bodies. In certain rare cases GBS can cause serious illness and even death in newborn babies.

Causes Approximately one third of us "carry" the GBS bacterium in our intestines without knowing. About a quarter of women also have it in their vagina. Most don't know it's there, but it can spread to your baby during birth and cause a serious infection.

Symptoms Because GBS usually causes no symptoms, pregnant women often find out that they have it by chance, perhaps when they have a vaginal swab taken to check for something else.

Most babies exposed to GBS before or during birth also suffer no ill effects. However, one or two babies in 200 born to GBS-positive mothers in the United States develop a GBS infection. Sadly, about one in 20 of these babies die. GBS infections in babies usually happen within seven days of birth, with 90 percent occurring within 12 hours of birth. Typical signs of GBS in newborns include: grunting when breathing, poor feeding, lethargy, irritability, low blood pressure, and an abnormally high or low temperature, heart rate, or breathing rate.

Treatment If you are found to be carrying GBS, talk to your obstetrician and agree to a pregnancy and birth plan that will protect your baby from the infection. Women are tested at 36 weeks and, if positive, will be given IV antibiotics either from the start of labor or from when their water breaks (whichever comes first) until their baby is born. They also might be prescribed oral antibiotics if they have diagnosed GBS prior to 36 weeks.

If your baby is at higher risk of developing a GBS infection, a pediatrician should examine him immediately after he is born. He may be put on intravenous antibiotics until he's given the all clear.

Hepatitis B

Hepatitis B is a virus that can cause chronic inflammation of the liver. It can also be transmitted to your baby at birth. If you have an acute attack of hepatitis B during pregnancy, or if you are a carrier, you will be at risk of premature labor.

Causes Hepatitis B is spread via the blood or body fluids from someone who has the virus. Many people with hepatitis B do not even realize that they

are infected. Because hepatitis B is transmitted through blood and body fluids and especially during sexual intercourse, those most at risk are people who have had unprotected sex with several different sexual partners, drug users who use intravenous drugs, people who have been tattooed with dirty needles, and health professionals who may come into contact with the blood of an infected person.

Symptoms An infected person may be jaundiced so that their skin and the whites of their eyes have a yellowish tinge. Sometimes the symptoms are simply loss of appetite and stomach pain, which are difficult to distinguish from the flu or a mild bout of food poisoning.

Treatment When you go for your initial blood tests, your doctor will probably take a blood test for hepatitis B. If it shows that you are a carrier, you may be referred to a specialist for advice. Since carriers are at risk of liver disease, you should continue to receive follow-up appointments after you have given birth.

Your baby will be washed thoroughly after he is born to remove all traces of your blood and he will be treated immediately with hepatitis B vaccine within 12 hours of birth. These precautions almost always prevent the infection from being passed to your baby. If he is not treated, your baby risks going on to develop serious liver disease.

HIV and AIDS in pregnancy

HIV stands for human immunodeficiency virus. Most people who have HIV do not have any symptoms and the only way of telling they are infected is by testing their blood for antibodies. AIDS stands for acquired immune deficiency syndrome. People develop AIDS when their immune system has been so damaged by the HIV virus that they

start to catch lots of other infections.

Causes The HIV virus is passed from person to person during sex and through body fluids, such as blood and breast milk. It can also be passed from a woman to her unborn baby during pregnancy and birth.

An unborn baby has about a one in four chance of catching HIV if his mother is HIV positive and does not receive any treatment or interventions to stop the virus.

Symptoms When you first catch the HIV virus you may experience symptoms such as a fever, sore throat, fatigue, and swollen glands. These symptoms are often very mild, so it is easy to mistake them for another condition, such as a cold. After these initial symptoms, you will probably have no other symptoms for years.

Eventually, though, the virus will damage your immune system, leading to symptoms such as chronic fatigue, night sweats, weight loss, diarrhea, and shortness of breath.

Treatment Most women who are HIV positive are identified before or during pregnancy. If you are HIV positive, you'll should have specialist care and regular checkups. You'll also be offered treatment in the form of anti-retroviral drugs. These interventions can greatly reduce the chance of your baby catching the infection from you during pregnancy and birth.

Having a cesarean reduces the risk of your baby catching HIV during the birth, but if your HIV is well managed then a vaginal birth may not increase the risk to your baby.

Rubella (German measles)

Rubella is a relatively mild illness for most people but it's very dangerous for pregnant women since it can lead to all sorts of problems in your baby.

Getting ready for pregnancy

Staying safe and healthy

Your pregnancy diary

Birth and beyond

Fortunately in the United States, the majority of women in their childbearing years are immune to the disease, either because they were vaccinated against it as a child or because they have already had the illness. Between 2001 and 2005, there were a total of 68 reported cases of rubella and five reported cases of rubella-related congenital problems in babies born in the United States.

Causes Rubella is a very infectious disease. The virus is passed on via droplets in the air from the coughs and sneezes of infected people. It used to be common in young children.

Symptoms Rubella causes a pinkish red rash that first appears on the face and then spreads elsewhere on the body. Other symptoms—which usually appear before the rash—include a temperature, conjunctivitis, and swollen glands. Up to half of people don't get any symptoms.

When an unborn baby is affected, it has what is called congenital rubella syndrome (CRS). This can lead to:
- Cataracts and other eye defects.
- Deafness.
- Heart abnormalities.

- Restricted growth.
- A smaller head than normal (microcephaly).
- Damage to the brain, liver, lungs, and bone marrow.

Luckily, due to the high rate of the rubella vaccine, CRS is now very rare.

Treatment If you know that you are not immune to rubella, you should, if at all possible, be vaccinated before you become pregnant. If your lack of immunity has been picked up from a blood test in early pregnancy, you'll have to wait until you've had your baby before you can be vaccinated.

Unfortunately, if you do catch the disease during pregnancy, there's nothing that can be done to protect your baby. Your doctor will talk to you about what tests can be done to find out whether your baby has been affected. Sadly, you may want to consider terminating the pregnancy.

Urinary tract infections (UTIs)

About 50 percent of women will have at least one UTI during their lifetime. If left untreated, UTIs can be quite painful—and even dangerous because the infection can travel upward and reach the kidneys. If a kidney infection is left untreated during pregnancy it could make you very ill and could lead to your baby being born with a low birth weight or being born prematurely.

Causes A UTI is caused when bacteria infect the urinary system. The changes your body goes through during pregnancy make you more susceptible to UTIs. Progesterone relaxes the muscles of your ureters, the tubes that connect your kidneys to your bladder. This slows down the flow of urine from your kidneys to your bladder. Your enlarging uterus has the same effect. This is an ideal opportunity for bacteria because they have more time to grow before they're flushed out.

Symptoms Signs of a UTI can include pain when passing urine, a feeling that you are unable to urinate fully, a raised temperature, and a frequent need to go to the bathroom. If the infection has spread to your kidneys you may have a high temperature and constant pain in the area of one or both of your kidneys.

Treatment UTIs can be safely treated with antibiotics during pregnancy. You will probably be prescribed a seven- to 10-day course. Talk to your doctor as soon as you notice any symptoms because an untreated UTI can lead to a kidney infection, which may in turn cause premature labor.

To reduce the risk of getting a UTI, wipe yourself from front to back after going to the bathrooom to prevent bacteria from the back passage being spread to the front passage. Drink plenty of fluids, and empty your bladder completely when you go to the bathroom. Wear cotton pants and avoid tights and pantyhose.

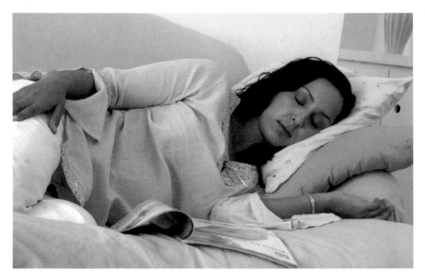

Certain infections don't put your baby at risk. You may just need to rest, drink plenty, and keep your temperature down. Check any medication is safe with your doctor.

Conditions in pregnancy

Anemia (iron deficiency)

During pregnancy, you need extra iron (see p.121) to keep you and your baby healthy. If you don't have enough iron for both of you, you may develop iron-deficiency anemia. One in five women develop this when they are pregnant.

Causes Women who have a diet that is low in iron (see p.149) are likely to become anemic. You are also more likely to have iron-deficiency anemia in pregnancy if your body's iron supplies have already been depleted, perhaps because you've had two or more pregnancies close together, or you had heavy periods before you became pregnant. If you're carrying more than one baby then the demands of each baby can also increase your risk of getting anemia.

Symptoms You may not be aware that you have become anemic, although fatigue and breathlessness are common signs. However, these are symptoms also experienced by many pregnant women who are not anemic.

Headaches, tinnitus, and palpitations are other symptoms of anemia, along with unusual food cravings. Your eyelids, nail beds and tongue may also look pale.

Unless you're severely anemic, you don't need to worry about your baby's health. Your body will make sure that your baby gets her quota of iron before you get yours.

Treatment You shouldn't need to take iron supplements if you make sure to have a diet rich in iron. This means eating lots of dark green leafy vegetables, whole-grain bread, iron-fortified cereals, lean red meat, raisins, prunes, and beans.

Vitamin C helps your body absorb the iron in your diet. Try drinking plenty of orange juice or eating fruit or vegetables that are rich in vitamin C when you have an iron-rich meal. This is particularly important if you don't eat meat since the iron in meat is easily absorbed, but iron in vegetables is not. Tea and coffee make it difficult for your body to absorb iron, so it's best not to drink them at mealtimes.

If your iron levels drop low your doctor will prescribe iron supplements.

Gestational diabetes

Gestational diabetes is diabetes that develops for the first time during pregnancy. It affects somewhere between 2 and 7 percent of pregnancies. Unlike other types of diabetes, gestational diabetes usually resolves itself after your baby is born.

Causes Diabetes develops when the body can't produce enough insulin, a hormone made by the pancreas. Insulin regulates the sugar in the blood. During pregnancy your body has to produce extra insulin to meet your baby's needs. If your body can't manage this, you will have too much sugar in your blood and may develop gestational diabetes.

You are in a high-risk group for developing diabetes in pregnancy if your body mass index (BMI; see pp.72–3) is above 30.

Symptoms Gestational diabetes often doesn't produce any symptoms, but you may experience the following:

- Fatigue.
- Excessive thirst.
- Passing a lot of urine.
- Blurred vision.

The main problem with having too much sugar in your blood is that it crosses the placenta to your baby, which means that there is a small risk that she could grow very large. A big baby may make labor and birth more difficult and you may end up needing to have a cesarean section.

Babies affected by too much blood sugar during pregnancy may have low blood sugar (hypoglycemia) or jaundice after birth. Babies born to mothers with diabetes are also more prone to obesity and type 2 diabetes later in life.

Treatment In most cases, you can manage the condition by changing your diet and getting regular exercise. In about 10 to 20 percent of cases of gestational diabetes, the condition can't be controlled by diet and exercise and you'll either need to take medication to control your blood sugar levels or to inject insulin.

Gestational hypertension

If you develop high blood pressure after 20 weeks of pregnancy and you don't have protein in your urine, you will be diagnosed with gestational hypertension (high blood pressure in pregnancy, as distinct from chronic hypertension). Gestational hypertension is usually diagnosed if you have two consecutive blood pressure readings of above 140/90.

Causes Caused by the extra stress that pregnancy places on your body, gestational hypertension is usually mild and probably won't cause any obvious problems for you or your baby. It is more common in women who are overweight. Around 10 percent of obese women (BMI of 30 or above; see pp.72–3) will have gestational hypertension, compared with around 4 percent of women with a BMI of 19 to 25.

Symptoms You probably won't notice any symptoms. However, the earlier in

Getting ready for pregnancy

Staying safe and healthy

Your pregnancy diary

Birth and beyond

pregnancy it sets in, the greater your risk of having a small-for-dates baby, or of it developing into preeclampsia (see p.233) The risk of preeclampsia is increased if you are obese or overweight, and have put on a lot of weight during pregnancy.

Treatment It's very important to go to all your prenatal appointments, because your doctor will take your blood pressure at each visit. If you have either gestational or chronic hypertension, she will monitor your health closely, and may prescribe drugs (which won't harm your baby) to lower your blood pressure.

If your blood pressure was normal before you became pregnant, it will most likely return to normal within 12 weeks of your baby being born. If it doesn't return to normal, then the original diagnosis of gestational hypertension will have been wrong. After performing tests, your doctor may then start treating you for chronic hypertension.

Hyperemesis gravidarum

Hyperemesis gravidarum literally means "excessive vomiting in pregnancy." Hyperemesis starts early, usually before week five of pregnancy. It may lessen around week 16 and end around week 20. Hyperemesis occurs in between approximately 0.5 and 2 percent of pregnancies.

Causes As with nausea and vomiting (see pp.237–8), a variety of factors are likely to be involved, including hormone changes. You are at greater risk of hyperemesis if you:
- Are expecting twins or more.
- Are the daughter or sister of a hyperemesis sufferer.
- Had hyperemesis in a previous pregnancy.
- Have a history of motion sickness or migraines.

- Have liver disease.
- Have thyroid abnormalities.

Symptoms You are said to have hyperemesis if you are vomiting many times a day, are unable to eat and drink without vomiting, and if you are losing weight. The usual treatments won't have helped, and you'll be struggling with normal life.

Treatment Your doctor may prescribe nausea medicine that is safe to use in pregnancy.

If you cannot keep food or fluid down, swallowing pills is also likely to be difficult. Some nausea medication is available as a suppository, in buccal form (dissolved between upper lip and gum), or it can be injected.

It can be a matter of trial and error to find the drug that works for you. Antihistamines are usually given first, since they have the strongest safety record in pregnancy. If these don't help, you may be offered Zofran. Steroids (such as dexamethasone) are rarely used for hyperemesis.

You may be admitted to the hospital to for rehydration and/or tube feeding if you cannot drink or eat, and continue to lose weight.

Low amniotic fluid (oligohydramnios)

Oligohydramnios means having too little amniotic fluid in your uterus. About 8 percent of all pregnant women are found to have low amniotic fluid at some point, usually in their third trimester.

Causes Experts don't always know what causes low amniotic fluid. The most common cause is your water breaking early. Oligohydramnios is more common in summer months so may be due to maternal dehydration. It has been found that drinking plenty of water may boost levels of amniotic fluid. You'll also want to make sure to eat well and rest.

There are other causes of oligohydramnios, each requiring its own treatment. These may include placenta problems and fetal abnormalities.

Symptoms Your doctor may suspect this problem if:
- You are leaking fluid.
- Your baby is "small for dates."
- On examination, the outline of your baby is easily felt.
- You have had a previous baby whose growth was restricted.
- You have chronic high blood pressure.
- You have diabetes (see p.23).
- You have lupus (see p.23).

To find out what's going on, she'll send you for an ultrasound.

Treatment Oligohydramnios is most commonly diagnosed later in the third trimester, when it usually requires nothing more than keeping a close watch on things. You may need to have your baby's heart rate monitored regularly and ultrasound scans to closely watch your baby's development until you give birth. If your water has broken early you may need antibiotics to reduce the risk of infection.

If your doctor is concerned about your baby's growth, it may be safer for your baby to be born early than to remain in the uterus. If you are near your due date and your doctor thinks your baby's growth is poor, she may decide to induce labor.

Obstetric cholestasis

Obstetric cholestasis, sometimes called OC, affects the liver and causes intense itching. This itching usually begins during the last 10 weeks of pregnancy, although it can start much earlier. Women describe it as constant and sometimes intolerable.

Causes It seems that, in some women, the liver is oversensitive to pregnancy hormones. Bile is produced in the liver and normally it flows down into the intestines. If you have OC, the flow of bile is reduced and so bile salts build up in your blood.

If you have a family history of OC and your mother or sisters were affected, you are more likely to suffer from it yourself.

Symptoms The main symptom is itching, which is usually worse at night so can result in fatigue and insomnia. It often begins on the palms of the hands and the soles of feet and can become generalized. Less commonly, women can develop jaundice. The itching completely disappears within a couple of weeks of giving birth.

Careful management of OC is important to prevent stillbirth. In the past, the stillbirth rate for women with OC was about 15 percent higher than in normal pregnancies but, if well managed, the risk can be reduced to about the normal rate of 1 percent.

Treatment Two drugs are currently used to manage OC. Ursodeoxycholic acid, also known by brand name Actigall or generic name Ursodiol, appears to eliminate or reduce the itching and can result in the liver function and bile acid results returning to normal. Steroids (in particular, dexamethasone) can also be considered, but need careful management.

Mothers with OC may be at risk of bleeding after the baby is born. This is because bile is needed to absorb vitamin K from food, and vitamin K helps the blood to clot. For this reason, in some hospitals, the mother is given vitamin K daily by mouth until delivery to protect her from this small risk of bleeding. The baby is also protected by the vitamin K.

Pelvic pain

The joint at the front of your pelvis may be more mobile during pregnancy, causing inflammation and pain. This is known as symphysis pubis dysfunction. This loosening may also lead to related conditions, including diastasis symphysis pubis, in which the gap in the pubic joint widens too far, and pelvic girdle pain, which is thought to be caused by instability of the sacroiliac joint at the back of the pelvic girdle.

Causes It's thought that pelvic pain in pregnancy is due to the effects of the pregnancy hormone relaxin. This softens the ligaments of your pelvis to help your baby pass through the birth canal as easily as possible. Unfortunately, this loosening effect can also cause instability, inflammation, and pain.

Symptoms Pain in the pubic area and groin are common symptoms. But you may also have:
- Back pain, pelvic girdle pain, or shooting pains in your buttocks or down the backs of your legs.
- Weakness in your legs.
- A grinding or clicking sensation in your pubic area.
- Pain down the insides of your thighs.
- Worse pain at night.

Treatment Treatment of pelvic pain in pregnancy may include exercises, especially for the abdomen and pelvic floor muscles. These are designed to improve the stability of your pelvis and back. You may need some gentle, hands-on treatment to correct any stiffness or imbalance. Exercise in water can sometimes be useful and a pelvic support belt can also give quick relief. You should also be given advice on how to make your everyday activities less painful and on how to make the birth of your baby easier.

Acupuncture, chiropractic, and osteopathy may also help, but you must make sure that your practitioner is trained and experienced in working with pregnant women.

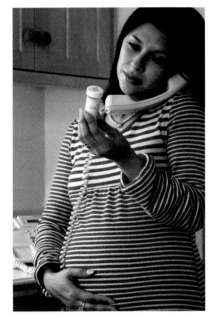

You should not take any medication during pregnancy unless you have checked that it is safe for you and your baby.

Placenta previa

Placenta previa (sometimes called low-lying placenta) is when the placenta covers part or all of the cervix after 20 weeks. About one in 200 pregnant women have this problem. If you have an ultrasound scan in early pregnancy and the placenta seems to be near, or even covering, the cervix, don't be too alarmed. As your baby grows, your expanding uterus usually pulls the placenta away from your cervix.

Causes Women who are having their second or subsequent baby are more at risk of placenta previa than women having their first. Also slightly more at risk are women who smoke, women who have had a cesarean, women who are expecting twins or more, and women who have previously had a pregnancy during which placenta previa occurred. However, most women with placenta previa do not usually have any obvious risk factors.

Symptoms Painless vaginal bleeding during the last three months of pregnancy is often a warning sign and you should call your doctor immediately if this happens. However, there may be no warning signs at all and the fact that you have placenta previa may only be discovered while you are having a routine ultrasound scan.

Treatment This depends on whether you're bleeding and how far on in your pregnancy you are. If the condition is diagnosed after 20 weeks, but you're not bleeding, you'll probably just be advised to take life easy. If you're bleeding heavily, you will be admitted to the hospital so that the bleeding can be monitored.

Uncontrolled bleeding (hemorrhage) is life threatening for both mother and baby, although this is rare. If the bleeding doesn't stop, or if you go into premature labor, your baby will need to be delivered by cesarean section even if your due date isn't for quite a few weeks.

Placental abruption

A placental abruption is a serious condition in which the placenta partially or completely separates from the lining of your uterus before your baby is born. Placental abruption happens in about one in 200 pregnancies. It is most common during the third trimester of pregnancy.

Causes No one knows exactly what causes placental abruption, but there are certain conditions that make it more likely, including cocaine use, having had an abruption in a previous pregnancy, high blood pressure (hypertension), preeclampsia, and too much amniotic fluid (polyhydramnios).

Symptoms Usually, you will have some vaginal bleeding, ranging from a small amount to an obvious and sudden gush. The bleeding is usually dark, without blood clots. Sometimes, though, the blood stays in the uterus behind the placenta, so you might not see any bleeding at all. You're likely to have some abdominal or back pain and your uterus will feel tender.

Call 911 immediately if you're losing a lot of blood or have any signs of shock—if you feel weak, faint, pale, sweaty, or disoriented, or your heart is pounding.

When you get to the hospital, your baby's heart rate will be monitored and you'll probably have an ultrasound scan.

Treatment If you're near your due date, your baby will need to be born immediately, even if the abruption is minor, because the placenta could separate more at any time. In most cases you'll have a cesarean. If the abruption is severe you may have lost a lot of blood. You'll be given oxygen, extra fluids and a blood transfusion through an IV in your vein.

If your doctor suspects that you have a minor abruption and your baby is very premature, you may be able to delay the birth a bit, as long as you and your baby are doing well and there is no further active bleeding.

Polyhydramnios

Polyhydramnios means having too much amniotic fluid in the uterus. It occurs in less than one percent of pregnancies in the United States.

Babies regularly swallow the amniotic fluid and it is passed out of their bodies as urine. In this way, your

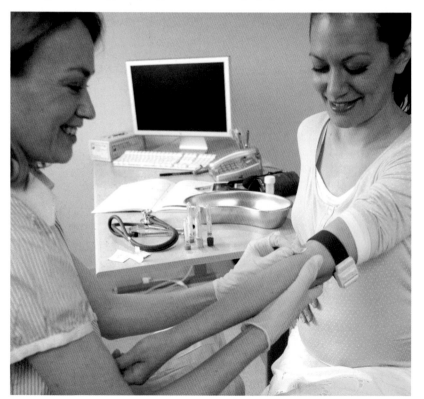

Some medical conditions don't have any symptoms, but are picked up during your regular prenatal examinations.

baby controls the volume of amniotic fluid around her. When this delicate balance is disturbed, the amniotic fluid can increase rapidly.

Causes It can be difficult to identify the cause of polyhydramnios and, sometimes, no cause can be found. It may be that the extra fluid is due to a problem with the baby, or with the placenta or with you, the mother. Possible causes include having diabetes, being pregnant with twins or infections, such as rubella.

Symptoms Polyhydramnios usually starts from about the 30th week of pregnancy. You may feel that your belly is getting too large too quickly and that your skin is stretched and shiny. You might feel so breathless that it is hard to climb a flight of stairs. Other symptoms include abdominal pain, severe heartburn and constipation, swollen legs, and varicose veins.

Treatment Your doctor will order a high-resolution ultrasound to check for abnormalities and possibly an amniocentesis to test for possible genetic defects.

You'll also need to have regular nonstress tests and ultrasounds for the rest of your pregnancy, and you'll be watched closely for signs of preterm labor. If you haven't yet been tested for gestational diabetes, you'll be tested now.

You'll need to head to the hospital early in labor, and right away if your water breaks.

Preeclampsia

Preeclampsia is a pregnancy-induced condition, which usually occurs in the third trimester. It is characterized by high blood pressure, swelling that happens suddenly along with rapid weight gain due to fluid retention, and protein in the urine. Since it reduces the flow of blood to the placenta, preeclampsia can be quite dangerous for your unborn baby.

Causes The cause of preeclampsia is not known but there are recognized risk factors. You're more likely to get preeclampsia in a first pregnancy or if there is a big gap, usually of at least ten years, between this and your last pregnancy. You are also more at risk if you are 40 or older, were very obese at the start of your pregnancy, or have a chronic problem that affects your blood system, such as kidney disease.

Symptoms Occasionally preeclampsia develops very quickly. Don't hesitate to call your doctor if you have any of the following symptoms in the second half of pregnancy or in the first few weeks after birth:

- Sudden swelling of your face, hands, or feet.
- Intense headaches.
- Blurred vision or flashing spots before your eyes.
- Severe pain in the upper part of your abdomen.
- Vomiting.

Treatment If your blood pressure is moderately raised, you will be advised to have as much bed rest as possible, lying either on your left-hand side because this improves the flow of blood to the placenta, or sitting well-propped up. Your doctor will check your blood pressure very often.

If your blood pressure becomes very high, you might be admitted to the hospital so that your condition can be monitored. You may also be given magnesium sulphate injections.

Rhesus incompatibility

People who are rhesus positive, or RhD positive, have a protein known as D antigen on their red blood cells. People who don't have the D antigen are known as RhD negative. Rhesus status only matters if an RhD-negative mother is carrying an RhD-positive baby. If some of your baby's blood gets into your own bloodstream, your immune system may react to the D antigen in his blood and produce antibodies against it.

If you become pregnant again and your new baby is also RhD positive, the antibodies you now have in your system can attack your baby's blood cells, causing anemia, jaundice, or, in severe cases, heart or liver failure in your baby.

Causes You may have antibodies in your blood if you have had a termination or an ectopic pregnancy (see pp.44–5), or if you have had vaginal bleeding or a miscarriage after 12 weeks of pregnancy. There is a chance that your and your baby's blood may come into contact during chorionic villus sampling (CVS; see p.136), amniocentesis (see p.147), external cephalic version (ECV; see pp.286–7)—performed to turn breech babies to a head-down position—or after a hard blow to your abdomen.

Your and your baby's blood will almost certainly come into contact with each other at the birth, particularly if you have a traumatic birth, a cesarean, or a manual removal of the placenta.

Symptoms You will not usually notice any symptoms.

Treatment Rhesus antibodies can be prevented by Rhogam, which is usually injected into your shoulder. The antibodies quickly destroy any Rh positive fetal blood cells in your circulation and prevent your body from making antibodies. All pregnant RhD-negative women should be offered a single dose injection at 28 to 30 weeks of pregnancy. You'll also need a shot within 72 hours if you have any reason to suspect your blood might have mixed with your baby's, in any of the scenarios described above.

Getting ready for pregnancy

Staying safe and healthy

Your pregnancy diary

Birth and beyond

Minor/temporary complaints

Backache and back pain

Backaches are a problem for many people, but during pregnancy it can be caused by pregnancy hormones that have a relaxing effect on your joints and ligaments. Supporting the weight of your belly also means there's more strain on your back.

What can I do?

- Avoid heavy lifting.
- Improve your posture.
- Don't sit or stand in one position for long periods.
- Wear a well-fitting, supportive maternity bra.
- Wear comfortable shoes.
- Avoid crossing your legs.
- Leave your desk regularly at work and get some fresh air.
- Make yourself comfortable when you are driving.
- Get gentle exercise, such as walking, swimming, and yoga.
- Do Kegel exercises.
- Use a hot pack.
- Try a support pillow in bed.
- Sleep on your side.
- Use a support belt.

What can my doctor do?

- Refer you to a physical therapist, if necessary.

Bleeding gums

Bleeding, sensitive gums are also known as gingivitis. During pregnancy, the pregnancy hormones play a part. They can make your gums swell and become inflamed. Then, when you floss or brush, your gums may bleed.

What can I do?

- Continue to floss and brush regularly, but gently.
- Use a soft brush.
- Brush your teeth twice a day for two minutes using fluoride toothpaste.
- Use an electric toothbrush—the action of an electric brush is more effective at removing plaque.
- Floss or use interdental brushes at least three times a week.
- See your dentist regularly.
- Quit smoking.
- Use a mouthwash (check with your doctor or pharmacist for one that's safe to use in pregnancy).

What can my dentist do?

- Arrange to have a dental hygienist have your teeth properly scaled and polished to remove plaque.

Breathlessness

During pregnancy you may find you are short of breath, particularly when you exert yourself physically. It is a problem that can start in the first trimester, but sometimes not until the second trimester. Later, as your baby grows, he pushes up against your diaphragm, which can also contribute to your breathlessness. Don't be alarmed. Breathlessness in pregnancy is normal and harmless. In the early stages, it is thought to be caused by changes in the levels of carbon dioxide that occur in your system during pregnancy.

What can I do?

- Try getting some light exercise— if you are out of shape, you are more likely to feel breathless.
- If you notice any other alarming symptoms, such as chest pain, palpitations, a racing pulse, or clamminess in your fingers and toes, call your doctor.

What can my doctor do?

- Test you for anemia.
- Adjust your asthma medication if you have asthma (see p.22).

Constipation

Difficulty in having a bowel movement can strike whether you are pregnant or not. During pregnancy, it's likely to be caused by the pregnancy hormone progesterone, which relaxes and slows down the movement of your intestines. In late pregnancy, it might be compounded by the pressure of your uterus on your rectum.

What can I do?

- Always go to the bathroom when you first feel the urge.
- When going to the bathroom, give yourself plenty of time and privacy.
- In the morning, or half an hour after a meal, are good times to try to have a bowel movement.
- Don't take iron supplements unless necessary.
- Avoid drinks that make you want to urinate more, such as tea or coffee.
- Drink eight glasses of water a day.
- Start the day with a cup of warm water with a slice of lemon in it.
- Begin each meal with a salad or fruit.
- Eat high-fiber foods, fresh fruits, and vegetables daily.
- Get gentle exercise, such as walking, cycling, and yoga.

What can my doctor do?

- Advise you on your prenatal vitamins, especially if they contain iron.
- Prescribe a laxative that is safe for you to use, if necessary.

Which complementary therapies can I try?

- Acupressure
- Acupuncture
- Aromatherapy
- Chiropractic
- Osteopathy
- Reflexology
- Tai chi

Dizziness

You may feel dizzy and possibly nauseous in the first and second trimesters of your pregnancy. This is caused by normal changes that occur in your circulation during pregnancy. In the second trimester, your growing uterus can put pressure on blood vessels and this can contribute to your dizziness. You might also feel dizzy if you haven't eaten for a while, if you've become overheated, or if you stand up too quickly.

What can I do?

- Sit down!
- If you're in a stuffy office or a crowded train, try to get some fresh air.
- If you haven't eaten for an hour or two, a quick, healthy snack will help boost your blood sugar levels.
- Try drinking some water or juice.
- Get up slowly and smoothly, instead of springing up from a chair or bed.

What can my doctor do?

- Check you in case you have an underlying problem, such as anemia or low blood pressure.

Fatigue

Fatigue and exhaustion are common during pregnancy as your body works hard to develop your baby. They are also caused by your changing hormone levels and metabolism. Low blood pressure and blood sugar levels can be factors, too.

What can I do?

- Basically, get as much rest as you can, when you can.
- Take catnaps and go to bed early.
- Eat a well-balanced diet with plenty of fruit, vegetables, and protein.
- Try not to skip meals, especially breakfast.
- Have regular, healthy snacks.
- Eat foods that are high in iron, such as red meat and dark green vegetables.

- Avoid energy-sapping junk food.
- Drink at least eight glasses of water a day.
- Ask your family to help you with the housework.
- Shop online.
- Get plenty of gentle exercise and fresh air.
- Socialize with your friends at lunchtime, instead of in the evenings.

What can my doctor do?

- Unfortunately, nothing, although he may check for anemia. The fatigue should pass after the first trimester, but may return in the third.

Which complementary therapies can I try?

- Aromatherapy
- Massage
- Reflexology
- Shiatsu

Finger pain and numbness (carpal tunnel syndrome)

You may feel some pain and numbness in your hands, fingers, and wrists. This is caused by swelling and weight gain.

What can I do?

- Don't sleep on your hands.
- Hang your hands over the edge of your bed at night.
- Shake your hands until the pain or numbness reduces.
- Flex your wrists and fingers regularly throughout the day.
- Dip your hands in ice cold water or apply an ice pack.
- Massage from your hands and wrists upward.
- Avoid jobs that require repetitive hand movements.
- Eat a well-balanced diet to avoid excessive weight gain.
- Drink at least eight glasses of water a day.
- Eat five portions of fruit, salad, and vegetables daily.

- Have a small amount of protein with every meal.
- Get wrist splints from the pharmacy.

What can my doctor do?

- Advise you on an prenatal vitamin rich in B6 that could help.
- Arrange for surgery after your baby's born, if necessary.

Which complementary therapies can I try?

- Acupressure
- Aromatherapy
- Chamomile tea
- Chiropractic
- Osteopathy
- Reflexology

Frequent urination

Needing to run to the bathroom a lot is a common early sign of pregnancy. It's mostly because the amount of blood in your body increases when you get pregnant. This leads to a lot of extra fluid getting processed and ending up in your bladder. In late pregnancy, and especially when your baby's head has engaged, your growing uterus leaves less room for your bladder, so its capacity is reduced. Pregnant women also often find that they have trouble emptying their bladder completely.

What can I do?

- Try drinking less for the hour or two before bedtime to cut down on nighttime trips.
- Keep drinking at least eight glasses of water during the day.
- Talk to your doctor immediately if you feel pain or burning when you urinate, or a sense of urgency while being able to produce only a few drops at a time.

What can my doctor do?

- Test you for a urinary tract infection (UTIs; see p.228)—if this is left untreated, it can lead to a kidney infection and this, in turn, can increase your risk of premature labor.

Getting ready for pregnancy

Staying safe and healthy

Your pregnancy diary

Birth and beyond

Headaches

We all suffer from headaches sometimes. If you find you get more headaches than usual during pregnancy, don't worry. They probably are caused by changes in your hormones and blood pressure. For most women, headaches diminish or disappear in the second trimester. There is a lot you can do to help yourself. Remember too that a headache is very different than a migraine. Migraines affect fewer people.

What can I do?

- Apply a compress.
- Take a cold shower.
- Get lots of fresh air.
- Ask your partner or a friend to give you a head massage.
- Get regular, gentle exercise, such as swimming, walking, or yoga.
- Improve your posture at work and when you're driving the car.
- Avoid bright lights and noise.
- Eat little and often.
- Eat a wide variety of foods of all types and all colors.
- Drink eight glasses of water a day.
- Cut down or avoid caffeinated drinks and alcohol.
- Get plenty of rest.
- Have an early night's sleep in every now and then.
- Acetaminophen is considered safe if taken in moderation.

What can my doctor do?

- Make sure that your headaches aren't a sign of something more serious, especially if you are still getting them in your third trimester.

Which complementary therapies can I try?

- Acupuncture
- Aromatherapy
- Chiropractic
- Osteopathy
- Reflexology
- Shiatsu

Heartburn

This common problem during pregnancy gives you a burning sensation that often extends from your lower throat to the bottom of your breastbone. It is caused by the pregnancy hormone progesterone, which relaxes the valve at the top of your stomach, allowing a small amount of stomach acid to surge upward.

What can I do?

- Eat small, frequent meals.
- Avoid spicy dishes, chocolate, citrus fruits, alcohol, and coffee.
- Take your time over food.
- Eat your main meal of the day at lunchtime.
- Don't drink with your meals.
- Wear loose and comfortable clothing.
- If you smoke, stop.
- Keep an upright posture, particularly during and after meals.
- Don't eat or drink anything in the three hours before going to bed.
- Sleep in a propped-up position.

What can my doctor do?

- Suggest an over-the-counter antacid.
- Recommend a different treatment if none of the above strategies works.
- Make sure that nothing else is wrong.

Which complementary therapies can I try?

- Acupuncture
- Chamomile, ginger, or peppermint tea
- Garlic capsules
- Osteopathy
- Reflexology

Hemorrhoids

These are varicose veins of the bottom. They can give you symptoms of itching, pain and sometimes bleeding.

What can I do?

- Don't wait when you get the urge for a bowel movement.
- Clean the affected area after a bowel movement (try baby wipes).
- Eat a high-fiber diet to avoid constipation.
- Drink fruit juices and at least eight glasses of water a day.
- Get regular, gentle exercise.
- Try deep breathing.
- Do Kegel exercises.
- Take a warm bath.
- Use an ice pack.
- Sit on an inflatable ring.
- Don't sit or stand for long stretches of time.
- Don't wear clothes or shoes that are too tight.
- If you smoke, stop.
- Avoid high heels.
- Sleep on your side, not your back.

What can my doctor do?

- Recommend safe topical anesthetics or medicated suppositories.
- Arrange minor surgery after pregnancy.
- Confirm that any bleeding is coming from the hemorrhoids and that nothing else is wrong.

Which complementary therapies can I try?

- Acupressure
- Aromatherapy oils in the bath.
- Osteopathy
- Reflexology
- Witch hazel

Indigestion and gas

During early pregnancy, high levels of the hormones estrogen and progesterone circulating in your body relax your gastrointestinal tract. The result of this is the slowing down of your entire digestive system. This is thought to benefit your baby because it gives your body more time to absorb essential nutrients from your food as it makes its (slow) way through your system. However, it may also give you bloating, indigestion, and heartburn, especially in the third trimester when your baby starts to push your stomach up toward your esophagus.

What can I do?

- Avoid putting extra pressure on your stomach while it's digesting: sit up straight and make sure you wear loose, comfortable clothing.
- Wait at least an hour after meals before lying down.
- Bend at your knees instead of from your waist.
- Don't eat big meals. Instead, eat several small meals throughout the day, take your time eating, and chew thoroughly.
- Avoid rich, spicy, and fatty foods.
- Avoid drinks containing caffeine or alcohol, which can aggravate your indigestion.
- Don't smoke, since this can relax the valve between your stomach and your esophagus.
- Avoid meals within three hours of your bedtime.
- Sleep with your upper body propped up with several pillows.
- Take over-the-counter simethicone after talking to your doctor.

What can my doctor do?

- Prescribe a safe remedy to help ease your symptoms.

Itchy skin

Many pregnant women suffer from some kind of itchiness of the skin. The experts believe that changes in your hormones, together with your stretching skin, are probably to blame. In addition, about two-thirds of all pregnant women will get red and itchy palms and soles, a condition that is believed to be caused by an increase in estrogen.

What can I do?

- Apply moisturizer or try a warm oatmeal bath (some pharmacies sell oatmeal bath products).
- Wear loose cotton clothing and avoid

going out in the heat of the day.

What can my doctor do?

- Prescribe a cream that will ease intense itching.
- In the third trimester, your doctor can test you for the rare liver problem, obstetric cholestasis (see pp.230–31), which causes itching.

Leg cramps

These are a type of muscle contraction that give you a sharp pain in your legs. They are probably caused by the extra weight you are carrying during pregnancy and the pressure that puts on your legs. It is also thought that too much phosphorus and too little calcium and potassium in the diet can be factors.

What can I do?

- Stay as active as possible by getting gentle exercise such as walking, swimming, and yoga.
- Incorporate foods into your diet that are high in magnesium, calcium, and vitamin C (see p.121).
- Eat plenty of fresh vegetables, fruit, and salad.
- Cut down on red or processed meat, and fast foods.
- Drink eight glasses of water a day.
- Eat a banana or drink a glass of milk before bed.
- Take a warm bath in the evening.
- Avoid processed soft drinks such as cola and carbonated drinks because they contain phosphorus.
- Stretch before going to bed.
- Avoid standing for long periods of time.
- Don't sit with your legs crossed.
- Rotate your ankles and wiggle your toes when you can.
- When a cramp strikes, massage the muscle and then walk it off.

What can my doctor do?

- Recommend a good pregnancy multivitamin and mineral supplement.

- Check for a blood clot, especially if your calf pain persists and the area is red and tender.

Which complementary therapies can I try?

- Aromatherapy

Nausea and vomiting

A feeling of queasiness, sometimes accompanied by vomiting, is the most common medical condition of early pregnancy. The condition—which can mar the joy of learning that you're pregnant—is caused by increased hormone levels together with a heightened sense of smell. Nausea and vomiting is different than severe sickness, in which you can't keep anything down. This is known as hyperemesis gravidarum (see p.230).

What can I do?

- Avoid any foods or smells that make your stomach churn.
- Avoid rich, spicy, acidic, or fried foods.
- Aim for high-protein foods and those rich in Vitamin B.
- Eat little and often, before you get hungry.
- Keep well hydrated.
- Drink ginger, peppermint, or spearmint tea.
- Sniff cut lemons.
- Wear acupressure or seasickness wristbands.
- Get as much rest and relaxation as possible.
- Keep some plain crackers by your bed to nibble on in the morning.
- Tell your family and friends how they can help you.

What can my doctor do?

- Recommend a safe pregnancy multivitamin.
- Prescribe medication, if necessary.
- Treatment becomes more difficult the longer you wait, so make an early appointment.

Getting ready for pregnancy

Staying safe and healthy

Your pregnancy diary

Birth and beyond

Which complementary therapies can I try?

- Aromatherapy
- Chiropractic
- Hypnotherapy
- Osteopathy
- Reflexology

Nosebleeds

Nosebleeds are a common pregnancy symptom. They are caused by your increased blood supply putting extra pressure on your nose's delicate veins. The membranes inside your nose may also swell and dry out, especially in winter, and this, too, can lead to nosebleeds.

What can I do?

- When your nose bleeds, remain seated and put pressure on the bleeding nostril for at least four minutes.
- Consult your doctor if you frequently have heavy nosebleeds.

What can my doctor do?

Not a lot. As annoying as nosebleeds can be, it's a temporary problem, likely to disappear after you have your baby.

Stomach cramps

Carrying a baby puts a lot of pressure on your muscles, ligaments, veins, and the rest of your insides, so it isn't surprising if you sometimes feel pains in your stomach. These pains on their own are rarely anything to worry about but if you have other symptoms, they may be a sign of a more serious problem.

What can I do?

- Most stomach cramps can be eased by getting into a new position or finding a way to relax.
- Mild cramps on one or both sides could be stretching ligaments—resting comfortably when the pain occurs usually clears it up.
- Cramps during and after orgasm can be eased by a gentle back rub.

- For cramps and persistent lower back pain in late pregnancy, resting on the sofa may help, or possibly going for a more active walk.

What can my doctor do?

- Examine you if you experience cramping along with spotting, heavy bleeding, fever, chills, vaginal discharge, tenderness, and pain, or if the cramps don't subside after several minutes of rest. These additional symptoms can be a sign of underlying problems, such as ectopic pregnancy (see pp.44–5), miscarriage (see pp.42–3), or premature labor (see pp.280-81).

Stuffy nose

What is it?

A runny or stuffed-up nose is a common condition during pregnancy, as early as the second month. It has a name—allergic rhinitis of pregnancy—but unfortunately there is no cure. There are measures you can take to help yourself, though.

What can I do?

- Fill a bowl with hot water, then cover your head with a towel and lean over the steaming bowl as if you were giving yourself an old-fashioned facial. Inhale and exhale a few times.
- A hot shower may also help.
- You might find a nasal spray provides relief (but only use one on your doctor's advice).

What can my doctor do?

- Advise you on nasal sprays and decongestants that are safe to use in pregnancy.

Swollen hands and feet (edema)

Swollen hands and feet are the result of a chain reaction in your body. First, you acquire extra blood during pregnancy. Second, your growing uterus puts pressure on your blood vessels, which causes your blood to pool. Third, pressure

from the trapped blood forces water down into the tissues of your feet and ankles—and that results in the swelling. Some pregnant women also retain excess water, which adds to the swelling. Some edema is normal, but if you have severe swelling in your hands and face, you should call your doctor.

What can I do?

- Raise your feet when possible.
- At work, keep a stool or pile of books under your desk; at home, try to lie on your left side when possible.
- Put on waist-high support hose before you get out of bed in the morning.
- Drink plenty of water to keep yourself hydrated.
- Exercise regularly, especially by walking, swimming, or riding an exercise bike.
- Eat well, and avoid sodium and salty foods like olives and salted nuts.

What can my doctor do?

- In the third trimester, test you for preeclampsia.

Vaginal discharge

All women have some vaginal discharge that changes according to the stage they're at in their menstrual cycle. During pregnancy, it is quite common for women to experience an increase in their vaginal discharge. It is almost always nothing more than leucorrhea—a mild-smelling milky fluid discharge that is caused by an increased blood flow to the area around the vagina.

For some women the discharge increases as they approach labor. The discharge can then be quite heavy. If this happens to you, it may be a sign that you are approaching labor.

What can I do?

- Keep your genital area clean.
- Wear cotton underwear.
- Avoid tight or nylon pants, perfumes,

and deodorant soaps.

• If you need to absorb the flow, use pantyliners, not tampons.

• Contact your doctor if you notice a brownish discharge.

What can my doctor do?

• Test you for a vaginal infection. A foul-smelling, thick, yellowish-green discharge, or one that causes itching or burning, could be a sign of a yeast infection or other infection. If you have these symptoms, check with your doctor.

Vaginal spotting or bleeding

Spotting is light bleeding from the vagina that can vary in color from red to brown. It is similar to, but lighter than, a period. About 15 to 25 percent of women experience some sort of bleeding in the first trimester. It is usually just "one of those things." However, it can be a sign of a more serious problem such as miscarriage (see pp.42–3). This is why it's always best to get it checked out.

In early pregnancy, severe, persistent abdominal pain with bleeding can be a sign of ectopic pregnancy (see pp.44–5) —go to the hospital immediately. In the third trimester, it can signal placenta previa (see pp.231–2), placental abruption (see p.232), or premature labor (see pp.280–81).

What can I do?

• Call your doctor or the hospital immediately for advice.

What can my doctor do?

• You may need a vaginal examination or an ultrasound to rule out any complications, such as fibroids or an inflamed cervix.

• In early pregnancy, your doctor will probably also do a urine pregnancy test and a blood test in order to check your hormone levels.

• An examination using "transvaginal"

ultrasound is often the best way to check whether or not all is well.

• Your doctor may refer you to a perinatologist so that any potential problems are monitored more closely.

Varicose veins

Varicose veins in the legs occur when the blood is unable to travel back up the legs to the heart.

Unfortunately, varicose veins are more likely to develop during pregnancy because the growing uterus increases blood pressure in the veins of your legs. On top of that, an increase in the hormone progesterone causes the walls of the veins to relax so they fail to push the blood through.

If you have varicose veins, you may just see the blue veins under your skin, or the veins may bulge; you may feel some pain, itchiness, or throbbing, or no discomfort at all.

What can I do?

• Exercise daily—even just a brisk walk around the block can help.

• Raise your feet and legs whenever you get a chance.

• Try to lie down on your left side with your feet raised on a pillow when you are at home.

• Before getting out of bed in the morning, put on special support hose.

• Don't stand on your feet for long periods of time.

• Don't cross your legs when you are sitting down.

• Be aware that excessive weight gain can contribute to the problem.

• If you have a tender, reddened area on the surface of a varicose vein, coupled with fever, leg pain, or a rapid heartbeat, report it to your doctor without delay. In rare cases, rapid heartbeat and/or shortness of breath could be signs of a pulmonary embolism (when the blood clot has traveled to the lungs). You

should go to the closest emergency department or call an ambulance.

What can my doctor do?

• If you have a major problem with varicose veins, your doctor can prescribe some support hose for you. If the problem persists several months after giving birth, you can ask for a referral to a specialist for treatment.

Yeast infection

This is a thick, white and creamy vaginal discharge, which can result in itching. It is caused by the vagina being rich in a sugar called glycogen during pregnancy. This promotes the growth of candida, which is the fungus that causes yeast infection.

What can I do?

• Reduce your consumption of sugar and sugary foods.

• Avoid getting too warm down below.

• Wear cotton underwear and abandon your tights and pantyhose.

• Wash your clothes in a nonbiological laundry detergent at 140° F (60° C) to kill the fungus.

• Don't lie in a hot bath for too long.

• Apply a cloth soaked in witch hazel or diluted tea tree oil to the inflamed outer area of the vagina.

• Press an ice pack to the inflamed, outer area.

• Eat natural live yogurt.

• Apply natural live yogurt to the affected area.

• Use garlic in your food.

• After using the bathroom, wipe your genital area from front to back.

• Do not use vaginal deodorants.

What can my doctor do?

• Prescribe some appropriate vaginal suppositories or creams.

What complementary therapies can I try?

• Acupuncture

• Probiotic supplements

Getting ready for pregnancy

Staying safe and healthy

Your pregnancy diary

Birth and beyond

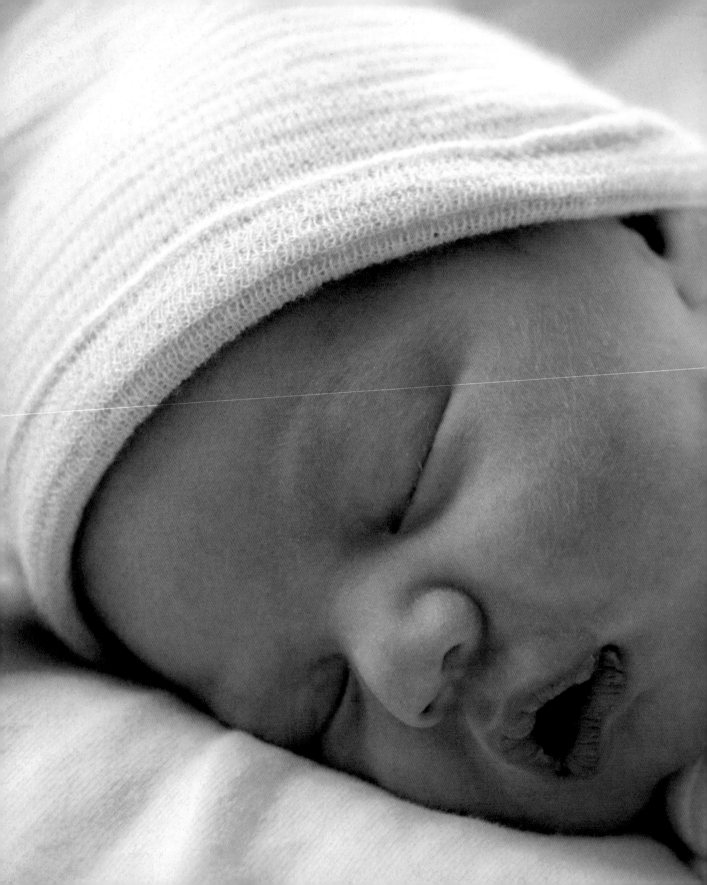

Birth and beyond

Becoming a parent

Labor and birth

You're going to be a parent

Your baby will arrive around 266 days after you conceive. Most babies arrive before or after, with only about 5 percent born on their due date. Each labor and birth is different, but knowing what's involved helps you understand and deal with any issues that may arise.

An overview

Some think labor begins when your body's hormones respond to triggers from the baby's adrenal gland. Your uterus starts to contract and your water may break. If you are overdue, you may be induced.

During the first stage of labor the contractions, which open the cervix become progressively stronger, longer, and more frequent. The cervix begins tightly closed and quite firm, but thins and stretches as labor progresses. So dilation starts slowly but speeds up as labor progresses. Once the cervix has dilated to 10 centimeters, it is fully dilated and the baby can move through it and down the vagina.

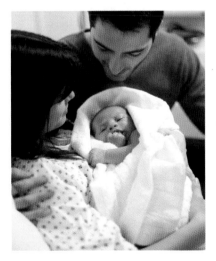

Labor is hard work but when it's all over and your baby has arrived, you and your partner can start enjoying being parents.

Now the second stage of labor begins. You will feel a very strong urge to push downward, unless you have opted to have an epidural, when the urge will be dulled. In this case your nurse or doctor will tell you when to push. The second stage of labor can take anything from a few minutes to a couple of hours or more, and it can be hard work! Your nurse doctor will guide you when to push.

Usually the baby's head comes out first and, after a few more contractions, the baby is fully born. If you are very tired or if the baby is in distress, either forceps (rather like large tongs) or a vacuum extractor may be needed to help the baby to be born. Occasionally, if the baby needs to be delivered very quickly, an emergency cesarean may be necessary.

After the birth

After birth, the umbilical cord is usually clamped and cut then, if all is well, you'll be able to hold your baby. The third and final stage of labor is the delivery of the placenta, which takes five to 30 minutes. You can have a medically managed third stage or, if you have no blood pressure problems and there is no risk of hemorrhage, the uterus can be left to contract naturally.

It's never too early to look into where and how you want to give birth. The majority of women in the United States have their baby in the hospital. However, midwife-led birthing centers are becoming increasingly popular.

Parents**Talk...**

"When we had visitors at the hospital, I was in such a tired, happy haze that I just let my husband take care of introducing everyone to our baby girl. He had a real look of awe and wonder in his eyes. That's something I'll never forget."
Melissa, 32, mom to month-old Jenny

"Everyone tells you about that baby smell, but until you have your own baby you really don't understand what they're talking about. The first time Em woke me up at night and I took her in my arms to comfort her, I was hit by it."
Jess, 30, mom to six-week-old Emma

Getting ready for pregnancy

Staying safe and healthy

Staying safe and healthy

Birth and beyond

Preparation and choices

There's a lot to think about when you're planning your baby's birth. Will you give birth in a hospital or at home? Who do you want with you? How will you manage the pain of contractions? Thinking your options through before the birth will help to give you confidence on the day.

Where to give birth: home or hospital?

The majority of American women— around 99 percent of them—give birth in the hospital. If you live in a big city, you may have a choice of two or three different hospitals. In rural areas, the possibilities are often limited, although you sometimes can choose between giving birth in a small, local midwife-led unit or in a large unit in your nearest town or city.

Hospitals have set ways of doing things, but it's your right to make it clear how you'd like to be treated when you're there. Talk to your doctor about what the routine procedures are during labor in the maternity unit where you'll give birth. If there's anything you don't like the sound of, say so. Talk through how you'd like things to go, and write a birth plan (see pp.174–5) to keep with you.

Make sure your birth partner is aware of what you want, too.

Birthing centers within hospitals are becoming increasingly popular in the United States. Some are staffed by midwives and others by both midwives and obstetricians. It is important to note, however, that you have to be prepared to be transported to the hospital if complications arise. If you'd like to know

---

Home birth versus hospital birth

This checklist sums up the pros and cons of home and hospital births. Home births are for low-risk pregnancies only.

Home birth pros

● You have your own bathroom. There is no risk of cross infection or hospital-acquired infections.
● You'll have one-on-one midwife care.
● You are more likely to have a straightforward, normal vaginal birth.
● Your own home comforts and distractions are always available.
● You are less likely to need pain relief.
● You can have as many people as you like with you at the birth.
● After the birth, you can relax at home in the comfort of your own bed.

Home birth cons

● Some pain-relief options are not available at a home birth, including an epidural. You'll need to discuss pain relief options with your midwife in advance.
● You may need to be transferred to a hospital. Be sure to have a backup plan.
● Birth can be messy. You will need to protect carpets and furniture.
● You may worry about noise disturbing the neighbors.

Hospital birth pros

● You may prefer knowing that doctors are there in case of an emergency.
● There is direct access to an epidural if you want one. Other forms of pain relief are also available.

● You may feel more comfortable making a lot of noise in a hospital.

Hospital birth cons

● You are less likely to know the staff who are taking care of you in labor and they may be caring for more than one woman at a time.
● You are more likely to have interventions such as forceps, vacuum, and a cesarean but this might be because you will be at a hospital if you have a high-risk pregnancy.
● You will need to get to the hospital in active labor.
● The hospital ward may be noisy and you may have to share a bathroom with other women.

more about a birthing center delivery, talk to your doctor or a midwife. The American College of Nurse Midwives in Washington, D.C., can direct you to resources in your area, including a list of certified nurse-midwives. The Midwives Alliance of North America is an organization for both direct-entry midwives and certified nurse-midwives. It can provide information about birthing centers, home births, and a list of members in your state.

If you rent a birth pool to use at home, you may like to get one that is large enough for your partner to get into and help you.

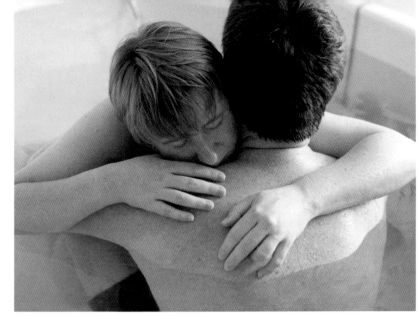

Standalone birthing centers

Birthing centers are small maternity units that are staffed and, mostly, run by midwives and nurses. They offer a comfortable, low-tech environment where birth is treated as a "normal" process rather than a medical one.

Most birthing centers are independent or "standalone," but some are affiliated with or even housed at hospitals.

Birthing centers are a kind of halfway house between home and hospital. They

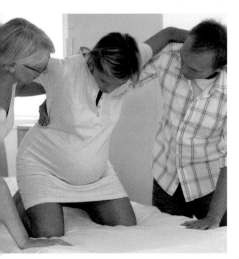

provide a homely, relaxed atmosphere, but they are also well-equipped and staffed with highly skilled midwives

Birthing centers can offer facilities that may not be available in your local hospital, such as family accommodation, water pools, complementary therapies, and comfortable, low-tech birthing rooms. You are more likely to have one-on-one care from a midwife throughout your labor in a birthing center than in a busy hospital unit.

Birthing centers also have a high standard of postpartum care. You'll probably have a private room with your own bathroom facilities, which will give you the opportunity to relax with your baby in peace. Other family members may be able to stay overnight and women are encouraged to stay until they feel ready to go home.

On the other hand, you are unlikely to have the full range of pain relief

A birthing center may be able to offer you a low-tech birthing room where you will feel more relaxed during the birth process.

available—you won't be able to have an epidural, for example. There is also no neonatal intensive care unit in the event of an emergency. However, midwives are generally skilled in life support and resuscitation techniques and in managing emergency situations.

There is also a chance that you may not be able to have an assisted delivery with forceps or vacuum extractor at a birthing center, although some birthing center midwives are now trained so they are able to use vacuum extraction.

If you do happen to get into difficulties during labor, you will be transferred to a hospital by ambulance, accompanied by your midwife. Despite the lack of medical facilities, evidence shows that giving birth in a birthing center is just as safe for you and your baby as having your baby in a hospital.

Eligibility criteria vary from one center to another, but you will generally only be able to book into a birth center if your pregnancy is low-risk and you have a good chance of having a normal birth at full term.

Getting ready for pregnancy

Staying safe and healthy

Your pregnancy diary

Birth and beyond

Hospital births

There's no shortage of information out there about the physical process of giving birth. But for those women who've opted for a hospital birth, they're not always sure what awaits them when they finally reach the maternity ward.

Some of your fears can be allayed and your questions answered if you visit the hospital where you plan to give birth to your baby. From about 34 weeks onward, you may be offered a chance to

taking care of you will ask you to tell her what has happened so far: have you had a bloody show (a brownish or blood-tinged mucus discharge), for example, or has your water broken?

Next she'll check your blood pressure, temperature, pulse, and urine. She'll measure and feel your belly to find out which way around your baby is and whether her head is engaged in your pelvis or not. She'll also assess how long,

"Women **are not** always **sure what will** happen **at hospital**."

visit. In addition to taking a tour of the labor, delivery, and recovery areas, your visit gives you the chance to become familiar with the layout and find out how things are done there.

On the day

When you arrive at the hospital, you'll be directed to the maternity ward reception. The caregiver who'll be

strong, and frequent your contractions are and how much pain you're in.

Checking your baby

The labor nurse or doctor will want to check that your baby is okay so she may ask to see your sanitary pad if you've had a bloody show, or if your water has already broken. She'll be checking for bleeding or meconium (your baby's first bowel movement) in the amniotic fluid. She'll also listen to your baby's heartbeat. Next, she may ask your permission to do an internal (vaginal) examination to see how many centimeters dilated you are. You don't have to have this examination if you don't want to.

Everything your labor nurse does is written down on your chart, which records every detail of your labor. This is important because it means that if your nurse goes off duty, the next labor nurse

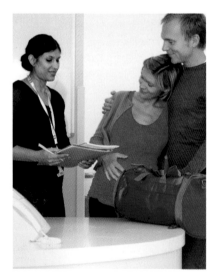

The receptionist on the maternity ward will welcome you and hand you over to your nurse to check how your labor's going.

on duty will be able to see at a glance how you're getting on.

If the labor nurse sees that you are in very early labor, you might choose to go home again and wait for the contractions to get stronger. If you're in active labor—more than three centimeters dilated—you'll be admitted.

In the delivery room

Many hospital delivery rooms are designed to look like a bedroom to help you feel more relaxed. In addition to the bed and a chair, there may be pictures on the walls and perhaps a TV.

At many hospitals, it's routine to start an intravenous (IV) drip when a woman in labor is admitted. You'll definitely need one to get antibiotics if you test positive for group B strep, for hydration if you can't keep fluids down, if you want a spinal or an epidural, if you need oxytocin (Pitocin), or if you have any health problems or pregnancy complications.

Your labor nurse or caregiver should also orient you, showing you where everything is in your room and on the unit (for example, where your partner can get ice for you) and explaining what she's doing and why all the time. Don't be shy about requesting anything you might need, like a rocking chair, a cool washcloth, or another blanket, and feel free to ask questions as things come up.

Your care providers should ask if you have a birth plan. If they don't ask but you have prepared one, be sure to bring it up as soon as possible.

Throughout your labor, your labor nurse will regularly check your pulse, temperature, blood pressure, urine, cervix, and the baby's position and heart rate. If you find that you do need some form of medical intervention— such as an epidural (see pp.277–9), an assisted birth (see pp.282–3), or an

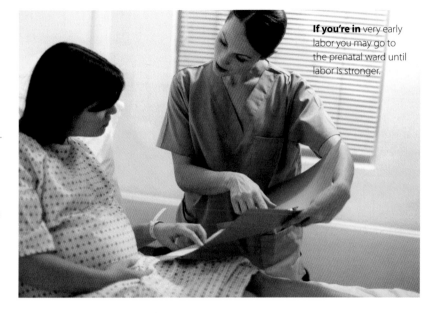

If you're in very early labor you may go to the prenatal ward until labor is stronger.

emergency cesarean (see pp.288–91) —all the specialist professionals will be on hand.

You don't have to get or stay in bed. In fact, being mobile in active labor can help your labor progress. Try to make your room comfortable: You may want to move the bed or adjust the lighting.

72%

of women say they plan to— or did—give birth in a hospital; 9 percent say they'd like to give birth at home. Another 18 percent plan to give birth in a birthing center.

ParentsAsk...

Can my partner stay with me during labor?

Yes, in fact it may be invaluable. One study showed that women meet an average of six or more unfamiliar professionals during their labor at a hospital, so a friendly face can make all the difference. A birth partner can be anyone you trust to be near you, who can provide you with emotional support during your labor, and who can also provide practical help. Another study found that a birth partner who offered encouragement in pain control made an epidural less likely and that meant that women in labor were less likely to feel panicky and exhausted.

Can I eat and drink in labor?

Drinking liquids is fine. It's okay to eat during early labor, but if you want to play it safe during active labor, you may want to skip snacking. On the off-chance that you need general anesthesia, a full stomach increases your risk of vomiting and aspiration, although this is rare.

Drinking liquids that have some calories in them, such as non-caffeinated sports drinks, will help to prevent ketosis. This is when the body breaks down its own fatty reserves for energy. Ketosis can make you feel nauseous, make you vomit, or can give you a headache. It's best to avoid ketosis during labor because you have a lot of hard physical work ahead of you.

Getting ready for pregnancy

Staying safe and healthy

Your pregnancy diary

Birth and beyond

Preparing yourself

Labor could start at any time now. As this reality hits home, it's normal to feel apprehensive, even a little scared. Being prepared on a practical level and mentally is the key to dealing with fear and pain during childbirth.

If you're still a bit hazy on the three stages of labor (see pp.262–5, 268–9, 270–71), now is the time to refresh your memory. When things get underway you

Make sure, too, that you have your birth plan (see pp.174–5) ready and review it one final time. Of course, no one knows in advance what sort of birth experience they will have, but a written plan will at least help explain to the labor nurse or medical staff what really matters to you.

Having a birth plan also helps you think through some of the options you might have to face, so that you

> "If you're a **bit hazy** about the **three stages of labor** now is the time to **refresh your memory**."

will feel much more in control if you recognize the early signs of labor and what to expect as it progresses. With your baby's birth perhaps only hours away, there's nothing like a time limit to focus the mind!

won't have to make certain decisions when you're in labor. But remember— your birth plan is not a list of demands. You need to acknowledge that things might not go according to plan on the day, so be prepared to be flexible.

ParentsAsk...

Can I try for a vaginal birth after a cesarean?

Just because you've had one cesarean doesn't mean that you'll have one next time. Guidelines recommend women be supported if they want a vaginal birth after a cesarean (VBAC), provided they are informed about all the pros and cons.

Though fewer VBACs are now done in the United States, there are advantages. After a vaginal delivery, for example, you are less likely to need a blood transfusion, your baby is less likely to have breathing problems, and your hospital stay will be shorter.

Disadvantages of VBAC may include perineal pain or stitches, more chance of stress incontinence in the first three

months after birth, and an increased chance of your uterus "dropping" (prolapse) in later years. One disadvantage that is specific to VBAC is that, very rarely, your uterus may rupture, which could put you and your baby at risk. Studies show that the rate of rupture in women having a VBAC after one previous cesarean section is less than 1 percent. The risk of uterine rupture is somewhat higher if your labor needs to be induced or augmented.

Your chances of having a successful VBAC are higher if you have delivered at least one baby vaginally in the past and if your last cesarean was for a breech baby.

About 60 to 80 percent of women who choose VBAC after a previous cesarean go on to have a successful vaginal birth.

What happens to my vagina and pelvic floor after birth?

Directly after a vaginal birth, the opening of your vagina will be bigger and not as neat as it was. But the area will regain its shape over time and if you do Kegel exercises (see p.135) regularly.

Your pelvic floor muscles may initially feel "switched off" due to pain and swelling. Start your Kegel exercises as soon as you can. Many health experts recommend waiting six weeks before exercising, but you can do these exercises as soon as you feel up to it. (Wait six weeks if you've had a cesarean.) The exercises increase blood flow to the area, aid healing, and tighten and strengthen the pelvic floor.

Mental preparation

Finally, it is useful to have some mental strategies ready to help you deal with the birth. Remember the breathing techniques (see below and p.274) that you learned at childbirth classes.

You might also use techniques like progressive or controlled relaxation, in which you release tension by zeroing in on a particular muscle, tightening it up, and then letting it go until it's as loose as possible. Some women also find visualization really effective—for example, repeating the thought "My body is strong and is working well for me." Many moms have used strategies like these to delay or avoid the need for additional pain relief or medical interventions during labor.

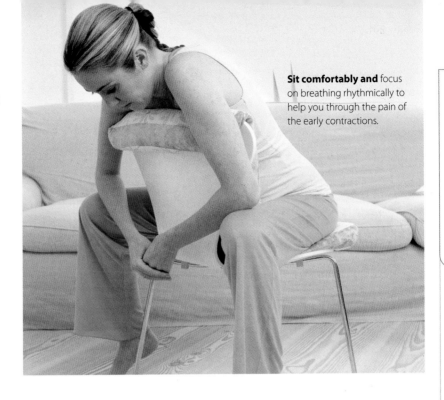

Sit comfortably and focus on breathing rhythmically to help you through the pain of the early contractions.

Breathing techniques

Practicing rhythmic breathing while you are in labor maximizes the amount of oxygen available to you and your baby. It can also help you deal with the pain of contractions.

It can be very hard to keep your breathing rhythmical and to relax every time you breathe out when you're having painful contractions. You're tired, and labor seems to be endless. This is where the support of your birth partner is essential. He can help you keep your breathing steady by breathing with you.

You need to be in eye contact with him, and he can hold your hands or place his hands on your shoulders. Then you can follow his pattern of breathing as he breathes in through his nose and blows out softly into your face. Practice this during pregnancy.

During the second stage of labor, you will be pushing your baby out into the world. Follow your urges and push as many times per contraction as feels right for you. You may find that you feel the urge to push briefly three to five times with each contraction, taking several breaths in between.

Sometimes women get the urge to push before their cervix is fully dilated. In this case, depending on how far dilated you are, your labor nurse or doctor may ask you to try not to push to give your cervix more time to open. This can be extremely difficult!

You can help by changing your position, perhaps onto your side or kneeling on all fours with your bottom in the air and your cheek resting on the ground. When a contraction arrives, give four short pants, then a quick in-breath, followed by four more short pants and so on. You can also repeat the phrase "I must not push" in your head as you pant. Try to breathe normally between the contractions.

Overcoming your labor fears

It's natural to have anxieties over giving birth, especially if this is your first baby. But there are strategies to help you overcome your fears:

● Talk to someone who knows you very well about how you have dealt with pain in the past. When you compare labor with other painful experiences, you may realize that you are stronger than you thought.

● If you have your baby in a hospital, you will have a range of pain relief options, such as an epidural. Talk to your labor nurse or doctor about these, and ask them to help prepare a birth plan, so that your wishes are clear to everybody taking care of you.

● If you have a strong fear of childbirth, talk to your doctor about counseling. This can help you to understand and come to terms with your anxieties.

Overdue babies

Your due date's arrived but your baby hasn't. What now? Don't worry too much—lots of babies arrive after their due dates. You may want to learn a bit more about induction in the meantime but, more importantly, put your feet up and get some rest.

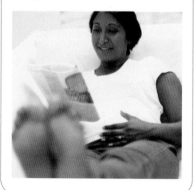

My baby's late

Lots of women go beyond their expected due date. About five to six percent have what is known as a prolonged pregnancy—a pregnancy that continues three or more weeks beyond the due date.

Babies born at 42 weeks and beyond can have dry, parchment-like skin and are often overweight. Waiting that long to deliver also increases your chance of developing an infection in your uterus that could be dangerous for your baby. It also increases your chance of having a stillbirth. What's more, your labor is more likely to be prolonged or stalled, both you and your baby have an increased risk of injury during a vaginal delivery, and you double your chances of needing a cesarean.

Research shows that membrane stripping (see opposite) increases the chances of labor starting naturally within 48 hours. But if membrane stripping doesn't work and your pregnancy has been straightforward, you should be offered the possibility of an induction (see opposite). Many women prefer to be induced at this stage, since they feel that they have had enough of being pregnant, but some others would rather wait and let nature take its course.

If, after talking to your obstetrician, you're not sure about having an induction, you could ask for a day or two to consider. If you decide not to be induced, it's highly likely that you'll go into labor spontaneously before 42 completed weeks (if your due date is based on a dating scan).

An alternative to induction is to have your pregnancy monitored on a regular basis (every two to three days) to check that your baby's okay. Your doctor may be able to listen to your baby with a portable ultrasound device, or you may be asked to have an ultrasound to check the levels of amniotic fluid.

Although the choice is up to you, your obstetrician will usually strongly encourage you to have be induced if you get to two weeks after your due date.

22% of babies per year is roughly the amount of induced births in the United States. An induction is usually done because the risks of prolonging a pregnancy are more serious than the risks of delivering the baby immediately. Most labors begin naturally, but sometimes the birth process may need a little help.

Natural ways to bring on labor

You're ready to go and nothing's happening? The following might be worth trying to get labor going.

● **Nipple stimulation** It's believed that this releases oxytocin, a hormone that causes contractions.

● **Sex** Orgasm may help to stimulate the uterus into action. Semen also contains prostaglandins to open the cervix.

● **Eating spicy food** There is no scientific evidence for this one! But it is said to stimulate the bowel, which is next to the uterus.

● **Eating pineapple** Fresh pineapple contains the enzyme bromelain, which is thought to help to soften the cervix.

● **Acupuncture** Limited studies suggest that acupuncture may be effective.

● **Walking** If your baby has not "dropped" or is still high in the pelvis, walking is thought to encourage your baby into a better position.

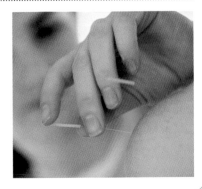

Induction

Although it's usually best to let nature take its course, sometimes the birth process may need a little help. When labor is started artificially, it is said to be induced. You may be offered an induction if:

● Your pregnancy has gone beyond 41 weeks.

● Your water has broken but labor hasn't started within 24 hours.

● You suffer from diabetes or another condition, such as preeclampsia (see p.233) or kidney disease, that could threaten your well-being or the health of your baby.

Some of the options used to try to get your labor started are:

Membrane strip The membranes that surround your baby are gently separated from your cervix during an internal examination.

Prostaglandin This hormonelike substance helps stimulate uterine contractions. Your labor nurse will insert a tablet, suppository, or gel containing prostaglandin into your vagina.

Foley catheter This is a small balloon inserted into your cervix. When inflated with water, it puts pressure on your cervix and stimulates the release of prostaglandins.

Rupturing membranes A small, plastic hooked instrument is inserted through your cervix to break your amniotic sac.

Pitocin This is the synthetic form of the hormone oxytocin. It is given via an IV and you are only offered it if your labor hasn't started after a membrane sweep or prostaglandin. Some women say the contractions brought on by Pitocin are more painful than natural ones.

There is some evidence that you are more likely to need forceps or vacuum to

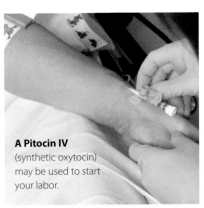

A Pitocin IV (synthetic oxytocin) may be used to start your labor.

help deliver your baby following any type of induction. This may be due to complications in the pregnancy that led to the induction and/or it may be due to problems caused by the induction itself.

Parents**Ask...**

How will I know if induction will work?

There are various methods of induction. Your doctor may suggest that one method is better than another, depending on how soft and ready for labor your cervix is.

The ripeness of your cervix is assessed using what's called the Bishop Score, which gives your cervix a mark out of 10 based on its condition. A score of eight or more indicates that your cervix is "ripe" and ready for labor.

About 15 percent of inductions started with an unripe cervix fail. In these circumstances, your doctor will discuss your options with you to help you decide whether to continue trying, either with stronger interventions at a later time, or to have a cesarean.

Getting ready for pregnancy

Staying safe and healthy

Your pregnancy diary

Birth and beyond

Home birth

Some research shows that, for women with normal pregnancies, a home birth is just as safe as a hospital birth. If you're expecting a straightforward birth and decide that a home birth is the right choice for you, find out if your doctor or midwife is supportive.

All you need to know

For women who have enjoyed a normal pregnancy and expect a straightforward labor, a home birth may be as safe as giving birth in a hospital.

If you've decided to go for a home birth and you're healthy and having an uncomplicated pregnancy, talk to your

Fact: Of the 1 percent of births that took place outside the hospital in 2006, 65 percent were in women's own homes. These percentages have remained largely the same since 1989.

doctor or midwife once your pregnancy has been confirmed. If your doctor isn't supportive, don't worry. You should be able to find a care provider who will support your decision, provided you're at low risk for complications. You will need a certified nurse-midwife (CNM), a certified direct-entry midwife (CPM or CM), or a physician with plenty of experience delivering babies at home. Your midwife might also be able to provide your prenatal care and offer support services after delivery.

You can change your mind at any time. Have a backup plan in place in case of complications and in case you

ultimately decide for a hospital birth instead. Opting early on for a home birth allows you the greatest possible flexibility, as you can decide to transfer to hospital right up to the delivery itself.

You need very little equipment if you are having a home birth. A few weeks before your due date, be sure you have whatever supplies your midwife or physician requires.

If you have older children, be sure to make arrangements for someone to watch them during your labor. Some older siblings may want to participate in the birth, but have a backup plan in case they reconsider.

Home birth checklist

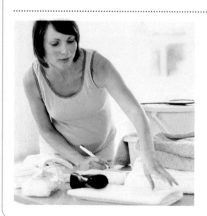

Your care provider should let you know what supplies she will need when attending your birth. You may also need:
- An adjustable floor or desk lamp, used to check your perineum.
- A plastic sheet, plastic shower curtain, or some old newspapers for the floor.
- A birthing ball.
- A birth pool if you want to use one.
- Some large, warm towels to put around you and the baby.
- Plenty of hot water if you want a bath.

- Energy-boosting snacks for you to eat, and drinks with bendy straws.
- A hand mirror so you can see your baby's head crowning.
- A fan to keep you cool.
- A portable heater if necessary.

Offer your midwives food and drink and make sure you're stocked up on beverages. Your birth partner can make sandwiches to leave out for them.

Finally, pack an emergency bag in case you need to be transferred to a hospital.

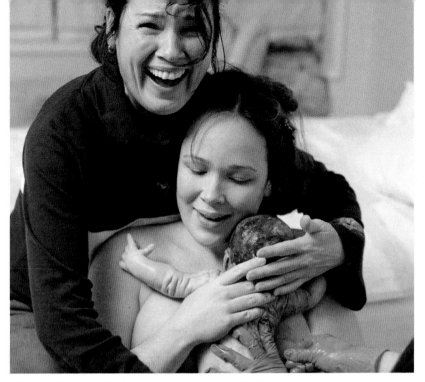

Having a home birth where your mother and other family members can be present can be a very moving experience for everyone.

You're in labor

Once you go into labor, your care provider may check on you by phone or in person to see how your labor is progressing. Once she thinks the birth is imminent, she'll remain with you and call in any assistants who will be part of your birth.

If your care provider thinks you need to be transferred to hospital, she'll discuss with you why she believes it would be a good idea. If you agree, she'll call an ambulance. You're far more likely to need to transfer to a hospital because your labor has slowed down than because there's a real emergency.

After the birth

Once your baby is born and the placenta (afterbirth) is delivered, your care provider may stay to check that everything's okay, then she'll probably leave you and your partner alone with your baby for a while. She will then check your baby over and weigh him, help you with

your first breast-feeding, help clean up any mess, and see you into bed. She'll return to check on you and your baby in the days after, and see how you're progressing. If her availability after the birth is limited, you may want to hire a doula for postpartum help. Your baby should see his doctor for a complete checkup within a day or so of birth.

A home birth is an intimate experience and allows your partner to participate more fully in what is going on.

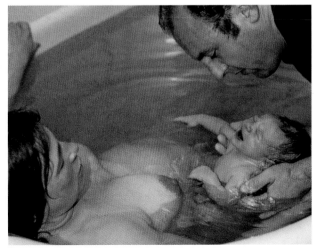

Your baby's position

Believe it or not, the position your baby is lying in when you go into labor is one of the key indicators of whether or not you'll have a straightforward birth. Find out which positions are likely to allow your baby a smooth birth and how to encourage her into them.

Lie, presentation, and position

Most babies get into the best position for birth before labor begins. This is in a head-down position, lying with the back of her head slightly toward the front of your abdomen. This is called an "anterior" position (see opposite, center).

During labor, most babies also curl their back over and tuck their chin into their chest. This is nature's way of helping your labor to progress and making birth easier. During contractions in the first stage of labor, the top of your baby's head puts rounded and even pressure on the cervix and helps it dilate. Then, in the pushing stage, your baby comes through the birth canal with the part of her skull that has the smallest diameter leading the way.

If your baby has her chin up or her head extended back, then her face or her brow will be coming first (see p.197). This doesn't happen very often, but when your baby's at this angle, the diameter of her head is much bigger, and this makes it more likely that she'll get stuck during the birth. Try putting on a tight turtleneck top using different parts of your head to push through and you'll understand why a tucked-in chin works best for birth!

Laid-back mom

Listening to your body in labor rather than pre-planning each detail is often the way to go.

"I really wanted to go with the flow during my labor, and listen to my body rather than plan everything too closely. And when it came to it, my body was saying 'Help, this really hurts!' It turned out my baby was in the posterior position (see opposite, right) so I had the most excruciating backache, and it slowed my labor down a ton. The pain went on forever, so I finally opted for an epidural. It took the pain away completely, so I could just relax, and push when the labor nurse told me to. I did end up having an assisted forceps delivery, though—he didn't want to turn and decided to be born with his face looking up at me!"

Parents**Talk...**

"My baby had his back next to my spine when I went into labor and it was really uncomfortable in the early stages. The only thing that helped was getting on all fours so he dropped away from my spine. He did eventually turn before making his grand entrance."
Meg, 28, mom to two-month-old Dylan

"My daughter was in a breech position right up until the week before my due date. I was willing her to get into the right position because I really didn't want to have a

cesarean with my first baby. I wanted to try to do it without any assistance first. Thankfully, she turned nine days before I went into labor and I delivered her naturally."
Julie, 30, mom to one-month-old Olivia

"My baby wasn't in the right position when I went into labor and I was terrified of having to deliver him with the help of forceps or vacuum. Luckily, though, he decided to do mommy a favor and turn just as I reached 10 cm."
Adriana, 31, mom to six-month-old Rafe

About one in 10 babies are head down but lying "back-to-back" at the start of labor. This "posterior" position (see below, right) means that the back of the baby's head is toward the mother's spine. Most babies in this position are born vaginally but your labor may be longer and you may need an assisted birth. It's rare, but your baby may be lying across your abdomen—called a "transverse" or "oblique" lie. If your baby stays in this position you'll need a cesarean birth.

Babies lying with their bottom down and their head up are in a breech position. If your baby is breech as you start the third trimester, don't panic. When labor begins at term, nearly 97 percent of babies are set to come out head first. Most of the rest are breech. Late term, an external cephalic version (see p.287) might get your baby in a better position. Most breech babies are born by cesarean section.

Common positions for your baby

As you approach your due date, you may notice that your doctor notes your baby's position. When she does her routine examination, she'll feel for the position of your baby's head and then try to figure out where her back is and where her arms and legs are. Below are the most common positions that your baby may be in during these last weeks:

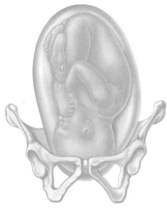

Left occipitolateral (LOL) Your baby is lying on your left side with her back toward your left side.

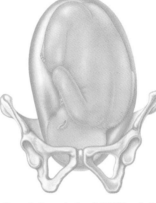

Left occipitoanterior (LOA) Your baby is lying on your left side with her back toward your belly.

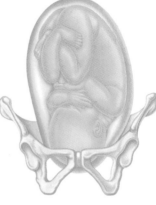

Left occipitoposterior (LOP) Your baby is lying on your left side with her back toward your back.

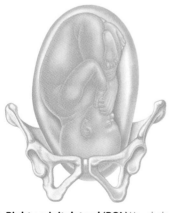

Right occipitolateral (ROL) Your baby is lying on your right side with her back toward your right side.

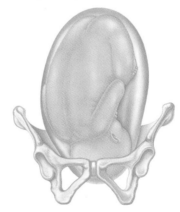

Right occipitoranterior (ROA) Your baby is lying on your right side with her back toward your belly.

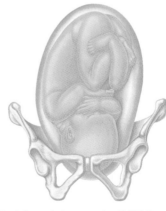

Right occipitoposterior (ROP) Your baby is lying on your right side with her back toward your back.

Getting ready for pregnancy

Staying safe and healthy

Your pregnancy diary

Birth and beyond

Signs of labor

It's the question that's uppermost in most heavily pregnant women's minds: "How will I know when I'm in labor?" Persistent lower back pain and breaking water are two possible signs. Read on to discover the other signs that say your baby's finally on his way.

Something's starting

Everyone's labor is different, and pinpointing when it begins is not really possible. It's more of a process than a single event. A number of changes

in your body work together to help deliver your baby. Signs of the approach of labor include:

- Lightening (when the baby's head begins to drop into position in your pelvis); you may notice that you can breathe more deeply and eat more, but you'll also need to urinate more often.
- Vaginal discharge becomes heavier and full of mucus.
- More frequent, and noticeably more intense, Braxton Hicks contractions (see box, left).
- Vomiting and diarrhea.

In early labor, also called the latent phase, you may experience some or all of the following:

- Persistent lower back or abdominal pain, often accompanied by a crampy premenstrual feeling.
- A bloody show (a brownish or blood-tinged mucus discharge). If you pass the mucus plug that blocks the cervix, labor could be imminent or it could be several days away. It's a sign that things are moving along.
- Painful contractions that occur at regular and increasingly shorter intervals and become longer and stronger in intensity.
- Broken water, but you're in labor only if it's accompanied by contractions that are dilating your cervix.

How you will feel in early labor depends on whether you've had a baby before, how you perceive and respond to pain, and how prepared you are for what labor may be like.

What you do when you are in early labor will depend on what time of day it is, what you like doing and how you're feeling. Keeping calm and relaxed will

True contractions or Braxton Hicks?

Most women who are pregnant for the first time will ask their doctor or friends how to tell the difference between Braxton Hicks contractions (see p.177) and real labor. The answer is usually maddeningly vague: "You'll know real labor when it begins."

Labor contractions are noticeably longer as well as more regular, frequent and painful than Braxton Hicks contractions. Also, labor pains are persistent, and they increase in frequency, duration, and intensity as time goes on, while Braxton Hicks contractions are always unpredictable and nonrhythmic.

If your contractions have become longer, stronger, more regular, and more frequent, then your labor may well be starting. Your doctor will probably have talked to you about what to do at this stage, but if you're in any doubt, give her a call.

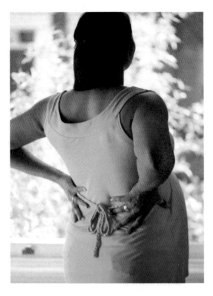

If you have lower back pain that just won't go away and a crampy feeling, you could be in the early stages of labor.

help your labor progress and will help you to deal with the contractions, so do whatever you like that will help you to stay relaxed.

Try to relax

Relaxing could mean watching a favorite movie, reading, or asking a friend or relative over to keep you company for a couple of hours. You could alternate between walking and resting, or try taking a warm bath or shower to ease any aches and pains. If you can, try to get some rest to prepare you for the work ahead. Some women are able to get in a nap between contractions. You may feel hungry so eat and drink if you feel like it.

Early labor is a good time to try out different positions and breathing techniques (see pp.249 and 274) to see if they help you deal with the contractions, now that you're having them for real.

Believe it or not, it is possible to have contractions and not be in labor. When you are in labor your cervix becomes progressively thinner (called effacement) and dilated (above, right). Some women are sensitive to the pain of contractions before the cervix has started to dilate.

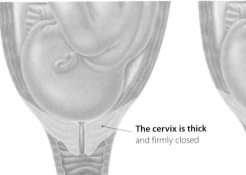

The cervix is thick and firmly closed

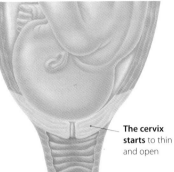

The cervix starts to thin and open

Before labor starts, the cervix is thick, tough, short and firmly closed. The baby's head is engaged.

When labor starts, the cervix begins to thin out, stretch and open. This is known as "effacement."

"The start of **labor** is a **process** not a **single event.** It's not possible **to pinpoint** it exactly."

A doctor or labor nurse will be able to confirm whether or not cervical changes have started by giving you an internal examination.

If your baby is in a posterior position (with his head down but his back to your back; see p.255) it can take longer for your baby's head to engage and for

labor to get started properly. Your contractions may come erratically and may not be very intense, and you may also have a lot of backache.

Your doctor will advise you on ways to manage at home until labor becomes stronger. You could try a warm bath or massage to relieve the pain.

Parents Talk...

"There was no mistaking it when my contractions started. They were very low down like period pains but with an extra strong 'sting' at the peak of them. Just enough to make you go 'Ooooh, something's happening and it hurts!'"
Shona, 24, first-time mom

"I was trying to get to sleep when I felt a weird, rippling sensation down on my left-hand side. I thought maybe the baby had turned his head and scraped against something. Anyway, I turned over to try and get comfy and felt a gush of fluid—I went to the bathroom and saw that I was leaking fluid. It smelled like honey and had very

small blobs of blood in it. My doctor said it sounded like my water had broken, so I called a taxi!"
Lesley, 30, mom to one-month-old René

"The night before my due date I kept waking up with what I thought were practice contractions, but I wasn't sure if I was in labor. I hadn't lost my mucus plug and my water hadn't broken. When the contractions jumped to being every three to six minutes and each one felt stronger than the last. I knew this was it. I never did spot the mucus plug, but I did have a beautiful baby boy on my due date!"
Mei, 27, mom to two-month-old Alex

Parents**Talk...**

"My water broke four weeks early while I was in the supermarket. I was so embarrassed that I told my husband to finish the shopping. I went to wait for him in the car."
Kelly, 27, mom to two-month-old Max

"A few days before my due date, my water started trickling out while I was out for dinner with my husband. I dashed to the bathroom to dry off. It was only when I saw the pink-colored liquid that I realized it couldn't be urine."
Maria, 30, mom to seven-month-old Angelina

"My water broke when my husband and I were lovemaking—so it kind of ruined the mood!"
Penny, 29, first-time mom

"When my water broke I was on the subway on my way home from some last-minute baby shopping—I quickly got off at the next stop, leaving a wet seat behind and hailed a taxi home as fast as I could."
Rebecca, 25, mom to year-old Leah

"When I was 9 cm dilated and they were encouraging me, I suddenly got the urge to push. I screamed, 'No, my water hasn't broken!' With that said, my water gushed out with a huge push, exploding all over my husband. I couldn't help it. I started laughing and kept laughing in between intense contractions. Just the look on his face was enough to set me off."
Fiona, 32, second-time mom

My water is breaking

During pregnancy your baby is protected and cushioned inside your uterus in a bag of membranes full of amniotic fluid. If a tear forms in the bag then the fluid leaks out via the cervix and vagina. This is known as your "water breaking." It is written in your records as SROM (spontaneous rupture of membranes).

Most women's water breaks toward the end of the first stage of labor. For about one in 10 women the water breaks at the end of pregnancy but before labor starts (prelabor rupture of membranes at term or PROM).

Prelabor rupture

If your water does break before you go into labor, don't panic. Put on a sanitary pad for protection. This will also make it easier to see the color of the fluid you are losing. The fluid is almost clear with a yellow tinge, and possibly a little bloodstained to begin with.

The amount of fluid you lose can vary. It may be a slight trickle or a large "gush." If there is a lot of fluid, a sanitary pad will not be enough and you'll be better off using an old hand towel. While undignified, it's more practical, especially if you need to travel by car to the hospital or the birthing center.

It's important that, regardless of how many weeks pregnant you are when your water breaks, you should call your doctor to see if you need assessment. Once your water has broken, there is less protection against getting an infection.

Once you have been examined, provided you are at least 37 weeks pregnant, you can choose to be induced. This will usually be done within 24 hours after your water has broken. Alternatively, the staff at the hospital might decide on a "wait and see" policy—to see if you go into labor after the 24 hours are up. About nine out of 10 women at full term give birth

naturally within 24 to 48 hours of their water breaking. If your water breaks earlier than 37 weeks—between 34 and 37 weeks—you may also have a choice of induction or to wait and see.

If all is well with you and your baby, you can go home if you want while you wait. A wait-and-see approach carries a slight risk of infection (about 1 percent of women compared to 0.5 percent of women whose water hasn't broken). In the meantime, it's safe for you to take a shower but don't have sex once your water has broken because this increases your risk of infection.

70% of women whose water has broken will go into labor within 24 hours, almost 90 percent within 48 hours, and 95 to 96 percent go into labor within 72 hours.

The "wait and see" approach

While you are waiting to see if you go into labor naturally, you will need to:

- Have your baby's heart rate and movements periodically checked by your doctor until you go into labor or are induced.
- Check your temperature while you are awake to make sure that you are not developing a fever.
- Check for changes in the color and smell of the amniotic fluid (water), which could indicate an infection.
- Check that your baby is still moving as usual.

If you have any signs of infection or fever (such as shivering and flushing), or you've noticed a decrease in your baby's movements, contact the hospital immediately. If an infection is diagnosed you'll need intravenous antibiotics and to be induced immediately.

If you have no signs of infection but your water has been broken for more than 24 hours, you're advised to give birth in a hospital. This is because your baby may need immediate access or transfer to a neonatal intensive care unit.

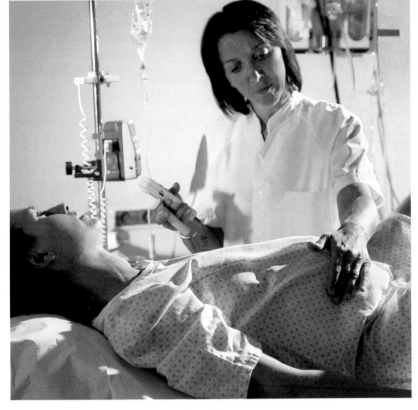

After your water has broken you might need an assessment. If everything's okay with you and your baby, you can choose to be induced, or wait to see if you go into labor naturally.

Parents**Ask...**

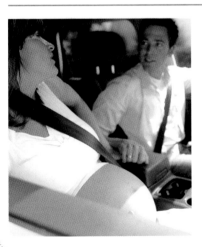

How will I know if it's too late to get to the hospital?

When you are having a first baby, it's very unusual for labor to progress so quickly that you'll wait too long to get to the hospital. First labors can be very long. The so-called latent phase (before the cervix has opened to 3 cm; see p.262) may last for many hours. Second and subsequent labors, however, tend to be quicker because your pelvis and vagina have already been stretched once and so are more elastic than last time around.

It's unlikely during a first labor that you won't have enough time to get to the hospital. The first phase of labor can take a long time.

If you are still at home, and you have an uncontrollable urge to push, then it might well be too late to go to the hospital. If you find yourself in this situation, call the hospital—or call 911 if you don't happen to have the hospital number on hand. The emergency services will arrange for a paramedic to come out to you at home. They'll also stay on the telephone with you until help arrives.

If you've had a previous labor that was fast and furious, it's important to be especially attuned to the signs of labor. Be prepared to make a mad dash for the hospital, because subsequent labors can go even faster.

False labor

You're having contractions, but they're coming and going. Are you in labor or not? Some women experience "false" labor at full term, in which contractions are sporadic and your cervix fails to open. Try to relax—it's a positive sign that your baby's birth is not far away.

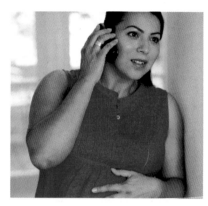

If you think labor may be starting don't feel embarrassed to call your doctor to check what you should do next.

Is this the real thing?

As you approach your due date, the Braxton Hicks contractions (see p.177) that you may have been feeling since mid-pregnancy sometimes become more rhythmic, relatively close together, and even painful, possibly fooling you into thinking you're in labor. But, unlike true labor, this so-called false labor doesn't cause significant, progressive dilation of your cervix, and the contractions don't grow consistently longer, stronger, and closer together.

Sometimes it's very hard to tell false labor from the early stages of true labor. Not every woman experiences bouts of false labor. And in some cases, the strong, regular contractions of true labor come on with little or no warning.

What might be happening

If you're 37 weeks or more, here are some clues to what's going on:
- False labor contractions are unpredictable. They come at irregular intervals and vary in length and intensity. Although true labor contractions may be irregular at first, with time they start coming at more regular and shorter intervals, they become increasingly more intense, and they last longer.
- With false labor, the pain from the contractions is more likely to be centered in your lower abdomen. With true labor, you may feel the pain start in your lower back and wrap around to your abdomen.
- False labor contractions may subside on their own or when you start or stop an activity or change position. True labor contractions will persist and progress no matter what you do.

If you're not yet 37 weeks, don't waste time trying to figure out what's going on. If you notice any signs of

When to contact your doctor

You and your doctor have probably talked about what to do when you think you're in labor. But if you're not sure whether or not the time has come, don't be embarrassed to call. Doctors are used to getting calls from women who need guidance; it's part of their job.

The truth is that they can tell a lot by the tone of your voice, so talking to her helps. She will want to know how close together your contractions are, whether or not you can talk through a contraction, and any other symptoms you may have.

If you are planning to have your baby in hospital or a birthing center, she may ask you to come in to assess you. If she

thinks you're still in early labor, depending on how you're managing and whether you've got a birth partner to support you, she may encourage you to go back home until you're in stronger active labor.

You should contact your doctor if:
- Your water breaks, or if you suspect you're leaking amniotic fluid.
- Your baby is moving around less than usual.
- You have vaginal bleeding (unless it's just a little blood-tinged mucus).
- You have a fever, severe headaches, any changes in your vision, or any abdominal pain.

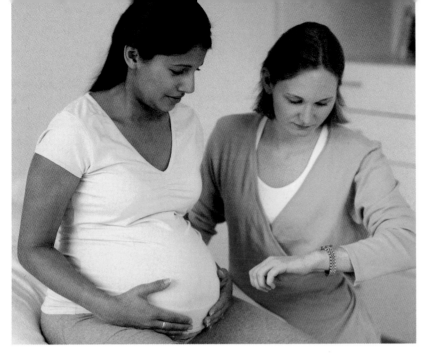

Time your contractions to see what is going on. If they become more regular, closer together, more intense, and longer-lasting, then your labor has started.

labor, call your doctor right away, especially if you have a watery or bloody discharge from your vagina.

After 37 weeks, you can sit out the contractions (whether they are false or from true early labor) at home and see what develops. The exceptions to this are if you think your water has broken (see pp.258–9), if you have any bleeding, or if you think your baby's movements have decreased.

False labor contractions can be a real drag, interfering with your sleep and making you tired and irritable. You might also feel anxious, wondering when true labor will start. If you feel discomfort, it sometimes helps to lie down or, conversely, to get up and take a walk—it's the change in activity that can help ease any pain you feel. A warm bath sometimes helps, too.

Now is a good time to practice staying relaxed during contractions, too. Take a deep breath and, as you breathe out, let your muscles relax so that they feel loose and soft. This way, by the time you eventually go into labor you will automatically be able to identify areas of tension in your body and to relax them.

If you have an older child, you might be constantly wondering whether it's time to call the babysitter. When in doubt, make the call—there's no harm done, even if you don't end up in labor, and you may be able to rest more easily knowing that help is at hand.

Time your contractions until you get a sense of what's going on. And don't hesitate to call your doctor to check in if you're concerned, confused, or just feel that you need a little encouragement or reassurance.

Dad's **Diary**

False alarm story

"1.00 am Emma wakes up, she has some sharp pains in her sides.

1:45 am Emma: 'I'm getting the BH contractions at seven-minute intervals, very regular.'

2:00 am Check pregnancy books—should BH contractions be random or what? Neither of us can remember. OK—it seems like they're just BH contractions. Attempt to relax.

2:15 am Emma: 'OK… brown mucus discharge. Looks like the "bloody show"'

2:16 am Me: 'DON'T PANIC! CALL THE HOSPITAL!'

I then panic and grab the bags for hospital. Emma calls the hospital who advises us to go straight there.

2:45 am 'RABBIT!' screams Emma as I swerve across the lane of the highway. Those suicidal rabbits are a nightmare! Luckily I avoid hitting him—karma remains balanced.

3:45 am After various discussions, samples, and examinations, Emma is hooked up to a machine to check her contractions. We're told that the figure needs to read 90 to 100 for it to be 'the real thing' but Em is peaking at 50. The nurse leaves us on monitor for more time to check contractions.

4:15 am The nurse checks Emma's cervix. It's confirmed that things aren't really happening but it was wise to check. She reassures us that, although the cervix isn't yet dilating, Em's body is getting ready for labor and that's a good sign. Doctor comes in and says Em can stay in if she chooses but we politely decline and head home.

5:45 am Finally get to bed! So it was our first 'false alarm.' It was a good test run, though."

"False **labor contractions** come at **irregular intervals** and vary in length **and intensity**."

First stage of labor

Early labor is an enjoyable, exciting part of your baby's birth. While contractions are still mild it's time to tune into your body and do whatever feels right. Taking a nap, eating a healthy snack, or just watching TV will help you to gather strength for the hard work ahead.

Latent and active phases of labor

The early phase of labor is sometimes called the latent period or pre-labor. The uterus starts to contract or tighten regularly and the contractions gradually become more painful. As the cervix begins to open, its position in your pelvis changes, moving forward. It softens and effaces, which means that it gets thinner and springier.

At this stage, you'll probably be able to putter around the house, go for a walk, watch a DVD, take a warm bath, or take a nap. Relax as much as you can and have lots of snacks to keep your energy levels up. Practice your breathing techniques and different positions to see what helps you cope with labor. Try some gentle relaxation exercises, if you feel up to it.

Doctors say you are in active labor once your cervix has dilated, or opened, to 3 to 4 cm. Your contractions will be getting stronger and more frequent. They will also be getting longer. Eventually they may be coming as frequently as every three to four minutes and lasting as long as 60 to 90 seconds.

Your doctor will probably ask you to wait to go to the hospital until you've been having contractions that last for about a minute each, coming every five

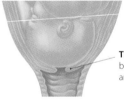

The cervix becomes springy and thinner

During the latent phase of labor, the cervix begins to stretch and thin. This is the start of effacement.

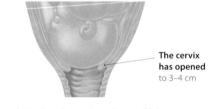

The cervix has opened to 3–4 cm

During the active phase of labor, contractions are stronger and the cervix thins to 3 to 4 cm.

Dealing with backache labor

If you are having a "backache labor," try one or more of these tactics to help relieve the pain:

● Get on all fours. This position may reduce the pressure of your baby's head on your spine.

● Do pelvic tilts (see p.151). These simple exercises may also help to minimize the pressure on your spine.

● Ask your labor coach to rub your lower back between or during contractions, or both—whatever feels best to you.

● Many women find that steady counterpressure on the lower back helps to relieve some of the pain. Ask your labor partner to push on this area with his fists during contractions or massage it with a tennis ball.

● Take a warm bath or shower, or apply warm compresses or a hot-water bottle to your lower back. Heat may ease the achiness and bring you some comfort. On the other hand, some women find cold packs more soothing, or that alternating hot and cold is helpful. You may want to give both a try. Just be sure to use a towel to protect your skin from direct contact with heat or cold.

● If you don't have your heart set on natural childbirth, consider getting an epidural. In most cases, it provides total pain relief.

minutes for about an hour. If you feel you'd be more comfortable at the hospital, call or head over. If you're having a home birth, call your midwife when you need some reassurance.

Contractions may start to feel as if they are coming one on top of another. Try to work with your body. What is it telling you to do? Would it help if you went to the bathroom?

This is the moment when breathing and relaxation techniques come into their own; your partner can remind you how to use them. Consider taking a warm shower or bath or getting into the birthing pool if you have one. Many women find the warm water relaxing and it's easier to change position in the pool. You hear stories of women who sink into a bath or pool when they're 5 or 6 cm dilated, relax, and are fully dilated an hour later!

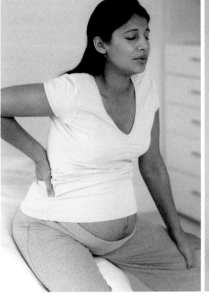

During the first stage of labor, try to find a position that's comfortable for you. This will allow you to focus on your breathing.

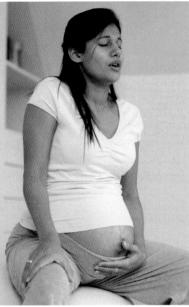

Using a birth ball can help to keep you upright and leaning forward, which is a good position for helping your baby descend.

Monitoring your baby in labor

Your doctor or labor nurse will listen to your baby's heartbeat during labor to get an idea of whether she is managing well with labor or is becoming distressed. There are two ways she can listen.

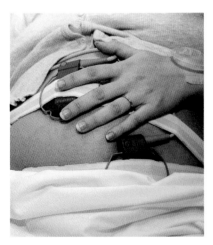

Using an electronic fetal monitor enables your baby's heartbeat to be checked while you are in labor.

Electronic fetal monitoring (EFM)

Most women who give birth in hospitals are hooked up to an electronic fetal monitor more or less continuously via two electronic disks called transducers strapped to their belly.

The transducers record both your baby's heartbeat and your contractions. They are connected to a machine (though some work wirelessly) that records this information on paper. If the monitor's volume is turned up, you'll be able to hear your baby's heartbeat.

Some moms-to-be find the monitoring uncomfortable. And being tethered to a monitor can limit your movement and may make it harder for you to deal with contractions.

Alternatively, your doctor may use internal fetal heart rate monitoring, in which an electrode is inserted through your cervix and attached to your baby's scalp with a tiny wire.

Intermittent monitoring

If you prefer not to be hooked up to a monitor and your labor is progressing smoothly, then your doctor may agree to check your baby's heart rate intermittently with a handheld Doppler device or fetoscope. Intermittent monitoring should be done at specific intervals, such as every 15 minutes in the active phase of the first stage of labor and every five minutes during the second (pushing) stage.

Getting ready for pregnancy

Staying safe and healthy

Your pregnancy diary

Birth and beyond

First stage of labor: transition

For lots of women, transition is the toughest part of labor. As your cervix dilates fully to allow your baby to pass through, your contractions become stronger and you may start to wonder if you can cope. Hang on in there—it won't be long until you can start pushing.

The cervix is now fully dilated so your baby can be pushed out via the birth canal.

The neck of the cervix now measures 10 cm

Now what's happening?

Transition is the last stage of the first phase of labor. It is the time when your cervix dilates from about eight to 10 cm. This stage of labor can be a stormy time, physically and emotionally, but the end is in sight.

Your contractions may now start to come one on top of another. Instead of peaking and fading away, a contraction may peak, start to fade, and then rev up again to a second peak. These contractions may be longer, but they may also be less frequent, giving you a bit of time to recover in between.

Transition may last for just a few contractions or it may feel like it's never going to end. The muscles of your uterus start to work differently during transition, and you may begin to feel some expulsive, pushing contractions. If you feel like pushing but your cervix isn't fully dilated, your doctor may ask you to not push, but to pant through these contractions instead.

How to deal with the transition phase

If you're laboring without an epidural, this is when you may fear you can't handle the pain. You'll need lots of support from those around you.

- Some women appreciate a light massage (effleurage), some prefer a stronger touch, and others don't want to be touched at all.
- A change of position can bring relief—for example, if you're feeling a lot of pressure in your lower back, getting on all fours may reduce the discomfort.
- A cool cloth on your forehead or a cold pack on your back may feel good, or you may find a warm compress more comforting.

On the other hand, because transition can take all of your concentration, you may want all distractions—music or conversation or even that cool cloth or your partner's loving touch—eliminated.

It may be useful to focus on the fact that those hard contractions are helping your baby make the journey out into the world. Try visualizing his movement down with each contraction.

The good news is that, if you've made it this far without medication, you can usually be coached through transition—one contraction at a time—with constant reminders that you're doing a great job and that the end is near.

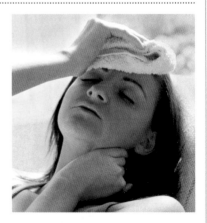

Ask your birth partner to put a cool cloth on your forehead to help to soothe you during the transition stage.

Dad's **Diary**

Our labor story

"Jenny was surprisingly calm and polite between contractions, but then I'd hear the most blood-curdling howl I'd ever heard in my life. You meet ultra-butch, Alpha-male dads who've fainted at this point, and you can understand why fathers used to be barred from births.

But the worst thing is that there's not a lot you can do. Your instinct is to embrace your wife and to try to make the pain go away but, of course, it won't. It's horrible. And the last thing she wants is the man who put her through all this telling her, 'Don't worry honey, it'll be all right.' Your main role is as an advocate—to convince overworked labor nurses that your wife's contractions really do hurt, that she's started dilating, that she still wants to stick to her birth plan and, no, she still doesn't want an epidural.

Like bare-knuckle boxing, labor is an endless barrage of noise, blood, and bodily fluids. And yes, chances are that there'll be some tearing involved.

I became an 'auxiliary nurse' as my wife was choreographed through more and more improbable birthing positions (on your knees, on your back, bend double, lean against me, try squatting, don't forget to breathe). Woe betide the man who hasn't done his homework."

Usually there is some sort of change in your behavior, which marks the transition phase. You might feel shaky, shivery, or sick. You may feel so out of control that you want to yell and scream, and demand pain relief. You may feel that you really can't continue any more! Or, you may feel sleepy and go within yourself during this stage. Some call this experience the "rest and be thankful" stage.

Partners are often quite worried by this stage of labor. You may feel the need to yell, cry out, or even swear as a way of coping, but your partner may see it as a sign that you need help and he may feel alarmed. Make sure he's well

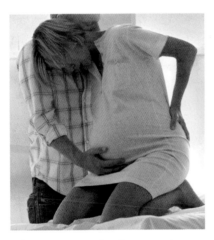

Your partner needs to be extra patient while you are in the transition stage, especially if you feel like shouting at him.

> "Some **call this** experience the **'rest and be thankful'** stage."

prepared for this stage. If he is aware of what is happening, he is more likely to be able to get through it himself—and to give you the support you need to help you get through it.

Recognizing that you're in transition, in whatever form it takes for you, can give you a boost. It means that you're nearly there! Think of it as a bridge you need to cross to reach your baby.

Parents**Talk...**

"Things weren't great for me during the transition phase—each contraction went on forever and was so painful. I was just screaming and gripping my husband's hand so tightly that I bruised him. (But despite him yelling from the pain, there's no way it came close to what I was going through!)"
Anna, 29, mom to month-old Owen

"For me, the transitional phase was the most physically difficult part of the whole of the labor process— I felt shaky and nauseous from the pressure and pain my body was enduring as the contractions were pushing my cervix to its limit before the big push."
Yoko, 31, mom to year-old Ricky

"The transitional stage had no effect on me—I couldn't feel a thing because of the epidural! The only problem came when I had to push. I had to wait for my nurse to give me the cue since I couldn't feel the contractions. That was a really odd sensation."
Frances, 24, first-time mom

"The pain was so intense, I felt like I was having an out-of-body experience during the transitional stage of my labor. I'd been doing my breathing through my contractions the whole time and, as they got stronger and longer, I just had the feeling that I was floating away on a cloud! It felt quite blissful."
Rachel, 30, mom to month-old James

Getting ready for pregnancy

Staying safe and healthy

Your pregnancy diary

Birth and beyond

Positions for labor

Forget those pictures you've seen on TV of women flopping around in bed during labor. Giving birth is a bit like running a marathon—it requires strength and stamina—and using active, upright positions is one of the things that will help your body to do its important work.

First stage positions

When labor starts, you'll probably feel restless. You'll want to move around but don't get overly tired before your labor is truly underway. Take short rests in a chair or lying down. If labor starts at night, try to stay in bed and relax for as long as possible.

As contractions get stronger, you'll need to concentrate on them and practice your breathing and relaxation exercises. Now is the time to find the positions that best help you cope with your contractions. Your nurse should help you find a comfortable position.

You might think that you'll be most comfortable lying down. However, keeping upright will help your labor to progress and help you and your baby to manage better during labor.

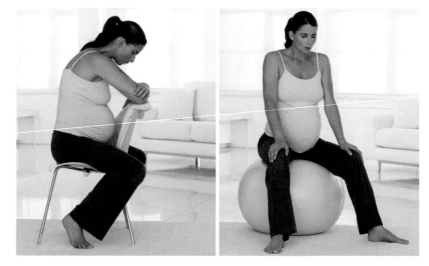

Sitting facing the back of a chair with your arms on the back for support gives you the chance to have a back massage.

Sitting on an exercise ball keeps you upright. This position helps you concentrate on your rhythmic breathing.

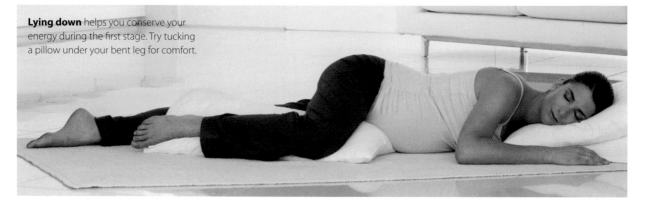

Lying down helps you conserve your energy during the first stage. Try tucking a pillow under your bent leg for comfort.

Transition stage

As you reach transition, upright positions can help lessen the pain of contractions and make it easier for your birth partner to massage your back or breathe with you. You could put your arms around your partner's neck and lean on him, or lean on a work surface or the back of a chair, Some women prefer to go onto all fours or kneel on one leg with the other bent. Rock your hips backward and forward or in a circle to help your baby through your pelvis.

You'll probably find that you don't want to move around a great deal. You'll need all your strength simply to deal with each contraction as it comes along.

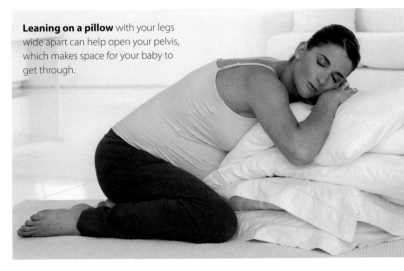

Leaning on a pillow with your legs wide apart can help open your pelvis, which makes space for your baby to get through.

Positions for pushing

Finding a comfortable upright position is recommended for the pushing stage of labor. You are less likely to need help with instruments to deliver your baby if you're upright. The combination of the muscular action of your uterus, your pushing efforts, a wider outlet through the pelvis, and gravity is a powerful one.

Alternatively, you could try kneeling on the mattress and leaning against a large pile of pillows placed at the top end. Some women find it very helpful to kneel on the bed and put their arms around their partner's neck as he stands at the bedside.

If your doctor is okay with you giving birth while on the floor, you could try kneeling. When it's time for your baby's head to be born, kneeling on all fours is an excellent position. Gravity is not so effective in this position, so your baby's head is able to emerge very gently from the vagina.

An all-fours position is good for giving birth gently since it reduces the effect of gravity.

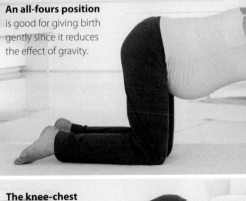

The knee-chest position helps slow things down while you adjust to stronger contractions.

Getting ready for pregnancy

Staying safe and healthy

Your pregnancy diary

Birth and beyond

Second stage of labor

Once your cervix is fully dilated, the work and excitement of the second stage begin. This is the stage of labor when your uterus pushes your baby down the birth canal and out into the world. The hard work is nearly over and you're about to meet your baby.

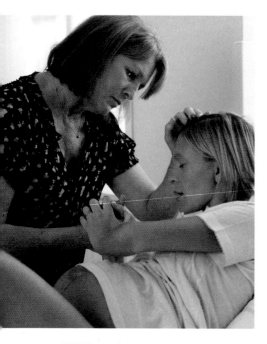

Descent and birth

During the second stage, your contractions change to expulsive, pushing contractions. You will feel pressure between your legs as your baby moves down your vagina.

As your baby descends you may get an overwhelming urge to push and hear yourself grunting deep in your throat with each contraction. For many women the urge to bear down and vocalize is instinctive and feels completely natural.

Not everyone feels "pushy," though. If you've had an epidural, the pushing urge

Seek reassurance and encouragement from your birth partner while you are doing the difficult job of pushing your baby out.

may be delayed for a while. Some women don't get the pushing urge at all. Your nurse or doctor may suggest you wait a while to see if the urge comes on or she may help you get into a good position for pushing and guide you to bear down with each contraction. She might ask you to push down into your bottom, as if you were having a large bowel movement!

The walls of your vagina are a bit like the folds of a concertina. Each contraction helps your baby stretch and move down the folds until his head appears at the entrance of your vagina. "Crowning" is when his head stays visible at your perineum and doesn't slip back at the end of a contraction. At this

ParentsAsk...

Will I need an episiotomy?

The vagina is designed to stretch around your baby's head as he moves down the birth canal. However, around 14 percent of women need an episiotomy during labor.

An episiotomy is a small cut made in the skin and muscle from the entrance of the vagina toward the back passage. Your doctor will give you a local anesthetic before the cut is made. An episiotomy will need to be stitched afterward using

dissolving stitches. You'll be given some more local anesthetic.

The most common reason for having an episiotomy is during an assisted birth with forceps or to allow your doctor more room to manipulate a large baby. An episiotomy may also be used if your baby is in distress and needs to be born quickly or if your baby is very premature (the episiotomy may help to protect his head). Other reasons why you might need an episiotomy include if you are

distressed or very tired, or if it is taking a very long time for the tissues of the vagina to stretch.

You may have feelings about having an episiotomy. It can be useful to discuss these with your doctor during your pregnancy and also during labor. Having a birth plan (see pp.174–5) will help to get the conversation started and ensure that your wishes are heard and noted by the staff who are caring for you.

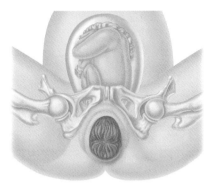

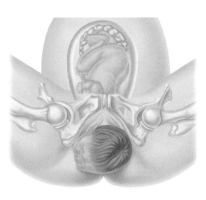

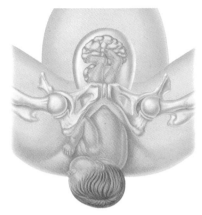

The head crowns, which means that it appears at the vaginal opening. When this happens, your doctor will tell you to pant instead of pushing to give the perineum time to stretch a bit more and to allow the head to emerge gradually.

The head emerges fully so it is free of the perineum. Your baby will extend his neck and automatically turn to face left or right to the inside of one of your thighs. His shoulders will now be in the best position for a smooth delivery.

The first shoulder slips under the pubic bone, quickly followed by the other shoulder. Now the rest of his body is free to slip out and he can be put on your belly.

point, you may want to reach down and touch the top of his head.

Listen to your body during this second stage and push when you get a strong urge. You'll probably want to push down several times during the course of a contraction, taking breaths in between, particularly when you start to push your baby's head out. Try not to hold your breath to push, since bearing down for long periods is more likely to result in you tearing, though it may work for some women. It's best not to hurry this stage.

Pant, don't push

You'll probably get a hot, stinging sensation as the tissues of your perineum and the entrance of your vagina stretch. Rather than pressing on through this "ring of fire," try to pant instead of pushing. Give the tissues of your perineum time to stretch a little more with each contraction.

When your baby's head is born you'll feel a sudden release. With the next contraction your baby's shoulders and body will be born. First-time babies usually take longer than second or later

babies, just because your body has done it all before.

Once your baby has emerged, he'll be dried and, if there aren't any complications, he'll be put on your stomach so you can touch and marvel at him. The skin-to-skin contact will keep him nice and toasty, and he'll be covered with a warm blanket—and perhaps given his first hat—to prevent heat loss. Your doctor will clamp the umbilical cord in two places and then cut between the two clamps—or your partner might like to do the honors.

The second stage can take from a few minutes to two or three hours. You'll feel proud, but relieved it's all over.

Fact: With each contraction and every push, your baby will move down through your pelvis a little, but at the end of the contraction, he'll slip back up again! Don't despair. As long as the baby keeps on moving on a little farther each time, you're doing fine.

Working mom

Work and being promoted are important, but giving birth is a unique experience.

"Ever since my first job, my work has always been really important to me. I've never resented doing overtime or putting the hours in at home if I needed to meet a deadline. Every promotion has meant the world to me because I know it's something I've earned on my own merits. My family have been really pleased with how far I've come, too.

However, that has all paled into insignificance now. When I gave birth to my son, after more than 20 hours of labor, I felt like I was going to burst with pride. Looking into his eyes, and at his perfect fingers and toes, I knew instantly that he was my greatest achievement. Nothing would ever top the feeling of pure satisfaction that I had made him. I've never felt happier or more content."

Getting ready for pregnancy

Staying safe and healthy

Your pregnancy diary

Birth and beyond

Third stage of labor

In the third stage, you deliver the placenta—the life-support system that has supplied your growing baby with nutrients and taken waste products away. Be prepared for a few more contractions and then, at last, the chance to relax and admire your beautiful new baby.

It's not quite over yet!

After your baby is born, contractions resume a few minutes later, but at much less intensity. These contractions cause the placenta to peel away from the wall of the uterus and drop down into the bottom of your uterus. You will probably feel as if you want to push. The placenta, with the membranes of the empty bag of water attached, will pass down and out of your vagina. Once this has happened, your doctor will carefully examine the placenta and membranes to make sure that nothing has been left behind. She will also feel your belly to check that your uterus is contracting, since this is nature's way of stopping the bleeding from the place on the uterus where the placenta was attached.

Delivering the placenta usually takes from five to 20 minutes, but it can take up to an hour. You may hardly be aware of the third stage, since your focus has probably shifted to your baby. Seeing and handling your baby, and offering her the breast will stimulate hormones that help the placenta to separate.

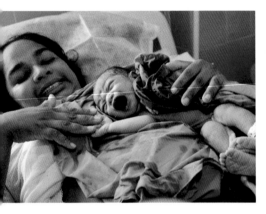

You may hardly notice the third stage of labor as you lie there with your newborn baby on your belly.

How you will feel

Now that the birth is over, you may feel shaky due to adrenaline and the adjustments your body immediately starts to make. Or you may simply be on a high, ready to pick up your baby and dance around the room.

Some women find it hard to pay attention to the baby if they have had a long labor, or if they've had Demerol or a similar drug. There's nothing wrong with their maternal instincts; they're simply exhausted. If this happens to you, take your time. After a rest, you'll be much more interested in getting to know your baby. A lot of women are hungry and ready for something to nibble on, while others want to telephone all their friends and family and tell them the wonderful news.

A natural or managed third stage?

You have the choice between a managed or a physiological (natural) third stage.

● A managed third stage involves administering Pitocin through an IV or, rarely, as an injection. The cord is clamped and cut immediately and the Pitocin makes the uterus contract strongly so the placenta comes away and is delivered quickly.

This is all over quickly, usually in five to 10 minutes. There is little blood loss and less risk of you having heavy bleeding. Pitocin can bring on heavy contractions or cramps.

● A physiological, or natural, third stage means waiting for the placenta to be delivered naturally. This can take around 20 minutes. If it's not out by 30 minutes, your doctor may have to help get it out. Cord clamping is delayed until the cord has stopped pulsating. This ensures that your baby gets the maximum amount of oxygenated blood from the placenta. There is a higher risk of blood loss.

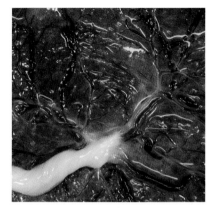

The placenta is attached to your baby's umbilical cord (yellowish-white). After the placenta has been delivered, the doctor will check to make sure it is all present.

ParentsAsk...

What is postpartum hemorrhage?

A primary postpartum hemorrhage (PPH) is heavy bleeding in the first 24 hours after the birth. It happens in about 5 percent of births with a managed third stage and in 5 percent of births with a natural or physiological third stage.

Most cases of primary PPH are due to the uterus not contracting down properly after the birth to shut off all the blood vessels where the placenta was attached. You may feel the blood trickling out or sometimes it builds up inside your uterus, so you may not be aware of the hemorrhage until signs of shock appear: a drop in blood pressure and a rise in your pulse rate, and you may feel faint and dizzy.

Your nurse or doctor regularly checks your uterus after birth to make sure it is firm and contracted. If it is soft she will massage the top of the uterus to encourage it to contract. She may give you another oxytocin injection and an intravenous drip to help your blood clot. If the bleeding is severe, you may need a blood transfusion.

Complications in the third stage

Retained placenta means that all or part of the placenta or membranes are left behind in the uterus during the third stage of labor. You'll be treated for a retained placenta if the third stage takes longer than usual or if there are signs that a small piece of placenta that was connected to the main part of the placenta by a blood vessel is still attached to the uterus.

The doctor will examine the placenta and membranes very carefully after delivery to ensure that they are complete. If she notices a blood vessel leading to nowhere, this should alert her to the possibility that part of the placenta has been left behind in the uterus.

Sometimes a part of the placenta may adhere to a fibroid or to a scar from a previous cesarean. Sometimes a full bladder will prevent the placenta from being delivered, so your doctor may insert a catheter to drain your bladder.

Normally after the placenta is delivered, your uterus contracts down to close off all the blood vessels inside it.

If the placenta only partially separates, the uterus cannot contract properly, so the blood vessels inside will continue to bleed. If small fragments of placenta or membrane are retained and are not detected immediately, this may cause heavy bleeding (see Parents Ask, above) and infection later on.

If the third stage is taking a while, you could try breast-feeding your baby or rubbing your nipples. This can make the uterus contract and may help to expel the placenta. If you're sitting or lying, try changing to a more upright position so that gravity can help.

If the placenta still cannot be removed, it may need to be removed manually. You will be given a local anesthetic or, if you prefer, you can ask for a general anesthetic.

Dad's **Diary**

My big thrill

"The nurses had me holding up one of my wife's legs at a bizarre angle while I tried not to look at what was going on between her legs. Jenny told me afterward that I proved to be a big, safe, chunky cushion to lean against.

After the most protracted scream I'd ever heard in my life, out it popped. I picked up our wonky-headed, blood-covered, prune-faced little baby, with a furry back and alarmingly hairy ears. The fruit of my loins. 'It's a girl!' I shouted excitedly. (This was a relief. Our boys' names were all horrible, but we both liked the same girl's name—Lilah.)

Then I was given the honor of cutting the umbilical cord. I hadn't really planned to do this. I thought I'd be too squeamish but, after everything I'd seen Jenny go through during the last few hours, this was a breeze. It was the first thing I did to care for my new baby daughter and it made me feel like a daddy for the first time."

Natural pain relief

We're lucky to live in an age when we can have effective pain relief during labor if we want it. Some forms of medical pain relief, though, can have side effects for you and your baby, so it pays to be clued in on natural pain-relief methods, too.

Your choices

Gone are the days when pain relief in labor meant using a magic charm. You now have a range of natural options to choose from.

Positioning and movement

When you're not medicated, you can try a variety of positions during labor, including standing or leaning on your partner, swaying in a "birth dance,"

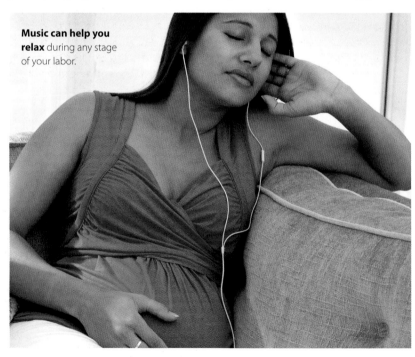

Music can help you relax during any stage of your labor.

sitting, and kneeling—either upright or on all fours.

You may find movement comforting, too. Try walking around, or rocking in a chair or on a birthing ball. Moving around can make you feel more in control, which may help to ease your anxiety and pain.

Even if you have complications that require continuous monitoring, you can

still try a variety of positions in bed. You may also be able to stand, sit, or pace at your bedside.

Some hospitals have wireless monitoring systems (telemetry) that enable you to move around freely. If a waterproof unit is available, you'll even be able to sit in the shower.

During the pushing stage, an upright position may help your baby descend, and squatting or kneeling may help open your pelvic outlet. That said, the best positions are the ones that work for you—so feel free to try a variety of positions and settle on the ones that make you most comfortable.

Acupuncture and acupressure

Acupuncture, which uses fine needles inserted into specific energy points of the body, may help to induce labor and reduce labor pains. You'll need to have a private acupuncturist with you in labor if you want to use it. Acupressure involves finger-tip pressure on these same energy points.

If your contractions are painful, ask your partner to massage very firmly into the small of your back. He can also use his thumbs to press firmly into the dimples on either side of your lower spine, starting at your coccyx (tailbone)

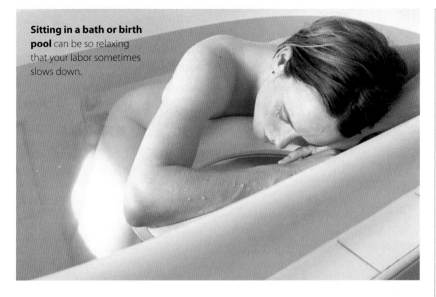

Sitting in a bath or birth pool can be so relaxing that your labor sometimes slows down.

and moving up to your waist. Ask him to apply pressure to each pair of dimples for two seconds, then move up to the next pair, and so on. When he reaches your waist area, he needs to start again at your coccyx. He can do this about four times during each contraction.

Reflexology

Reflexology is based on the idea that your feet represent a map of your body. Reflexologists believe that putting pressure on particular points of the feet will alleviate symptoms in the corresponding part of the body.

If you are finding contractions hard to deal with, ask your birth partner to squeeze your heels several times during a contraction. Your heels are supposed to represent the reflexology zone for the pelvis. Squeezing your heels is a way of "hugging" the part of your body that is doing all the work during labor.

If your contractions slow down, your partner could massage the back of your big toes. There's a reflexology point here which is believed to relate to the pituitary gland in your brain, from which labor hormones are produced.

Hypnotherapy

Hypnotherapy can help reduce pain by preparing you mentally for labor and birth, and by using the power of suggestion to help you relax. It may also help to alter your perception of pain.

You can learn self-hypnosis techniques from special CDs, or take a special hypnotherapy course while you're pregnant. Some women find their own registered hypnotherapist. She may use traditional hypnosis techniques both before and during your labor.

Hypnosis may shorten the first stage of labor but it can lengthen the second stage slightly. If you choose to have medical pain relief in addition to hypnotherapy, you might find that you can deal with much lower doses.

Water and water births

It's becoming more common for women to get into a shower, bath, or special birthing pool to help deal with labor, and many nurses are experienced and skilled in supporting this.

If you are using a birth pool in a hospital, you may not be able to get into the pool until your labor is well

---

Natural pain relief methods

This handy summary of natural pain relief shows what you—and your partner—can easily do to help ease those labor pains.

- ask for information: the more you know, the more relaxed you'll feel
- breathe rhythmically
- cuddle your partner
- drink sips of isotonic drinks or water in between contractions
- eat carbohydrate-rich foods little and often if you feel hungry
- fan yourself with a small electric fan
- groan and moan
- hold your partner's hand
- imagine your baby moving down through your pelvis with every contraction
- joke with your partner and your doctor or labor nurse
- kisses (from your partner, mom, sister, friend)
- listen to music
- move around
- nestle down in a large pile of pillows
- open your pelvis as wide as possible, for example, by kneeling on one leg with the other out to the side
- think positively
- question what you don't understand
- rock your pelvis
- sigh out gently with every breath
- trust your body
- understand the treatment offered
- visit the bathroom regularly; a full bladder will slow your labor
- walk around to ease the aches and pains
- more kisses!
- yell, loud and long
- zzzzzzz: doze off in between contractions

Getting ready for pregnancy

Staying safe and healthy

Your pregnancy diary

Birth and beyond

established. This is because getting into the pool may cause labor to slow down. Once you get in, you might find either that your contractions are less intense for a while, or that they suddenly become more frequent and stronger. Either way, you will benefit.

Remember that the pool is there for you to use as it suits you. This may mean getting in and out several times, or staying in all the time, or getting out completely if it doesn't seem to help.

As the end of the first stage of labor approaches and contractions are coming thick and fast, you might want to get out of the pool, even if you had originally intended to give birth in it. Or, alternatively, you might feel that you simply cannot get out, although your

plan had been to give birth on dry land. Unless your hospital has a strict policy about women not giving birth in the pool, you are free to choose what you want to do when the time comes.

Breathing techniques

In labor, you need to conserve your energy as much as possible and give your baby plenty of oxygen to help him deal with the birth process. Rhythmic breathing can help you do this and focusing on your breathing is a great way of getting through each contraction.

Take a deep breath at the beginning of the contraction and, as you breathe out, re-lax. Then breathe in through your nose and breathe out through your mouth, keeping your mouth and cheeks very, very soft. Don't worry too much about how deeply you're breathing, just keep a good rhythm going. Breathe in through your nose, and out through a

soft mouth. And again. And again. Concentrate as hard as you can on your breathing as the contraction builds up, and as it fades away. When the contraction's over, re-lax.

Or you can try counted breathing. As you breathe in, count slowly up to three or four (or whatever number seems comfortable for you) and, as you breathe out, count to three or four again. You might find that it's more comfortable to breathe in to a count of three and out to a count of four.

Massage

Massage stimulates the body to release endorphins, which are natural pain-killing and mood-lifting substances. Childbirth experts recommend it because it has been shown to ease pain and reduce anxiety in the first stage of labor. The use of massage may possibly be connected to shorter labors and a lower risk of postpartum depression.

Massage can also bring you closer to the person who is caring for you: your labor nurse or your birth partner. Tell them where you'd like to be massaged. You might like massage at the very base of your back during contractions. Or you might like your shoulders massaged in between contractions to help you relax. Give feedback when you can, so that you get the best out of it.

A massage that starts slowly is best—frantic rubbing will simply make you feel panicky rather than relaxed! And it's firm pressure that's needed. This will help stimulate your body to release endorphins, which is what makes massage such a positive and relaxing experience.

Aromatherapy

Aromatherapists believe that essential oils—extracts of certain plants and flowers—can stimulate and balance

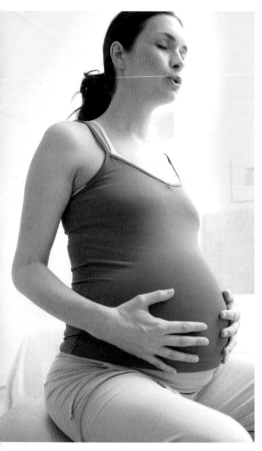

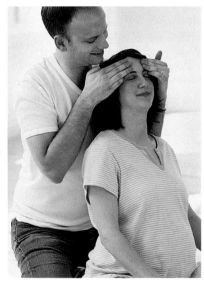

Ask your birth partner (above) to massage your temples or shoulders to help you relax between your contractions.

Focusing on your breath (left) when in labor helps you through contractions and gives your baby plenty of oxygen.

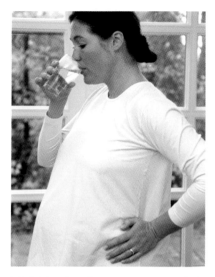

Drinking sips of water or an isotonic drink can help you to relax between contractions, and also keep you well hydrated.

hormone levels and soothe stress. Massage with essential oils during labor can help reduce anxiety and increase our levels of "feel good" hormones such as oxytocin, which help labor to progress normally. If you don't like the idea of massage, you can just inhale the scents of the oil by putting one or two drops on a tissue.

Grapefruit, bergamot, ylang ylang, mandarin, and lavender essential oils can all help to relieve tension in labor. Frankincense is particularly recommended: it is especially useful for easing any feelings of panic you may experience when contractions are getting difficult to cope with.

Warmth
Using warmth is a traditional way of relaxing tense muscles. It can also be used to provide relief from labor pain.

You can warm your back, belly, or groin using a wheat bag or a hot-water bottle. A wheat bag is filled with wheat husks. You heat the bag up for a few minutes in the microwave, then apply it.

The wheat bag will drape and shape itself to your body and will stay warm for an hour or more. You can buy wheat bags online or in pharmacies. Some hospitals sell them also.

If you are planning to use a hot-water bottle, you should fill it with hot (but not boiling) water, and carefully wrap it in a towel or soft cover before using it. Do this to make sure you don't get burned by the hot rubber.

Don't forget that massage provides warmth as well. Having someone rub your back will warm your skin as well as stimulate your body to release natural pain-killing endorphins. Using a birth pool is yet another way to envelop yourself in all-encompassing warmth.

When your baby's head is being born, a soft warm washcloth or compress placed over your perineum (the tissue between the back of the vagina and the back passage) may make you feel more comfortable as the perineal tissue stretches. However, the warmth won't necessarily prevent any tears.

Homeopathy
Homeopathy uses minute, highly diluted doses of substances which, if taken as a full dose, would actually cause the same symptoms that the diluted dose attempts to treat. There is no scientific evidence that homeopathic remedies are safe or effective. Please consult your healthcare practitioner before taking them.

Homeopathic remedies, like other complementary therapies, are best administered by an experienced homeopath who is trained in this method. Some homeopaths will prescribe a "birthing set" of remedies which are specially designed to suit you for your labor.

Homeopaths often recommend taking arnica to treat the shock, trauma,

or bruising you may experience during and after giving birth vaginally or by cesarean. If you're interested in trying homeopathy after childbirth, see a professional homeopath who can prescribe a specific remedy and dose based on your symptoms. Strong tinctures can be dangerous.

Green mom

If you're planning a natural labor, research some natural methods of pain relief.

"I knew the decision not to have any pain relief would be tough, but I was ready for the challenge. I'd prepared some natural pain-relief techniques— some of which required a lot of help from my husband! To keep me relaxed and ease tense muscles, I had a couple of hot-water bottles for my belly and lower back. Joe gave me a slow, firm massage on my lower back during contractions, and kept me calm in between with a soothing shoulder massage. My breathing really helped carry me through, too. At the start of each contraction I took a deep breath through my nose, then breathed out slowly through my mouth while trying to stay as relaxed as possible. I also found that leaning on Joe, rocking my hips back and forth, kneeling on all fours, and walking around the room were a few movements that kept me comfortable when the contractions became very painful. And I'm pretty sure they helped to speed my labor up, too."

Getting ready for pregnancy

Staying safe and healthy

Your pregnancy diary

Birth and beyond

Medical pain relief

Nobody knows exactly how labor will feel for them until it starts. Some of us find that labor is bearable with little or no pain relief, although many of us are likely to want help at some point. Either way, it's useful to read up about your choices early on.

ParentsAsk...

I'm really scared of labor. What if the pain relief I'm offered doesn't help?

There are many strategies you can adopt. All labor involves some pain, which can be frightening, but thinking about it beforehand, and accepting it, can help you deal with it better.

Talk to someone who knows you well about how you have dealt with pain in the past—you may have managed better than you thought.

Having good one-on-one support can help you, too. Think about who would be the best person to help you in labor: it may be your partner, a friend, or relative, or you may be able to employ a birth supporter or a doula.

Remember that there are very effective methods of pain relief available to you in the hospital, such as an epidural. Talk to your doctor about these and other options, and ask them to help you prepare a birth plan, so that what you want is clear to everybody taking care of you.

Make sure you understand what happens during labor. Knowing how your body works can help with the fear. Try to figure out which aspects of labor are worrying you. Is it the fear of losing control? Do you worry that something might go wrong? Once you have put your finger on the key worry you can talk it through with your doctor or childbirth class teacher.

Your choices

We've moved on since the days when women turned to ether to ease their pain in childbirth. Women today have more—and safer—options.

Most moms-to-be in the United States choose some kind of pain medication (most commonly an epidural) to help them deal with labor.

Some decide well before delivery day that they want pain medication, some ask for relief when they find that labor isn't what they imagined, and some end up opting for medication if nature throws them a curve ball and they find themselves having a long or complicated labor. You must keep in mind that the intensity of the discomfort during labor varies from woman to woman and birth to birth.

In any case, you'll usually need to make a decision about whether you want drugs while you're still in the first stage of labor. By the time you're pushing, it's generally too late to be given any drugs.

It's a good idea to find out in advance what options are available at the hospital or center where you plan to deliver your baby. If you have any questions about pain relief options, discuss them with your care provider before you're dealing with contractions!

Systemic medications

Systemic painkillers such as narcotics dull your pain but don't completely eliminate it. You may also be given a tranquilizer—alone or in combination with a narcotic—to reduce anxiety or nausea, or to relax you.

Systemic drugs are either delivered through an IV line to your bloodstream or injected into a muscle. They affect your entire body rather than concentrating pain relief in the uterus and pelvic area. They may make you feel sleepy, but unlike the general anesthesia that's often given for surgery, they won't make you unconscious.

Systemic pain relief may help if you can deal with some pain but need something to take the edge off and help you relax. It's easier and less invasive to be given an IV or an injection than it is to have an epidural or a spinal block, and it usually doesn't require an anesthesiologist. Doses are typically small and available during active labor.

Disadvantages of systemic medication

• Systemic medication is much less effective than an epidural or a spinal block for pain relief. (The dose that can be given must be relatively small, because these drugs cross the placenta and can affect your baby.)

• Narcotics can cause a variety of unpleasant side effects, such as drowsiness, dizziness, and disorientation. Because of this, you'll have to stay in bed. Some of these drugs may also cause nausea and itchiness.

• Sometimes, especially if they're given too soon, narcotics slow labor.

• In large doses, narcotics can interfere with your breathing. (This very rarely happens, in part because it's unusual to get high doses of narcotics during labor. If it does happen, you'll need medication to reverse the effects of the narcotic.)

• Systemic pain medication can affect your baby's heart rate in such a way that your doctor or labor nurse will have trouble interpreting the results of fetal heart rate monitoring.

• Narcotics sometimes make it harder for your baby to start breathing by himself after birth, particularly if you've had multiple doses during your labor or you're given a relatively large dose within a few hours of delivery. For this reason, your doctor will be stingy with narcotics late in your labor.

Sometimes, though, labor will progress much more quickly than expected. If that happens, your baby will need medication to counteract the effects of the narcotic. (If your baby is premature or otherwise at risk, your doctor may recommend an epidural instead of systemic pain relief.)

• Systemic narcotics may make your baby less alert at birth and may cause him to nurse less effectively early on, making your first attempts at breastfeeding more difficult.

Common drugs
You may have some choice in which systemic medications you can take advantage of, but the availability of specific drugs depends on the hospital or birth center where you deliver.

Commonly available narcotics include Stadol, Demerol, Nubain, fentanyl, and morphine. They generally have similar potential side effects for both mother and baby. Stadol may make you sleepier than other drugs. Fentanyl, which takes effect quickly but doesn't last as long as other drugs, is less commonly available; in most hospitals it must be administered by an anesthesiologist. Morphine is longer-acting and is more commonly used to help women get a few hours of deep rest.

Patient-controlled analgesia
With patient-controlled analgesia (PCA), you can control the medication by administering it yourself. This is becoming increasingly available as an option during labor.

With PCA, a fine tube is inserted into your vein and the other end of the tube is attached to a pump. You can operate the pump to give yourself small amounts of medication.

A relatively new drug that can be administered by PCA but is not widely available is remifentanil, or Ultiva. It is a fast-acting drug that carries less risk of prolonged sedation. It is not available everywhere.

Epidural
An epidural is where painkilling drugs are passed into the small of your back via a fine tube. The drugs are injected around the nerves that carry signals from the part of your body that feels pain when you're in labor. The result is very effective pain relief.

When you have an epidural, your anesthesiologist will first give you an injection of local anesthetic in your lower back. She then guides a hollow needle between the bones of your spine

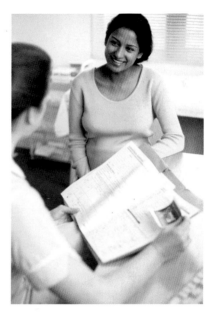

Your doctor will be able to give you information about the various methods of pain relief, so discuss them beforehand to help you decide.

into the space between the layers of tissue in your spinal column (the epidural space). A fine tube is then passed through the needle. Once the tube is in place, the anesthesiologist removes the needle. The tube is taped up your back and over your shoulder. Once your epidural is in place, it should stay in until after your baby is born and your placenta is delivered.

Most hospitals use low-dose epidurals. These contain a mixture of painkilling drugs, usually a local anesthetic, bupivacaine, and an opioid—fentanyl. Having a low-dose epidural means that you may still have some sensation in your legs and feet.

You can have an epidural at any point during your labor, but most women choose it when their contractions are getting pretty strong, which is often when their cervix has dilated by about 5 or 6 cm. You'll also be offered an epidural if your labor has to

Getting ready for pregnancy

Staying safe and healthy

Your pregnancy diary

Birth and beyond

be speeded up with a Pitocin IV, because this can make your contractions difficult to deal with.

An epidural can provide excellent pain relief during labor and is typically on a continuous pump, which means you don't usually need to wait for an anesthesiologist once the epidural is in place. Another advantage is that your mind remains clear. You may still be aware of your contractions, but feel no

---

Organized mom

Knowing that pain relief is on hand can help you through the worst of labor.

"I felt that it was much better to be prepared and make a definite decision beforehand about pain relief, instead of deciding at the last minute and then feeling flustered and panicked. I knew I wanted my birth to go as smoothly as possible, and to be controlled but relaxed.

I did as much research as I could about all the methods of pain relief and what would be best for me. My final birth plan was to have Demerol during the first stage of labor, as the contractions started. Then, as the contractions grew stronger and more painful, I intended to have an epidural. When I actually went into labor, knowing that pain relief was definitely on the way stopped me from panicking. And I knew exactly how the Demerol and an epidural would be administered, and was prepared for how I would feel when the pain relief took effect. In the end, I was so happy that I'd made this decision— I don't think I'd have dealt with the pain easily, since my labor ended up being a long one!"

---

pain. Another bonus is that only a tiny amount of medication reaches your baby.

One disadvantage is that the epidural may not work properly at first. You may find that you are numb in only parts of your abdomen. If you are not free of pain within half an hour of being given the epidural, ask for the anesthesiologist to come back to adjust it or to try again.

Epidurals have other disadvantages, too. Once you have had one you will have to stay in bed. With a low-dose epidural you may be able to shuffle around on the bed but you won't be able to walk around. You could lose some sensation in your legs and be unable to stand. You may also need to have a catheter inserted to empty your bladder, and your baby's heartbeat will be monitored continuously for at least 30 minutes when you're first given the epidural.

There's also more chance of your baby needing to be born with the aid of forceps or vacuum (see pp.282–3). This may be because an epidural can make it difficult for your baby to move into the best position to be born. An assisted delivery means you will have more bruising, stitching, and postpartum pain, as well as an increased risk of long-term incontinence

There is a small risk of you having a severe headache. This can happen if the epidural needle punctures the bag of fluid that surrounds the spinal cord, causing a leak of fluid. There is about a one in 100 chance of this happening.

Even maternity units equipped to give epidurals may not offer a 24-hour service, so be prepared for the possibility that you may not be able to have one.

Walking epidural

A walking, or ambulatory, epidural is similar to a standard low-dose epidural; it gives excellent pain relief, but also

allows you to retain some sensation in your legs so you may be able to move around somewhat, but you will need help to do so. The main goal of this kind of epidural is to relieve pain; keeping you mobile is only a secondary concern. Some women find that they're not really mobile at all.

A walking epidural uses the same combination of drugs as the low-dose epidurals that most hospitals offer as standard. It is a regional anesthetic, which means the drug is injected around the nerves that carry signals from the part of your body that feels pain when you're in labor.

Hospitals that offer walking epidurals have procedures in place to ensure that it is safe for you to move around with an epidural in place, and that they have enough staff to support you while you're doing so. If the medical staff agree that you are safe to walk, you must always be accompanied and monitored while you are moving around.

You may find that you only have a very limited amount of movement. Some women can manage to move from the bed to a chair, and a few can walk with help. You may also find the extra monitoring you'll need intrusive.

Check in advance whether or not your hospital offers walking epidurals.

Spinal block

A spinal block (or "spinal") quickly delivers pain relief to your lower body for a limited period of time. You will have a needle inserted into your lower back and guided through the membrane surrounding your spine. You will then have an anesthetic, with or without a narcotic, injected into your spinal fluid. This effectively eliminates pain from your waist down. Unlike an epidural, it's a one-time injection: Relief is rapid and complete but lasts only a few hours.

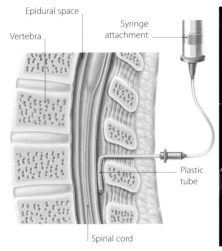

Epidural space
Syringe attachment
Vertebra
Plastic tube
Spinal cord

In an epidural, anesthetic is injected via a fine tube inside a hollow needle that has been positioned in your back.

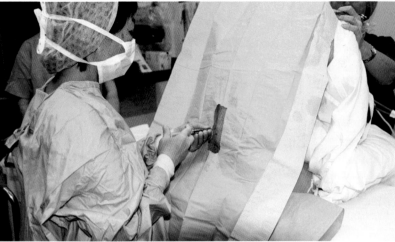

When you have an epidural, a sterile cover is put over your back and you are given a local anesthetic. The hollow needle is then guided between the bones of your spine.

Getting ready for pregnancy

Staying safe and healthy

Your pregnancy diary

Birth and beyond

A spinal may be an option if you want pain relief late in labor, or if you need to have a cesarean.

Only a tiny amount of medication reaches your baby. As with an epidural, you'll have to stay in bed after getting a spinal block. The reduced sensation can make it harder for you to push your baby

An anesthesiologist or nurse anesthetist injects your back with numbing medicine and guides an epidural needle into your lower back. Then she puts the narrower spinal needle inside the epidural needle, guides it through the membrane surrounding your spine, and injects a small dose of medication

hour or two (which allows you to continue to walk around). Then you have the epidural to fall back on once the spinal starts to wear off. In more active labor, you may opt for a combined spinal/epidural so you get immediate relief from the spinal while you're waiting for the epidural to work.

"A spinal block **effectively eliminates pain** from the **waist down** but relief only **lasts a few hours**."

out, increasing your odds of needing a vacuum extraction or forceps delivery. The anesthetic drugs that are used may temporarily lower your blood pressure, reducing blood flow to your baby, which in turn slows his heart rate. If this happens, you will be treated with fluids and sometimes medication.

Combined spinal/epidural
A combined spinal/epidural block is a newer technique that offers the rapid pain relief of a spinal and the continuous relief of the epidural.

into your spinal fluid. After removing the spinal needle, she passes the epidural catheter through the remaining epidural needle. Then she removes that needle and tapes the catheter in place, so medication can be administered through it as needed. You can lie down at this point without disturbing the catheter. Complete pain relief kicks in after only a few minutes.

In early labor, this technique can work like a walking epidural because you rely primarily on the narcotics in the spinal injection for pain relief for the first

The epidural provides a route for very effective pain relief that can be used throughout your labor, and it offers the advantage that you'll remain awake and alert during labor and birth. It can also be used to provide anesthesia if you need a cesarean or if you're having your tubes tied after delivery. Another advantage is that only a small amount of medication reaches your baby.

However, a disadvantage is that you might find it harder to push, making it more likely you might need a vacuum extraction or forceps delivery.

Premature labor

About 12 percent of babies are born prematurely (at less than 37 weeks), and about one percent arrive very prematurely (at less than 32 weeks). Here's how to spot the signs of premature labor and what to expect if you deliver your baby early.

What is premature labor?

A premature birth is when a baby arrives before 37 completed weeks of pregnancy. Twelve percent of babies in the United States are born prematurely each year. A baby who arrives at 34 weeks is unlikely to have any problems, although he may be a bit small and may have breathing difficulties.

However, babies who are born earlier than this still have a lot of growing to do and their internal organs need to mature (see opposite). They may be quite weak and find sucking and breathing difficult.

It is still very difficult for doctors to predict whether a healthy woman will

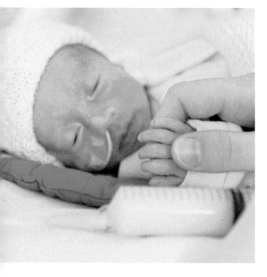

A baby born before 34 weeks will have to go immediately into intensive care. You'll be able to visit and sometimes touch him.

go into labor prematurely. There is evidence to show that the presence of certain bacteria in the urine makes premature labor more likely. Because of this, it is now recommended that all women have their urine tested for bacteria early in pregnancy.

There are a number of other risk factors for premature labor:
- Infections of the vagina and of the urinary tract.
- Expecting twins or more.
- Smoking.
- Using recreational drugs, such as marijuana, ecstasy, or cocaine.
- Some abnormalities of the uterus.
- Previous premature birth.

If your water breaks, or you start having contractions before 37 weeks of pregnancy, contact your doctor or hospital immediately, even if it's the middle of the night. You will almost certainly be asked to go to the hospital. Don't drive yourself. If you have nobody to give you a ride, the hospital will send an ambulance for you.

At the hospital, you will be given a vaginal examination to see if your cervix

is shortening and opening. A number of tests may be done to check for infection, including a urine test and vaginal swab. You may be offered a vaginal ultrasound scan to see how long your cervix is. A short cervix may indicate that labor has started. Another test is for a substance called "fetal fibronectin" in the fluid in your vagina. Finding this substance often indicates that the baby will be born soon.

If labor's underway

Unfortunately, doctors can't stop labor if it's really underway and resting won't help either. However, if you are less than 34 weeks pregnant, your doctor can give you a drug to delay the birth for a while so there's time to transfer you to a hospital with a neonatal intensive care unit (NICU). You'll also be offered steroid medication to help your baby's lungs mature. If you are more than 34 weeks pregnant, your doctors will probably allow labor to continue at its own pace.

You will naturally feel very worried, and perhaps out of control because of all the medical attention you are receiving. Ask your labor nurses and doctors to explain everything that's happening.

Your baby's heartbeat will be monitored throughout labor. Although labor is premature, you won't necessarily need a cesarean. However, you might have to have one if you've gone into labor following a hemorrhage or if your baby is severely distressed.

If your baby is born before 34 weeks, he may need to go immediately to the neonatal intensive care unit (see p.297). This can be frightening but staff will give you the support you need. A baby born between 34 and 37 weeks may not need medical treatment and may be able to go to the postpartum ward with you. You may be encouraged to carry him close to your breasts. This seems to provide the right physical and emotional conditions for your baby to grow quickly.

Future risk

If you've had a second-trimester loss or a spontaneous preterm birth and are carrying only one baby, you might be treated with a progesterone compound called 17 alpha hydroxyprogesterone caproate, or 17 P for short. Studies have shown that weekly injections of this compound significantly reduced the risk of a repeat preterm delivery.

If you have already had one premature birth you are at an increased risk of having another premature baby. There is about a 15 percent chance that your next baby will also be premature.

At the moment, doctors don't know how to prevent a woman from giving birth prematurely. However, if you smoke or use recreational drugs, quitting will reduce the risk. At least, if you've had one premature birth then, next time, you'll be able to prepare for the possibility that your baby may arrive early. During a subsequent pregnancy, your doctor will monitor you and your pregnancy closely and will help you deal with the anxiety you are bound to feel.

If your baby is born prematurely

Number of weeks	Possible problems	Treatment
Pre 28 weeks	Most of these babies weigh less than 35 ounces. They can't suck, swallow, and breathe at the same time. They have little muscle tone, and most don't move much.	All need oxygen and mechanical assistance to help them breathe. They must be fed through a vein (intravenously) until they're able to suck and swallow. They have a high risk of one or more medical complications and may face an extended stay in the neonatal intensive care unit.
28 to 31 weeks	These babies usually weigh 2 to 4 pounds. About 90 to 95 percent survive. If they weigh less than 3 pounds 4 ounces they are at risk of serious disabilities.	Most require oxygen and mechanical assistance to help them breathe. Some can be fed breast milk or formula through a tube placed through their nose or mouth into the stomach, although others will need to be fed intravenously.
32 to 33 weeks	More than 95 percent of babies born at this time survive. Most weigh 3 to 5 pounds. Some can breathe on their own, and many just need supplemental oxygen to help them.	Some can be breast- or bottle-fed, but those who have breathing difficulties will probably need tube feeding. These babies are less likely than babies born earlier to develop serious disabilities, although they remain at a slightly increased risk for learning and behavioral problems.
34 to 36 weeks	Babies born at this time are almost as likely as full-term babies to survive. They have a higher risk than full-term babies for health problems, including breathing and feeding problems, difficulties regulating body temperature, and jaundice. These problems are usually mild, and most babies make a quick recovery.	Most of these babies can be breast- or bottle-fed, although some (especially those that have mild breathing problems) may need tube feeding for a brief time. It's estimated that, at 35 weeks' gestation, the weight of the brain is only around 60 percent that of full-term babies. Late preterm babies, which is what babies born at 34 to 36 weeks' gestation are called, are unlikely to develop serious disabilities resulting from premature birth, but they may be at a slightly increased risk for subtle learning and behavioral problems.

Getting ready for pregnancy · Staying safe and healthy · Your pregnancy diary · Birth and beyond

Assisted birth

Chances are you'll push your baby out into the world with nothing but a bit of encouragement from those around you. Now and again, though, babies need a helping hand to be delivered—what's known as an assisted delivery. The two main methods are forceps and vacuum.

The whys and hows

About 1 percent of all US births use forceps in assisted or operative vaginal deliveries, and a little over 4 percent use plastic vacuum or suction cups. Forceps look like and have sometimes been described as "stainless steel salad servers" or "large sugar tongs." They have two intersecting parts and a pair of curved ends to cradle your baby's head. There are many different types and makes of forceps.

The vacuum extractor has a suction cup attached to a small vacuum pump, and a handle for pulling on. The cup fits on top and toward the back of your baby's head.

Your labor nurse and doctor might recommend an assisted birth if:

Avoiding an assisted birth

It's not always possible to avoid an assisted birth, but the following factors can help reduce your risk. These include:
- Having continuous support during labor from a birth partner or doula.
- Using upright positions during labor.
- Avoiding an epidural (see pp.278–9).
- If you've had an epidural, waiting for at least an hour after you are fully dilated or until you feel the urge to push, before trying to push your baby out.

"Some factors **can reduce** your **risk of** having an **assisted birth**."

- Your baby has become distressed during the pushing stage of labor.
- You are very tired and just can't push any more.
- Your baby isn't making any progress through your pelvis.
- There's a medical reason why you shouldn't push for too long (for example, if you have heart disease).

Forceps may also be used during a vaginal birth of a breech baby (see pp.286–7) if your baby's body is born and then there is difficulty delivering her head.

Although it may sound frightening, in experienced hands an assisted delivery is considered safe as long as your baby's head is low enough in your birth canal and there are no other complications.

If your water hasn't already broken, your doctor will rupture your membranes and a catheter will be inserted to drain your bladder. And, unless you already have an epidural, you may be given a pudendal block—a local anesthetic injected into your vaginal wall that numbs your entire genital area. You may also need an episiotomy (a small cut in

---

Dad's **Diary**

My vacuum baby's head
"I'd seen the pictures in books. I knew that newborn babies came out looking a bit blue or gray, and covered in greasy white stuff. But I wasn't prepared for how ours looked after his vacuum-assisted birth. A vacuum is basically a suction device. His head was bruised and a bit swollen, and his scalp was scratched. It was very worrying at first, but our doctor was quick to reassure us that this was entirely normal and that the marks would clear up within a week or so. The next day, we noticed that he had a blood blister on his head where the suction cup had been attached. He was jaundiced, too, which they said may have been related to the blister. He was a little tender for a couple of weeks, so we were careful to be especially gentle with him. The blister took a few weeks to go away, but there were no lasting problems. Now, at 12 weeks, his head looks perfectly normal."

the tissue between your vagina and your anus), particularly for a forceps delivery so that there's room to insert the instrument. Finally, it is routine for a pediatrician to be on hand for any delivery that requires instruments.

Vacuum birth

Many doctors prefer to use a vacuum for an assisted birth because it's often less painful. You're less likely to need an episiotomy, and there's less risk of perineal tearing. The doctor or specially trained midwife will place the cup on your baby's head inside the vagina, then suck the air out of the cup using a foot-controlled or handheld vacuum pump. Once the cup is securely fixed on your baby's head, the doctor will ask you to push when your next contraction comes along, and she will pull on the cup to help your baby out.

Forceps birth

Your doctor may need to give you an episiotomy through the back of your vagina to enlarge the opening so that the forceps can be placed around the sides of your baby's head.

Once the forceps are in place, the doctor will gently pull while you push during a contraction to help your baby move down through the birth canal and be born. If your baby is not moving down with each pull or is not born after three contractions/pulls then normal practice is for the forceps to be abandoned and for your baby to be born by cesarean section (see pp.288–91).

Vacuum and forceps

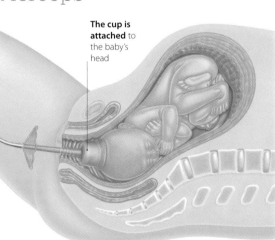

In a vacuum birth, a cup is attached to the baby's head and the air is pumped out of the cup. This creates a vacuum that holds the cup in place. Pulling gently on the cup helps the baby through the vagina.

The cup is attached to the baby's head

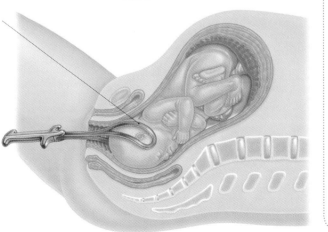

The curved blades of the forceps cradle the baby's head

In a forceps birth, the baby's head is cradled by the forceps, which are inserted into the mother's vagina. Pulling on the forceps in time with the contractions helps the baby out.

ParentsAsk...

How will I feel after an assisted birth?

After an assisted birth, you may have:

● Soreness and bruising from a tear or episiotomy.

● Pain or numbness in your perineum when you go to the bathroom.

● Problems with leaking urine when you're not on the toilet.

Your nurse should give you pain relief and check to ensure that you're able to urinate properly after the birth.

How will my baby feel after an assisted birth?

Your baby may have some bruising or marks after an assisted birth.

● Forceps babies tend to have marks or bruising on the face or side of the head.

● Vacuum babies may have a bruised swelling or slight scraping to the scalp, or a blood blister.

● Very occasionally the facial nerve is damaged, causing a palsy, so that your baby's mouth droops at one corner; this is usually temporary.

These marks usually clear up within a week or so, although a blood blister may take several weeks to disappear. Bruises and trauma may cause your baby some discomfort, so handle her gently.

Getting ready for pregnancy

Staying safe and healthy

Your pregnancy diary

Birth and beyond

Twin/multiple birth

As you probably already know by now, there are some additional risks linked with giving birth to twins or more. The trick is to discuss your babies' birth fully with your doctors so that, together, you can make sure it is as safe and positive as possible.

ParentsAsk...

What are the chances my twins will be born prematurely?

Twins and higher multiples do tend to arrive ahead of schedule. Although some twin pregnancies go to 40 weeks or even longer, 37 weeks is considered to be full term in a twin pregnancy. Anything earlier than this is considered premature. Around 30 percent of twin pregnancies go into premature labor, and around half of all women expecting twins give birth before 37 weeks.

Premature labor is more common in identical (monozygotic) twins, especially if the babies are sharing the same placenta, membranes, or amniotic sac.

Premature babies born between 34 and 37 weeks generally do very well. Extremely premature babies born before 28 weeks may survive, but they'll need intensive medical care and a little luck. However, advances in neonatal care mean the outlook for premature babies is improving all the time.

The factors behind whether you will go into labor prematurely have little to do with your behavior or lifestyle. While you shouldn't get too anxious about whether this may happen, it's important to familiarize yourself with the signs of preeclampsia and premature labor.

Eating healthily during your twin pregnancy is also important, since it gives your babies the best chance of being born healthy and at a good weight.

Delivering more than one

If you are expecting more than one baby, it's very likely that you'll give birth in hospital, because of the potential risks associated with giving birth to twins or more. It may be possible for you to have your babies in a birthing center, although this happens very rarely.

Some doctors argue that it is safer to plan for your twins' birth at about 37 to 38 weeks of pregnancy, either by induction or by planned cesarean. This limits your place of birth to a hospital, since neither induction nor cesarean can be done at home or in a midwife-led birthing center. Ultimately the choice is yours, and if you do want to consider having your babies in a birthing center, you should discuss your options with your doctor and midwife. Home births are extremely rare for twins and not recommended because of the chances of needing a cesarean.

The chances of a cesarean

You don't automatically have to have a cesarean, although your chances of having one are higher than if you were pregnant with just one baby. Whether you have a cesarean or not will most likely depend on the position of your first twin. If she's in a head-down position and the placenta isn't in the way of the cervix, a vaginal birth is generally possible. Many doctors and labor nurses will also do their best to deliver your second baby vaginally rather than by cesarean, even if he is in a breech position (see pp.286–7).

Of course you may need to have a cesarean for the same reasons any other pregnant woman would—for example, if:

- There is a complication with your labor.
- The babies don't fit through your birth canal.
- One or both babies' heartbeats drop drastically.
- You have severe preeclampsia (see p.233).
- There is placental abruption (see p.232).
- There are other signs that your babies could be in danger—for example, if they are small for their gestational age.

50% is the approximate percentage of twins born before 37 weeks' gestation. Some twin pregnancies go to 40 weeks or more, but 37 weeks is considered full term.

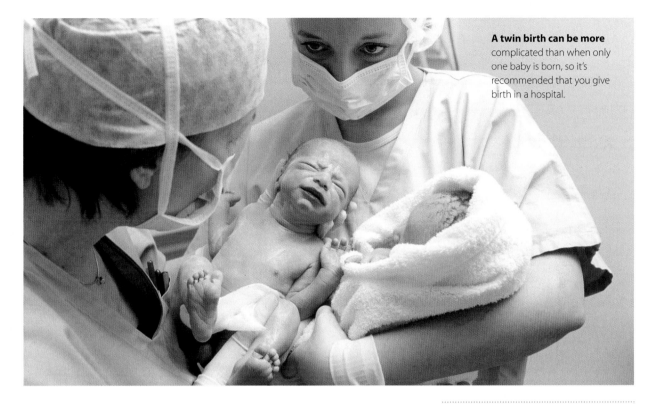

A twin birth can be more complicated than when only one baby is born, so it's recommended that you give birth in a hospital.

Unfortunately, all of these potential complications are actually more common in the case of multiple births.

It may help you make a decision about the kind of birth that you want if you can choose a doctor who has experience of delivering twins. If you don't want an unnecessary cesarean, discuss your birth options with her. Ask if she's comfortable delivering twins if one is in the breech position, and what she'll do in order to avoid a cesarean.

Although some things are beyond your control, such as your babies' positions in the uterus and any complications you may have developed, you can take steps to stay as healthy as possible during pregnancy by eating well (see pp.48–51, 120–21, 148–9, and 182–3). You should also try to remain active during labor. This may, in turn, improve your chances of avoiding a cesarean. When you're in labor, also try to use positions that will help your babies to turn if necessary.

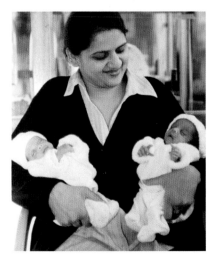

Most twins are born early, often by induction or planned cesarean. However yours are born, you'll be thrilled to hold your two new little ones in your arms.

ParentsAsk...

What will my recovery be like?
That depends on whether you've had a vaginal birth or a cesarean and whether or not you've had other complications. If everything goes well, you can be discharged from the hospital within two days after a vaginal birth and within four days after a cesarean. Some babies aren't able to go home right away.

Because twins tend to have more complications, particularly those related to being born earlier and smaller, it's not uncommon for them to be admitted to the neonatal unit. All mothers can use lots of help taking care of a new baby, but you'll be even more exhausted if you're taking care of multiples. Arrange to get as much help as you can. Many dads of twins save up some annual leave and combine it with their paternity leave, so they have more time at home.

Breech babies

As labor approaches, most babies settle into a head-down position. However, a few end up bottom down—a breech position—which can make birth more difficult. That's why a doctor should offer to turn your breech baby before she is born.

Planning for a breech birth

If your baby is breech, it means that she is in a bottom-down position. When labor begins, 96 percent of babies are lying head down in the uterus, but a few settle into a breech position.

If your baby is breech at 36 weeks, your doctor may offer you the chance to have your baby turned manually into a head-down position. This is called external cephalic version (ECV; see Parents Ask, opposite). ECV is more likely to work if you have given birth before. Sometimes, however, a baby just refuses to budge or she will rotate back after ECV into her breech position.

Most breech babies in the United States are currently born by cesarean. A review of the research on breech births in 2004 suggested that it is safer for breech babies to be born by cesarean section. But some doctors challenge this. They feel that a normal birth is just as safe, provided that the doctor has the special skills needed to help a woman give birth to a breech baby vaginally.

A vaginal birth
If you want a vaginal birth with a breech baby, your doctor may be more likely to be supportive if:
- You've given birth vaginally before.
- A doctor who is trained and

Breech-baby positions

There are several types of breech presentation. Your doctor will be able to tell your baby's position when she examines you toward the end of your pregnancy. You may also be able to tell by your baby's movements. If you feel strong kicks on your bladder and you can feel something hard and uncomfortable under your ribs, your baby may be breech.

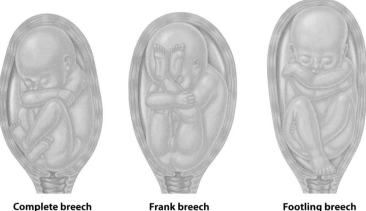

Complete breech　　**Frank breech**　　**Footling breech**

Complete breech This is one of the most common of the breech presentations. Your baby has her feet tucked beside her bottom, and her knees and arms are close to her body. A vaginal birth is sometimes possible.
Frank breech This is another of the most common of the breech presentations. Your baby sits bottom down with her legs fully extended, straight up toward her head. This is the best position for achieving a vaginal breech birth.
Footling breech This is the rarest breech presentation. Your baby is bottom down with one or both feet extended below her bottom. A vaginal birth is unlikely.

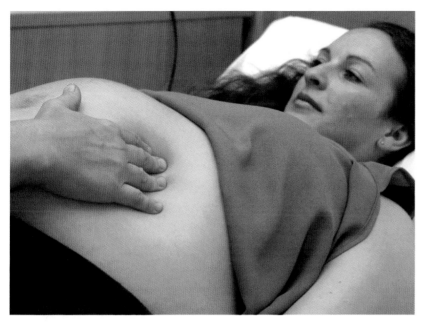

If your baby is in a breech position, once you've reached 36 weeks of pregnancy, you may be given the chance to have your baby turned by hand.

experienced at breech birth will be present at the birth.
- Facilities for a cesarean (in case one is needed) will be available nearby.
- There are no other features of your

situation and discuss the risks and benefits of both a cesarean section and a vaginal birth so that the two of you can choose what's likely to be best for you and your baby.

"Sometimes a **breech baby** refuses **to budge** or rotates **back**."

pregnancy that would make having your breech baby vaginally more risky for you or your baby.

Before making a final decision, you and your doctor should evaluate your

As the number of breech vaginal births continues to fall, it may be more difficult for you to find an obstetrician with the skills and knowledge needed to deliver your breech baby vaginally. If your local hospital doesn't have an obstetrician with this experience, you should ask to be referred to a hospital where this option is available if you want.

If you still want to give birth to your breech baby vaginally and your doctor isn't okay with this, you could consider going to an independent midwife at a birthing center attached to a hospital.

Fact: A breech labor is usually slower than a normal one because a baby's bottom doesn't exert as much pressure on the cervix as a baby's head. Some breech labors are quick and straightforward, though.

Getting ready for pregnancy

Staying safe and healthy

Your pregnancy diary

Birth and beyond

ParentsAsk...

Are there any safe and proven methods available for turning a breech baby?
Many breech babies spontaneously turn around before, or even during, labor without any assistance. Some babies who remain in the breech position can be turned by hand, using a technique called external cephalic version (ECV).

This technique has been practiced by doctors for thousands of years and a great deal of research has been carried out to test its safety.

ECV can be done at any point from 36 weeks of pregnancy; there is no upper limit. Sometimes, it is even done at the beginning of labor, if the water hasn't already broken. ECV has about a 58 percent success rate in turning breech babies (and a 90 percent success rate if the baby is in a transverse lie).

The procedure should be performed in the hospital, where there is equipment to monitor your baby's heartbeat and ultrasound to check your baby's position. You may be given a medication to make the muscles of your uterus relax. If you are rhesus negative, you will have an injection of Rh immune globin (see p.233). The procedure is not painful, so you will not need to have a general anesthetic.

Why are some babies breech?
A lot of babies are breech before 30 weeks, so if your baby is premature she may be in the breech position. Sometimes a baby cannot turn because something is in the way—a fibroid perhaps. Sometimes there is a problem with the umbilical cord—it may be too short for the baby to be able to turn. If you have a small or unusual-shaped pelvis, and your baby can't fit her head through it, she may turn around and put her softer and smaller bottom there instead. In most of these cases, where turning isn't possible, the baby would need to be born by cesarean.

Cesarean section

Cesareans, or C-sections, are done for a wide variety of reasons and more than 29 percent of women have them in the United States. While cesareans are very safe, it is a major operation, and you will take longer to recover after the birth than if you give birth naturally.

The lowdown on C-sections

Some women know that they will need a cesarean before they go into labor. This is called an elective or planned cesarean. In other cases the decision to opt for a cesarean is made during labor. This is called an emergency cesarean. The risk of you needing a planned cesarean is greater if:

- Your baby is in a breech (bottom first; see pp.286–7) or transverse (sideways; see p.197) position.
- You are having three or more babies.
- Your baby has a fetal illness or abnormality.
- You have an infection such as herpes (see p.226) or HIV (see p.227).
- You have placenta previa (see pp.231–2) and the placenta is so low in the uterus that it's blocking the baby's exit.
- You have preeclampsia (see p.233) and it is rapidly worsening, making it dangerous to delay delivery.

Organized mom

Choosing an elective cesarean may suit you since it can bring certainty and peace of mind.

"When I reached 36 weeks, my baby was showing no signs of moving from the breech position. My doctor offered to try to turn the baby manually but, because this was my first, it had less chance of working than if I'd given birth before. We did try and my baby refused to budge!

I could have gone ahead and had a vaginal birth anyway, but I felt that the best thing for me was a cesarean, seeing as this was my first baby and I was worried about the risk of complications. I admit I was slightly disappointed at not having a vaginal birth, but I also felt relieved knowing that my baby would arrive safely—and I had the date written on the calendar so I could prepare for his arrival!"

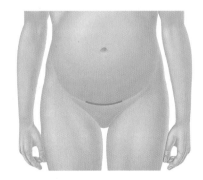

For a bikini incision the doctor makes a horizontal cut just above the public hairline. After healing, the scar is hardly noticeable.

- You have a history of invasive uterine surgery or multiple cesarean sections.

You may also need an unplanned cesarean during labor if:

- Your baby's heart rate has become irregular.
- The umbilical cord prolapses, or slips, through the cervix.
- Your baby is not moving down the birth canal.

What happens in a cesarean?

During a cesarean, the doctor will make a cut in your abdomen and uterus and will remove your baby through it. In most cases, your partner will be allowed to be with you for the birth. He will only be asked to leave in a true emergency, or if you need a general anesthetic.

Most cesareans are performed using an epidural or spinal block so you can be awake and see your baby immediately after the birth. In addition to having the epidural in your back, you will have a catheter to drain your bladder, and an IV in your arm or hand to give extra fluid or pain relief if needed. You will also have to wear a heart monitor, and the top section of your pubic hair will be shaved.

A screen will be put up while the cesarean is taking place. Once you are numb, the doctor makes a straight cut in

ParentsAsk...

I'm having a planned cesarean since my baby is breech. Will I be able to hold him right after he is born?

As soon as your baby has been lifted out, he will be checked over, then shown to you. Your partner will probably hold him while the placenta is delivered and you are being stitched up. After this, you may be able to hold him or you may be moved to a side ward, where you will be able to breast-feed him if you want to. The only circumstances in which you won't be able to hold him are if he is very small or very sick and needs to go immediately to the neonatal intensive care unit (see p.297).

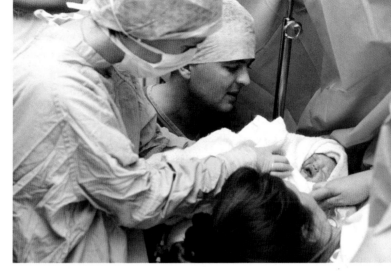

After your baby is born you should be able to hold him once the placenta has been delivered and he's been checked over.

your skin above your pubic bone (this is called a bikini cut; see opposite), and then makes a second cut in the lower section of your uterus. Your baby is then lifted out. It takes only a few minutes.

Your baby will be checked by the pediatrician, then you or your partner can hold him while the placenta is being delivered and you are stitched up using a double layer of stitches. The wound will be closed with stitches or staples.

Reducing the risk

Cesareans can be life-saving for both mothers and babies, so not all should be avoided. But there are some ways you can reduce your chances of having one. These include:

● Staying healthy during pregnancy, eating well (see pp.48–51, 120–21, 148–9, 182–3), exercising safely (see pp.56–7, 134, 184), and getting plenty of rest (see pp.162–3, 198–9).

● If you have a choice of hospitals, check out the cesarean rates at each and compare them. You may want to avoid hospitals that appear to have a high rate. You can call hospitals to inquire, consult with your doctor, or check statistics on record with your state board of health.

● Having a female birth partner, as well as your labor nurse, to support you during your labor can reduce your chances of having a cesarean. You'll need good, solid support from the moment your labor starts. You could ask a female friend or relative, or a doula, to be there for you.

● If your baby is in a bottom-down, or breech, position as you near the end of your pregnancy, you could talk to your doctor or midwife, if you have one attending your delivery, about trying to move your baby into a head-down position (see p.286).

● If your pregnancy is considered to be low risk, your baby should be monitored now and again during labor rather than continuously. Continuous electronic fetal monitoring (EFM; see p.263), which stops you from moving around during labor, is linked with an increase in cesarean section rates.

 Single mom

Choose a birth partner who can truly sympathize with you when you're giving birth.

"When I found out that I'd have to have an elective cesarean, it confirmed to me that my sister really was the best choice to be my birth partner. Her second baby was delivered by emergency c-section, and knowing that she'd been through the same experience gave me confidence that she'd be the most supportive and sympathetic person to have at my side during the birth. Also, knowing that she'd made a great recovery afterward was a great help.

She knew exactly what to do and say to me: she kept telling me I was doing great and that it was all going well. I couldn't have done it without her. She knew just what to say and when because she'd been there herself. We're closer than ever now."

Getting ready for pregnancy

Staying safe and healthy

Your pregnancy diary

Birth and beyond

ParentsAsk...

How many cesareans can I safely have?

Although vaginal delivery after a previous cesarean is now common and safe (VBAC; see pp.221 and 248), sometimes another cesarean section is your only option. Your doctor will give you individual advice on the health of your uterus and any risks to you of another surgery. There are many things that need to be considered, including your weight, age, medical history, fertility history, childbirth history, as well as personal choice. The choices you make will also depend on why you needed to have a cesarean with your first baby, so you should be sure you understand what happened last time.

If you have a cesarean birth, you should always seek advice from your doctor about the best way for you to have your next baby.

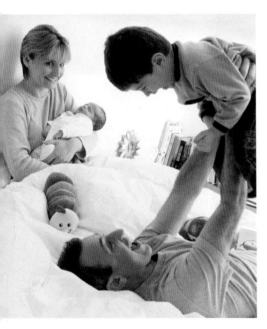

As a precaution after a cesarean you shouldn't lift anything heavy for six weeks—not even your toddler.

After a cesarean

Everyone knows a cesarean is major surgery, but you may be surprised by how much it hurts afterward. You may feel you can't do anything by yourself—even to move up the bed a little you'll probably need something to hold on to. Trapped gas is another problem, especially by about day three—tightening the abdominal muscles on an outward breath helps expel the gas. The nurse may give you some over-the-counter medication containing simethicone, which makes the gas easier to expel.

It will hurt when you cough or laugh, but less if you support the incision (with your hands or by holding a pillow over your stomach) when you do. Wearing panties a size bigger than you really need (or boxer shorts or disposable maternity underpants), may make you feel more comfortable, and you'll need to use sanitary pads because the lochia, or bleeding from the uterus, is the same as after a vaginal birth.

If you had an epidural, you'll probably have the catheter left in place for a few hours afterward so that top-ups of painkiller can be given when you need them. If you had a general anesthetic, you'll be offered pain-killing injections in the hours and days after the birth. Doses of painkiller you can control yourself, or patient-controlled anesthetic

(PCA; see p.277), is often used soon after a cesarean. This gives you pain-relieving drugs through a fine tube into a vein in your arm. You can control the dose by pressing a button.

Getting out of bed

At first you'll probably feel as though you'll never walk again but, as soon as six hours after the birth, your nurse will probably cajole you out of bed. However hard it seems, try to move—the earlier you can, the better for your circulation and general recovery. Also, you'll have to try it sometime—and when you've already made it out of bed once, the next time will be easier. In addition to moving around out of bed, you'll be encouraged to do ankle exercises while you're in bed, to improve blood circulation to your legs and help prevent clots.

You'll probably have to stay in the hospital for about four days. You'll be encouraged to start gentle postpartum exercises the day after your surgery to help speed your physical recovery. A physical therapist will show you what to do. You should not start a more strenuous exercise program until six to eight weeks after delivery.

There's no reason why you shouldn't breast-feed after a cesarean. But the pain from your incision may make it a bit difficult in the early days (see below).

Precautions after a cesarean

A cesarean is major surgery. Once you have had one, you need to take a few commonsense precautions.

● You'll probably be warned not to drive for five or six weeks, since turning and twisting may cause pain and having to make an emergency stop would be extremely painful.

● You shouldn't lift anything heavy—

including, unfortunately, a toddler if you have one—so if you have a willing helper, do enlist his or her help.

● You will need help to breast-feed at first. Your partner can hold your baby while you lie on your side. Put two or three pillows on your lap so the weight of your baby doesn't press on your incision.

ParentsTalk...

"I had an emergency cesarean and I hate it when people say I gave birth the easy way. Believe me, the pain afterward is not easy! I needed help on hand to do everything for the first couple of days afterward. Just moving in my bed was excruciating."
Sara, 23, mom to six-month-old Joe

"I had a lot of leftover adrenaline after my cesarean. There was such a huge build-up of excitement for nine months, and then—within a few hours—the baby was here. Being confined to bed with stitches in my belly really didn't help, either!"
Emily, 31, first-time mom

"My nurse persuaded me to get out of bed for a walk a few hours after my cesarean. Despite the pain, it was nice to spend quiet time holding and feeding my baby."
Lizzy, 32, mom to one-month-old Aaron

In some ways life will be easier once you're home—your bed, for example, will almost certainly be lower than the hospital bed and easier to get in and out of—but you can't expect to be back to normal immediately and there are some precautions you should take (see opposite). In fact, it may take your body

your partner, need to ask the nurse who was at your baby's birth, and maybe the obstetrician involved, to talk to you about it.

If you feel it would be helpful, you can request a copy of your labor records by contacting the medical records department at the hospital.

"It may **take your body** up to **six** months **to recover** after a section."

up to six months to recover and many women say they don't feel completely themselves for up to a year.

Following a cesarean, most of us are just glad it's over and grateful we—and the baby—have survived. You may feel elated and delighted—or you may be weepy, and disappointed that you didn't give birth to your baby vaginally.

If things changed quickly during your labor, you may still feel traumatized by what you have been through. It may help your emotional recovery to go over again, and perhaps again and again, the reasons why a cesarean section became necessary. To do this you, and maybe

Talk to your partner about how you feel as well. If your relationship with your partner or your baby is affected, you may need to seek professional help. Your partner may also be affected after witnessing what happened to you and may be in need of as much help as you.

Speak to your doctor and find out if there are any support groups near you or women who have had similar experiences that she can put you in touch with. If you are really struggling to come to terms with the cesarean, speak to your doctor. It may be that you are in need of counseling or that you are suffering from postpartum depression.

Dad's **Diary**

Coming to terms with a cesarean

"After our baby was born by cesarean section, Sally felt really disappointed that she hadn't been able to give birth naturally. She had high hopes for an active labor, with no medical pain relief, but after 18 hours, we were told that the baby was in a very awkward position and that a vaginal birth would be extremely difficult. Sally eventually agreed that a cesarean would be the best option. As I walked down to the operating room with her, she kept saying that she felt like a failure—which, of course, she absolutely wasn't. I was proud of her for going through so much for so long. I'm sure I couldn't have done it. James was born 20 minutes later.

Sally recovered well physically, but it took longer for her to get over her disappointment. I found it hard to understand why—I was just relieved that it was all over and they were both safe and healthy. A week or so after the birth, we were able to meet up with the doctor to talk about it. It helped Sally to come to terms with the decision once she knew exactly why she'd had to have a cesarean. She quickly saw that it really was the only option."

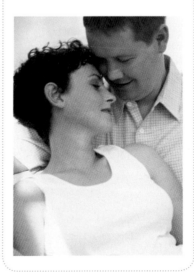

Emergency deliveries, fast labor

If you've planned to have your baby in a hospital, chances are she will arrive safe and sound once you're there. Sometimes, though, babies have other ideas and arrive on the way to the hospital or even before you're out the door! Here's how to manage if it happens to you…

No time to get to the hospital

It's unlikely that you'll find yourself unexpectedly giving birth at home or in the backseat of a taxi—particularly if it's your first baby—but it can happen. In less than 1 percent of births, a woman who's had no labor symptoms or only intermittent contractions suddenly feels an overwhelming urge to push, which may signal the imminent arrival of her baby. Still, it's always wise to be prepared, so here is your quick guide to emergency home birth.

If you think your baby is coming too quickly for you to get to the hospital:
- Don't panic! Women are made to have babies. Babies are meant to be born. If your baby has been nine months in the uterus, and she's coming quickly, it's probably because she's finding it very easy to get out. Your pelvis is clearly a nice spacious one with lots of room to help babies be born easily!
- Call 911. Then, if you're by yourself, call someone who can come over quickly—perhaps your mom, friend, or neighbor.
- Make sure the front door is unlocked so that all the people coming to help you can get in. Then find a large clean towel ready to wrap the baby in, and more towels and sheets for you to lie on.
- If you've got an overpowering urge to push, you may simply have to go with it. However, if you can, try panting instead. Give three quick pants and a long blow. Three quick pants and a long blow, and so on. This might just delay your baby's arrival for a few minutes.

If your baby insists on putting in an immediate appearance, don't worry. When her head is delivered, if there's a loop of cord around her neck, if you can do so gently, ease it over her head. Then leave the cord alone. You don't need to do anything else with it. Don't pull on it! Wait for your baby's body to be born with the next contraction.

Your baby may well be screaming lustily. If not, breathe on her face and stroke down the sides of her nose to press out any mucus or fluid that's trapped inside.

Pick her up, dry her, and hold her. She's probably just as amazed as you at this sudden transition from being inside you to being outside.

Above all, keep her warm. Place her against your skin and drape a towel or blanket over her. Being warm and held close to you will help her to calm down.

If you are planning to breast-feed—or even if you're not—place your baby against your breast so that she can

A previous fast labor? Be prepared

If you've had a previous labor that was fast and furious, it's important to be especially attuned to the signs of labor. Be prepared to make a mad dash for the hospital or birthing center, because subsequent labors can go even faster. And as your due date nears, be sure you and your partner have gone to childbirth preparation classes and know what to do in case of sudden, quick labor.

For more information, you should review the American College of Nurse-Midwives' Guide to Emergency Preparedness for Childbirth. This offers advice on how to deliver a baby at home and care for the baby and mother through the first few days.

1%

or fewer women who have had no symptoms of labor or who have only had intermittent contractions, suddenly feel an overwhelming urge to push. This may signal the imminent arrival of the baby.

Parents**Talk...**

"My midwife arrived 10 minutes after Mia was born! I thought I would be in labor for hours, but after only an hour, I realized I was ready to push. That's when I phoned her. Luckily David had been to my childbirth classes."
Lynda, 29, mom to two-month-old Mia

"They say second babies are often quick, but it took less than an hour from start to finish for me. I wouldn't have made it to the hospital, so luckily I'd planned a home birth—although it did end up taking place in my parents'

home rather than my own. They weren't too pleased about the mess I'd made of their spare room!"
Jennifer, 36, mom to Joely and Laura

"I gave birth in the ambulance on the way to the hospital. When I started pushing I demanded that the driver stop by the side of the road, because I was being bumped around in the back. My husband told me later that our son was officially born outside a Chinese restaurant—cool!"
Christine, 27, mom to three-month-old Andrew

---

nuzzle. If she manages to suck just a little, this will stimulate the release of the hormone oxytocin, which helps the placenta to be delivered.

After the birth

Probably pretty soon after your baby is delivered, you will feel the urge to push again. This is your uterus contracting to expel the placenta. The placenta will feel quite soft and slithery as it slips through the vagina. You might be

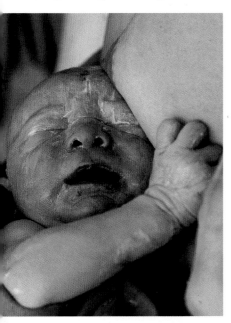

Keeping your baby warm after the birth is most important. Put her against your skin and lay a blanket or towel over her.

surprised by how large it is (about the size of a dinner plate). If you don't want to look at it, get whoever's with you to pop it into a plastic bag or bucket. So now you have your baby in your arms with the cord still attached to her, which is still attached to the placenta, which is in a plastic bag or bucket. Relax. The ambulance crew will deal with the cord and placenta when they arrive. After you deliver the placenta, firmly massage your uterus by vigorously rubbing your belly right below your navel. This helps your uterus contract and stay contracted.

Congratulations! You've managed to do it all on your own. And as your baby grows up, she will be able to tell her friends the amazing story of her unexpected arrival.

If you have been upset by this unexpectedly quick birth, talk it over with your doctor. When you have your next baby, you may decide to have a home birth again (planned this time!) or, if you choose a hospital birth, you'll know to go in at the first sign of labor. Planned home births are great, but unplanned ones are best avoided.

Don'ts in an emergency

You probably know the "do's" about an emergency home birth—but what about the "don'ts"?

- Don't panic—stay calm, get comfortable, phone the doctor and the hospital and, if you're alone, phone a friend or family member who can come over immediately to help.
- Don't try not push if the urge is overpowering. Your baby wants to get out!
- Don't cut or pull on the cord when your baby has been born. The ambulance crew can deal with it when they arrive.
- Don't hold back if you need to push again after your baby has arrived—this is your uterus contracting to expel the placenta. Stay where you are until you've delivered it. Ask whoever is with you to pop it in a plastic bag or bucket when it comes out.
- Don't give birth standing up—without professional help, your baby could fall and be seriously injured.
- Don't lift your baby up high. Lay her on your belly or thigh and cover her with a blanket.

Getting ready for pregnancy

Staying safe and healthy

Your pregnancy diary

Birth and beyond

Life with your new baby

A life's begun

You're exhausted, emotional, and feel like a wreck. But you've also never felt so happy. Welcome to the confusing but wonderful world of parenthood. Most of your hours are now spent caring for the new little person in your life, but don't forget to take care of yourself, too.

New parents sign on here

Depending on how the birth has gone, you may be feeling alert and happy, even exhilarated, or you may feel bruised and exhausted. Either extreme—or anything in between—is perfectly normal. Remember that you're recovering from a huge physical upheaval (and major abdominal surgery, if you had a cesarean). So be kind to yourself and allow yourself time to rest and recover.

If you're both fine, you may be discharged the same day or within a day or two. Whether at home or in the hospital, sooner or later you'll want to

Breast-feeding will help your uterus shrink back more quickly—you may feel a few contraction-like "afterpains" as it happens. Any minor scrapes and tears to the neck of the uterus, vagina, and perineum usually heal within days but, if you've had stitches, these may take a little longer.

As you hold your newborn, the realization that you are responsible for this precious new life can feel daunting, but don't forget that every mom and dad was a new parent once. Relax—no one expects you to be perfect.

"**Responsibity** for this **precious new life** can feel **daunting**."

freshen up. Make sure someone is near as you shower or wash, in case you feel a bit wobbly. Take a plastic bottle into the bathroom with you and pour some warm water over your vagina as you urinate, to stop any sore bits from stinging. You'll also need to put on a sanitary towel to absorb the lochia (postpartum bleeding).

Holding your newborn may feel strange but you have a whole lifetime to get to know each other better.

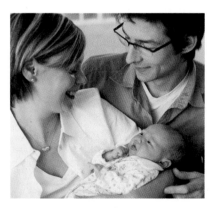

Green mom

Now you're a mom, thinking about the future of the planet is even more important.

"There are so many things us moms can do to help the environment. To start, I'm breast-feeding, which is completely natural. And I'm also using reusable cotton diapers as well as specially designed reusable wet wipes. All these can be washed carefully and dried on the line. Recycling's even more important to me, too, and it's not just baby jars and toy packaging— I've been buying as many things as I can secondhand, like clothes, toys, and nursery furniture.

When my baby starts on solids, I plan on making everything myself from scratch using fresh ingredients and, if I've got time, I'll even try my hand at growing some of my own vegetables. My husband's talking about getting a couple of chickens so we have an unlimited supply of eggs! And I've been walking as much as I can with the stroller. It not only saves on using the car, but also gives me some much-needed exercise."

After the birth: your baby and you

As you'll soon discover, newborns don't need much. All your baby needs to thrive is regular feeding, cuddling, and diaper changes. For now, try to sleep when he sleeps and ask for help whenever you need it. Don't be shy about calling a doctor if you have any questions.

ParentsAsk...

Will it be love at first sight?
Bonding is a very individual experience. Some parents feel an intense love for their baby within minutes of the birth. For others, it may take days, weeks or even longer. However, parents who are separated from their newborns for medical reasons or who adopt their children when they're several months old can still develop enormously close, loving relationships.

Your stay in the hospital

Make the most of your time in the hospital to recover from the birth and bond with your baby. If there haven't been any problems, you and your baby may be able to go home on the same day. If not, you may stay in the hospital for a day or two. If you had a cesarean you'll probably stay three or four days.

You'll be feeling very tired after giving birth. Postpartum wards can be noisy with other babies and mothers, so remember to bring earplugs with you to the hospital. Try to sleep when your baby sleeps—it's harder to bond when you're physically exhausted.

If you need to stay in the hospital for a while, remember that the nurses are there to help you. If you need help with breast-feeding, don't struggle alone, your hospital may have a breast-feeding specialist, or one of the nurses can come to see you.

Newborn tests and checks

After the birth, your baby will have examinations to check that he is healthy. The first is the Apgar (see right; the name is an acronym for Appearance, Pulse, Grimace, Activity, and Respiration). It is done at one minute, then again at five minutes, after birth. Shortly afterward, your baby will be weighed and the circumference of his head measured.

A full examination is done between four and 48 hours from birth. Among other things, your baby's ears, eyes, spine, mouth, genitals, and feet will be checked.

Before your baby is one week old, a heel-prick blood test is also done to check for conditions such as sickle-cell disorders and cystic fibrosis.

Apgar scoring system	Score of 0	Score of 1	Score of 2	Component of acronym
Skin color	blue all over	white at extremities; body pink	pink all over	Appearance
Heart rate	absent	slow	fast	Pulse
Reflex response	no response to stimulation	grimacing when stimulated	crying and coughing	Grimace
Muscle tone	limp or stretching of limbs	some bending movement	active	Activity
Breathing	absent	weak or irregular	good and your baby is crying	Respiration

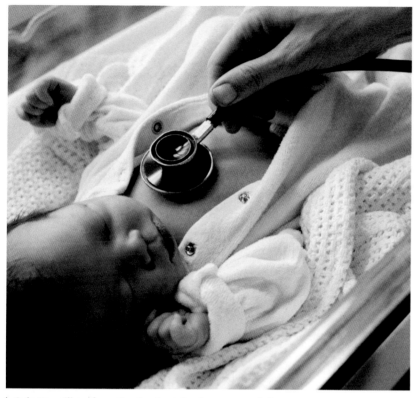

A doctor will perform the standard checkups on your baby, both right after birth and before you take him home.

ParentsAsk...

My newborn's got jaundice. Should I worry?
About half of all normal, healthy babies develop a yellowish tinge to their skin, or jaundice, in their first few days of life. If your baby does, it's probably nothing to worry about, but mention it to your doctor. In rare cases it can be a sign of something more serious, such as a liver problem. Breast-feeding should help to clear up the jaundice, but some babies may need treatment in the hospital with ultraviolet light.

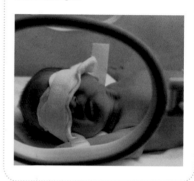

(see opposite)

During your time in the hospital you'll learn how to keep your baby clean and how to care for his umbilical cord stump. Don't worry if you don't bond with your baby immediately—everyone is different.

Before you leave the hospital to go home a doctor will do some checkups on your baby (see opposite). He'll have a physical examination and his weight will be noted. He may also have a hearing checkup.

Your baby in special care

A neonatal unit is specially designed to provide expert, around-the-clock care for newborn babies who are ill or are born prematurely. Between 6 and 10 percent of all newborns spend some time here, so it is not all that unusual.

However, most parents do not expect that their baby might have to go to the neonatal unit, and it usually comes as a real shock to them.

Some hospitals may not be equipped to provide the care your baby needs. Your baby might therefore have to be transferred to a unit far from your home. This could also happen if your local hospital does not have enough room.

On the neonatal unit, a skilled team from different professions will care for your baby. Some of the people you may meet include neonatal nurses, a pediatrician or neonataologist, and other specialist doctors, such as surgeons.

Last but not least, there's you, the parents. Your special-care baby needs all the things that other babies need from their parents. Your touch, voice,

and presence all help a great deal. The professionals will recognize this and treat you as part of the team.

If you're eager to breast-feed, let the nurses know and they should make every effort to help you. They will help you express your milk if your baby is not well enough to breast-feed. The expressed milk may be given to him via a feeding tube or will be stored and used to feed him when he is ready.

Most hospitals have an "open policy," which means parents can visit their neonatal unit 24 hours a day. Others have more restricted visiting hours. Don't forget that, if you're not at the hospital, you can call the neonatal unit anytime, day or night. Always ask questions or talk to the staff about any worries you may have.

Getting ready for pregnancy

Staying safe and healthy

Your pregnancy diary

Birth and beyond

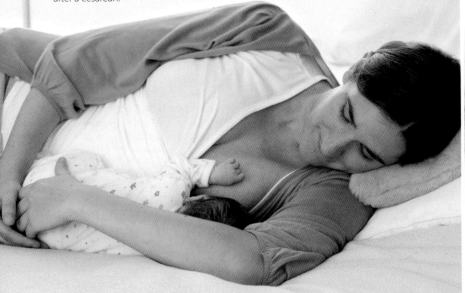

Breast-feeding while lying down can give you some much-needed rest, especially at night. It's also comfortable after a cesarean.

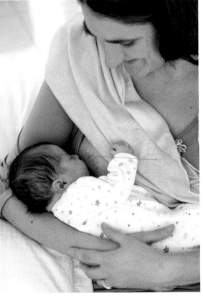

For breast-feeding while seated, make sure your back and arms are well supported and you are relaxed. It will make you more comfortable if you use a pillow on your lap to bring your baby up to the right height.

Avoiding sore nipples

Sore nipples are common in newly breast-feeding mothers. You well may feel some tenderness at the beginning of a feeding during the first few days. But if the pain is intense or lasts longer than a few days, it is a sign that you may need to make some changes.

The most likely cause is that your baby isn't latching on well or that she's incorrectly positioned at the breast. She needs to take a large mouthful of breast—not just the nipple—into her mouth before she begins to suck. If she is just sucking on the nipple, it will probably hurt. It is important for you to get expert help from a lactation consultant or from an infant feeding specialist to figure out your baby's latching-on technique.

Feeding your baby

Whether you decide to breast- or bottle-feed your baby, giving that first feeding can be an emotional experience. If you've never given birth before, the maternity support staff will give you practical advice on how to go about it.

Breast-feeding

Offer your baby the breast soon after she's born—babies are sometimes very alert at this time and they feed well. But it doesn't matter if all your baby wants to do is to lick a little and enjoy the loving, close cuddling she gets when you hold her in your arms this way.

The nurse should help you find a comfortable position and will talk to you about how you can help your baby to get "latched on" (see left) so she

nurses effectively and doesn't make your nipples sore.

Your baby needs a wide open mouth to take in your breast. Remember to bring your baby onto the breast. Don't try to "slot" your nipple in. You and your baby will get better and better at this, and you shouldn't be discouraged if you don't get it right at first.

Feed your baby as often as she seems to want it. Keep her close to you—next to you in bed, snuggled up against your skin. That way you will both get plenty of "feeding practice" and you can rest a little in between. It's not helpful to wait until your baby is yelling loudly before you feed her. No one learns well when they're upset, and your baby will find it hard to get a good mouthful of breast if she is crying, because her tongue will be in the wrong position. It needs to be forward to feed correctly. If she's crying, it's too far back in her mouth.

Bottle feeding

As with breast-feeding, most experts agree that you shouldn't follow a rigid schedule in the early weeks. Instead, you should offer the bottle every two to three hours, or when your baby seems hungry. Until she reaches about 10 pounds, she'll probably take 1 to 3 fluid ounces per feeding. Your baby's doctor will advise you.

Before you first use new bottles, nipples, and rings, you should sterilize them by submerging them in a pot of boiling water for five minutes. Then allow them to dry on a clean towel.

After that, a good cleaning in hot, soapy water or a cycle through the dishwasher is sufficient. (You can find some handy bottle gear, such as dishwasher baskets for nipples, rings, and bottle caps, and bottle drying racks, at most baby supply stores.)

A lot of formulas come pre-made. Some don't. To make up formula, follow the instructions on the package carefully. Fill the bottle with water to the marked level and measure the milk powder with the scoop provided. Use a knife to level off the scoop, but avoid packing the powder down. Add this to the water in the bottle. Put the nipple and cover on and then shake well. Don't be tempted to add extra scoops of powder since this can make your baby sick. If you choose to warm the bottle, heat it in a pan of warm water, run it under the tap, or use a bottle warmer. Don't heat bottles in the microwave.

Mix only what you think you'll use in the next 24 hours. Once you've mixed formula, refrigerate it immediately.

Green mom

After the birth you may have afterpains—especially if this isn't your first pregnancy.

"I had afterpains for several days after the birth of my second baby, as my uterus began contracting back to its pre-pregnancy shape. My doctor told me that each pregnancy stretches the uterus more so it has to work harder to get back to its original size. The pains got a bit worse when I was breast-feeding. They felt like very bad period pains. I was offered analgesics, but I'd survived labor with no pain relief, so I wasn't about to start now! I put hot-water bottles on my belly and lower back and found that rocking my hips and moving around helped. Stu did a great job massaging my back and he also did practical things like taking care of our new baby and toddler while I had a rest."

How to bottle-feed your baby

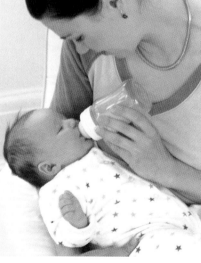

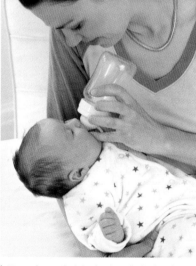

Stroking your baby's cheek before a feeding helps stimulate the sucking reflex and encourages her to open her mouth ready for the bottle.

Hold the bottle at an angle to keep the nipple full of milk and free of air. If you hold the bottle firmly, she can pull against it slightly to get a good sucking action.

Near the end of the feeding tilt the bottle so the last drops fill the nipple. To stop your baby from sucking on an empty bottle, slide your finger into her mouth to release the suction.

Getting ready for pregnancy

Staying safe and healthy

Your pregnancy diary

Birth and beyond

Going home with your newborn

After nine months of growing your baby and several hours of giving birth, you're finally at home with your newborn. Feeling overwhelmed, confused, and ever so slightly terrified? We can help. Our survival guide will lead you through these first few hectic days.

The first few days at home

Some women feel completely at ease and can't wait to get home with their new baby; others are overwhelmed by the responsibility—especially when they're still recovering physically and emotionally from labor. Either way, as a new mom you'll need lots of support and help. You will get some of it automatically, but sometimes you may need to ask. You shouldn't think that asking for help is a sign of weakness;

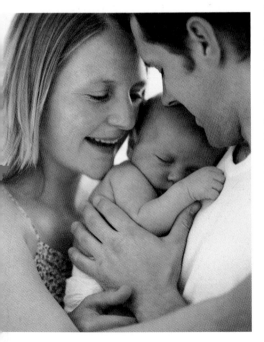

it's simply acknowledging the fact that you need to get enough rest so you are able to care for your new baby.

Now's the time to forget housework and anything else—just focus on recovering from labor and bonding with your baby. Get your partner, family, and friends to take care of everyday chores and ensure any visitors are the type that will take care of you, rather than expect to be entertained. In the early days you'll very likely stay in close contact with your doctors, to check that you are healing okay, continue your baby's medical care, help establish feeding, and provide other advice and support.

After three or four days your milk will arrive, making your breasts feel hot, swollen, and tender. At first your nipples may feel very sensitive, and the first 10 to 20 seconds of each feeding may be uncomfortable. This usually begins to ease off after about the fifth day.

It's common for women to feel weepy around this time—a combination of raging hormones and exhaustion—so don't feel guilty if you're not feeling elated every minute of the day.

Hand your baby over to your partner as often as you can. You need plenty of rest if you are to care for your baby properly.

ParentsAsk...

Is it okay to have my baby in bed with me?

The nurturing and closeness that co-sleeping brings can help create a stronger relationship between you and your child.

Studies have shown that sleep-sharing babies breast-feed more, yet disrupt their mothers' sleep less, than babies who sleep alone. Mothers who co-sleep also tend to breast-feed their babies longer.

Co-sleeping babies also stay awake for shorter periods of time during the night than solitary sleepers, and they may cry significantly less, too. Sleeping close to your baby allows you to respond quickly if he coughs or cries in the night.

However, it is not safe to take a premature baby into bed with you. Also, to reduce the risk of SIDS, you should never share a bed with your baby if you or your partner have been drinking alcohol, have taken drugs or medication, or if either of you are a smoker. Never sleep with your baby on a sofa or armchair, nor in a waterbed. And you shouldn't ever share a bed with more than one child.

An alternative to sharing a bed with your baby is to use a co-sleeper crib that attaches to your bed. Its mattress is the same level as your mattress, so it creates a level surface. Many mothers find the cost well worth it.

Bathing your baby

You don't need to wait for your baby's umbilical cord stump to fall off, or for the area to heal completely, before you give him a bath. For the first week or so, you may find it easier to stick to sponge baths (see below). The most important thing when bathing your baby is to make sure you keep him warm.

Newborns don't need a daily bath. Until he is crawling and getting into messes, a bath isn't really necessary more than once or twice a week.

While he is tiny, you can bathe him in a small baby bath. Fill it with about 2 in of water, at a temperature that is warm but not hot—about 100.4° F (38° C).

Always test the water with your forearm, since the skin is more sensitive there than on your hands. Never put your baby in the bath while the water is still running in case the temperature changes. Also, you should avoid using strong cleansers, because they may damage your newborn's skin.

How to give your baby a sponge bath

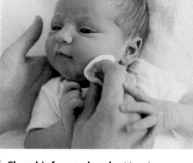

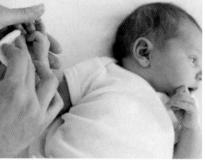

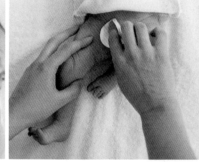

Clean his face and neck with a damp cotton pad. Don't forget the neck creases. Wipe the eyes from the inner to outer corners. Pat dry with a soft towel.

Gently uncurl his fingers and use a fresh damp cotton pad to wipe the fronts and backs of his hands and in between his fingers. Pat dry with a soft towel.

Take off his diaper and use fresh damp cotton pads to wipe around his genital area. Clean in between the skin creases, then pat dry with a soft towel.

How to give your baby a bath

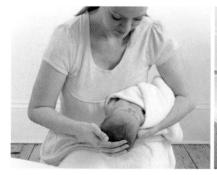

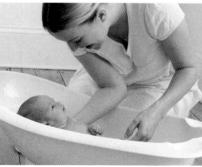

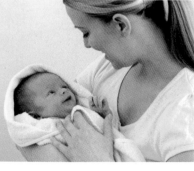

Undress your baby and wrap him in a towel. Tuck him under your arm, support his head with your hand, and gently wet his hair. Dry his hair with a soft towel.

Unwrap the towel and lower him into the water, supporting his shoulders with one hand. Always hold him securely. Slowly splash water over him with your free hand.

Lift him out with your free hand under his bottom, then wrap him gently in a towel. Pat him dry thoroughly, making sure you have dried in between the skin creases.

Getting ready for pregnancy

Staying safe and healthy

Your pregnancy diary

Birth and beyond

The first two weeks

You'll probably spend the first two weeks of your baby's life in an exhausted but happy haze. In between feedings and diaper changes, you'll be welcoming visitors eager to see your little bundle and the house will be filled with cards and flowers. Lie back and enjoy the fuss!

Fatigue

While you can't change your baby's around-the-clock schedule, some strategies help you survive the bleary-eyed days and get more sleep at night.

● Simplify your daily routine—keep household chores to a minimum and don't take on anything overly ambitious, such as trips with your baby to packed shopping malls.

● Say no to caffeine in the late afternoon and evening.

● Nap or rest during the day when your baby sleeps. This isn't a good idea in the long run, but for now it's an important way to keep your energy up.

● Get some gentle exercise and fresh air—a stroll in the park with the carriage is perfect.

● If you're falling asleep on the sofa or in the chair in your baby's nursery, make yourself get into bed. Getting into the habit of sleeping anywhere but the bed can lead to sleep problems.

● Avoid heavy meals near bedtime. But if you need an evening snack, choose a high-carbohydrate food, such as a bowl of cereal. It can actually help you sleep.

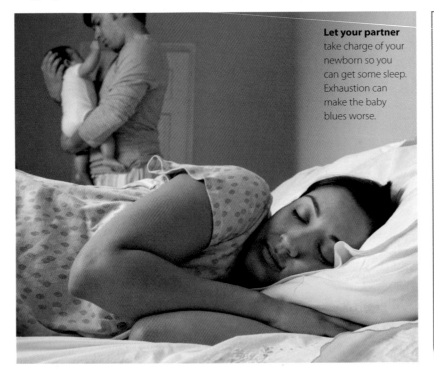

Let your partner take charge of your newborn so you can get some sleep. Exhaustion can make the baby blues worse.

Active mom

Take every opportunity you can to get a nap in while your newborn is sleeping.

"A couple of days after having my baby, the natural high started to wear off and I was hit by a brain-numbing exhaustion! I just felt so physically tired from giving birth and my daughter was waking up several times a night to feed. I started to feel like I'd never catch up on my own sleep. That's when I decided that if she was sleeping, then I needed to be, too. Even though this meant I was napping in the day and still suffering from broken sleep at night, I started to feel so much more human again. Finally she was sleeping through. Bliss!"

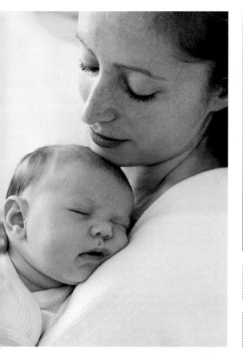

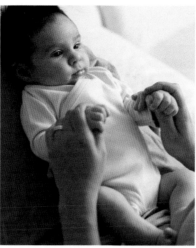

Your baby will enjoy it *(above)* if you play with her and talk to her while you are getting her dressed.

Support your baby's head *(left)* as you pick her up, then bring her close to your chest and hold her gently but firmly.

Handling your newborn

Until about four weeks, your baby won't have any head control. Be sure to support her head firmly at all times, but especially when picking her up and putting her down. Use your other hand and arm to cradle her bottom and back, and draw her near you in a fluid motion.

Then you can embrace her gently against your chest. Or hold her up, with her head resting on your shoulder, her bottom in the crook of your arm and your forearm supporting her back. Reverse these steps to put her down.

When your baby is next to your chest, be sure her head is slightly higher than her body. You can also use a sling, as long as her neck and head are well supported and she fits securely in it.

Getting your baby dressed can feel daunting at first. Newborns seem very fragile, and often cry when they are undressed. You can make the process much simpler by choosing clothes for your baby that are quick and easy to put on and take off, and having everything on hand before you start.

Your baby's one-piece goes on first, over her diaper. Your newborn baby's neck muscles aren't properly developed yet, so support her neck gently as you carefully place her one-piece over her head. Pull it down over her body and do up the snaps at the crotch. Then lay your baby carefully on top of her sleepsuit, ease her arms and legs in gently, and fasten the snaps all the way down the front.

As you get your baby dressed, enjoy talking to her—tell her what you're doing—or singing to her. Don't worry about sounding silly—your baby will love to hear your voice.

Dad's **Diary**

Where does dad come in?
"Fathers often feel that there's nothing useful they can do when there's a newborn in the house. This is hogwash. Starting with the basics, we can:

- Change diapers.
- Burp the baby.
- Rock baby to sleep (important because, unlike your breast-feeding partner, you won't smell of milk and so won't have your fully fed baby demanding more).
- Read stories (baby won't understand a thing, but it's important to introduce the concept early).
- Keep baby occupied through play (we're the fun parents, remember).
- Talk to baby (she can't talk back yet but it gets her familiar with grammar and vocabulary).

Even helping around the house is useful—and earns us dads extra brownie points. The following easy tasks might provide light relief:

- Doing the dishes.
- Cooking for your partner.
- Doing the laundry.
- Cleaning up the house now and then.
- Doing the shopping.
- Waiting on your partner unquestioningly, hand and foot."

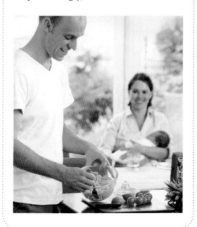

The signs of PPD

It is generally thought that about 10 percent of new mothers suffer from postpartum depression (PPD). If you have a lot of the symptoms that are listed below and you are suffering from them all the time, you should talk to your doctor just in case you are one of that 10 percent. You may be feeling:

- Miserable most of the time and especially bad in the mornings and/or evenings.
- That life is not worth living and you have nothing to look forward to.
- Guilty and very ready to blame yourself.
- Irritable and snapping at your partner or other children.
- Tearful.
- Constantly exhausted, yet not able to sleep.
- Unable to enjoy yourself.
- That you have lost your sense of humor.
- That you can't cope.
- Terribly anxious about the baby, so that you are constantly seeking reassurance about your anxieties from health professionals.
- Worried about your own health, perhaps frightened that you have some dreadful illness.
- Unable to concentrate on anything.
- That your baby is a stranger and not really yours.

You may also be suffering from:

- Loss of sex drive.
- Low energy levels.
- Memory problems.
- Difficulty making decisions.
- No appetite *or* comfort eating.
- Anxiety.
- Disturbed sleep, including early-morning wakefulness.

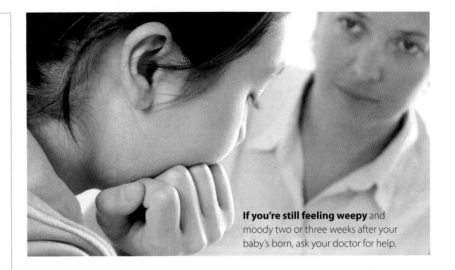

If you're still feeling weepy and moody two or three weeks after your baby's born, ask your doctor for help.

Still feeling blue?

Soon after giving birth, many women have what's commonly called the "baby blues"—weepiness and moodiness. These are often linked to hormonal changes three or four days after delivery, when pregnancy hormones dissipate and milk production starts. They're also linked to the physical and emotional anticlimax after the birth. Returning home from hospital can also increase a new mother's sense of uncertainty.

Baby blues affect 60 to 80 percent of women shortly after labor, and many find themselves exhausted, unable to sleep, or feeling trapped or anxious. Your appetite can change, or you can feel irritable, nervous, worried about being a mother, or afraid that being a mother will never feel better than this.

All these feelings are normal, and they usually last only a few days. Few women find that their sadness persists for longer. Remember—the responsibility that comes with a baby can be overwhelming, and the reality of what parenthood involves doesn't really hit many women until these first few days at home.

Baby blues are often confused with postpartum depression (PPD) because they share common symptoms. But in the first few days after delivery, some emotional upheaval is to be expected. If you continue to feel this way beyond two to three weeks after the birth, you should seek professional support.

 Organized mom

Many moms experience the baby blues in the first few days after their baby is born.

"I had a week of baby blues when my son arrived. I was overwhelmed with the love I felt for him, and spent hours gazing at him. But I felt weepy and emotional at the same time. Being so tired didn't help, either. He's three weeks old now and I feel much more back to my old self and we're starting to form a little routine. My husband and my family were so supportive—they really helped me in those early days."

Colic

About 20 percent of all babies develop colic. This is a catch-all phrase for uncontrollable crying in an otherwise healthy baby. A baby who has real colic will be crying for more than three hours a day, and for more than three days in one week.

Generally, a baby becomes colicky around two to four weeks and is over it by about three months. In addition to persistent crying, a colicky baby looks truly uncomfortable. He may alternately extend or pull up his legs and pass gas, as well as turn red in the face. Colic usually occurs between late afternoon and late in the evening, although it can occur around the clock, generally becoming worse in the evening.

Colic is often blamed on a baby's immature digestive system or, according to some people, it's the baby's still-developing nervous system simply tensing up. Others subscribe to the theory that the baby is tired or overstimulated, and that colic is his way of blocking everything out so he can sleep. Yet another theory is that babies who are exposed to cigarette smoke are more likely to develop colic.

One theory is that breast-fed babies become colicky because of something in their mother's diet, although there's no evidence to support this. Some moms find that if they stop drinking cow's milk and other dairy products, the situation improves. Some breast-fed babies seem to be bothered if mom indulges in a lot of spicy food, wheat products, or cruciferous vegetables such as cabbage and cauliflower. To test if these foods are making your baby uncomfortable, try avoding them for a few days and see if it makes a difference.

If your baby is bottle-fed, you might try a faster flow nipple to see if that improves things. Make sure that you're burping him during and after feedings—it helps to relieve the pressure that builds up when he swallows air. If colic doesn't improve, see your doctor.

ParentsTalk...

"Sara had colic from week five to week eight. She'd cry from 6 pm to 10 pm every night and nothing would soothe her. Since I was breast-feeding, my doctor advised me to stop eating spicy foods and dairy products for a while, but that didn't work. I eventually tried a natural colic remedy suggested by my doctor and that seemed to help."
Vanessa, 34, mom to Sara and Ashley

"My doctor showed me how to do baby massage when Damian had colic. She thought he might be a bit constipated and massage, especially on the tummy, can get things moving. A warm washcloth on his tummy at bathtime soothed him, too."
Kate, 31, mom to Damian

"I was really upset when George had colic. He'd scream between midnight and 3 am most nights. My doctor suggested using a faster flow nipple in his bottle, and it worked immediately. He was obviously swallowing too much air with the old nipple."
Nadia, 29, mom to George

Laid-back mom

You'll get lots of advice about caring for your new baby. But it's okay to go with your own instincts.

"My daughter's eight months now and a couple of my friends have babies of a similar age. Francesca wakes up several times a night. I always go to her to see if she's hungry or needs her diaper changed, but I have a feeling that it's just a case of her wanting to hear my voice and know that I'm still there for her.

I don't mind losing sleep to comfort her, but my friends think I'm crazy! They both opted for the crying-it-out method and said that, after a few difficult nights, their babies realized that they wouldn't be getting mommy's attention just for the sake of it. They now both sleep through. I just can't bear to hear my daughter cry, though, and despite my friends nagging me for spoiling her, I'm going to keep doing what I'm doing.

We're all different as parents and, as long as we're confident that we're doing our best and the right thing, then I think that's all that matters."

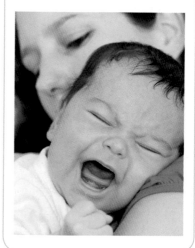

Getting ready for pregnancy

Staying safe and healthy

Your pregnancy diary

Birth and beyond

Diet during breast-feeding

Your body is highly efficient at producing milk, so you shouldn't need to take in lots of extra calories while you're breast-feeding. It's best to be guided by your appetite and to eat when you are hungry. There's no right answer about how many calories a day you should have. The amount you need to eat depends on your weight and how active you are.

It's important to get your vitamins, though. Focus on eating whole grains and cereals, fresh fruit and vegetables, as well as foods that provide plenty of protein, calcium, and iron. Opt for nutritious snacks such as yogurt, sandwiches made with whole-wheat bread and filled with leafy greens and canned salmon, tuna, or cheese, a baked potato with baked beans, or fruit. The occasional "naughty" treat is fine.

What to drink

You only need to drink enough to satisfy your thirst while you're breast-feeding. Drinking lots of water, or indeed going a bit thirsty, won't affect the amount of milk you make. It's a good idea to have a drink nearby when you are breast-feeding, though. While you are feeding, your body releases the hormone oxytocin, and it makes you feel thirsty.

If you want to drink alcohol, don't have more than one or two units once or twice a week. The Department of Health says if you're breast-feeding, it's best to follow the same rules that apply to drinking in pregnancy. Alcohol enters your bloodstream—and then your breast milk—at different speeds, depending on how much you weigh and whether you drink alcohol with food or on an empty stomach. The amount of alcohol in your blood usually peaks 30 to 45 minutes after you drank it. You'll need to allow a couple of hours for your body to be clear of one unit of alcohol.

Weight loss

You may have put on a bit of weight while you were pregnant, and it's fine to shed some while you're breast-feeding. Losing about 2 pounds a week shouldn't affect the amount of milk you make. It's not a good idea to go on a strict diet when you're breast-feeding, but eating healthily and getting gentle exercise will help you get in shape.

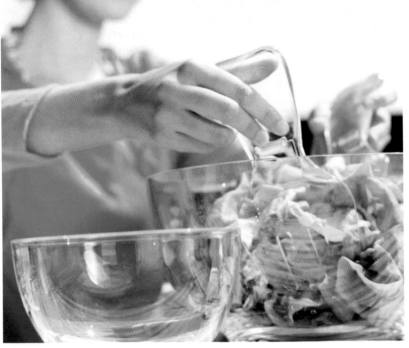

Keep up the healthy habits of your pregnancy by eating plenty of fresh fruit and vegetables as well as whole grains and cereals.

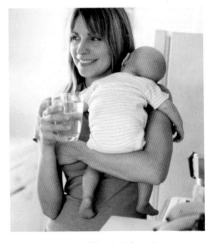

Drinking lots of fluids (above)— especially water—will help you to quench your thirst while you're breast-feeding.

Changing a diaper

Your baby will be wearing diapers day and night for the next two to three years. And, believe it or not, she will need eight to 10 diaper changes a day to begin with. Changing her diaper regularly is important, since urine combined with the bacteria in stool can make her skin sore and lead to diaper rash. Wetness doesn't bother most babies so don't expect her to cry every time she needs changing.

Before you change her, be sure you have everything you need nearby. Don't leave her unattended on a changing table for even a second. Lay her on a safe changing area with a hygienic, washable surface to clean her. For a girl, always wipe from front to back. This helps reduce the possibility of any bacteria causing an infection.

The clean diaper's top half (the one with the tabs) should go under your baby's rear, and the bottom half should come up between her legs. Try not to bunch the diaper up between her legs—this can cause chafing and discomfort. If you are changing a newborn's diaper, you should avoid covering the umbilical cord. For boys, tuck the penis down; that way moisture will be less likely to escape. Fasten the diaper at both sides with the sticky tabs, making sure it's snug, and voilà!

How to change a diaper

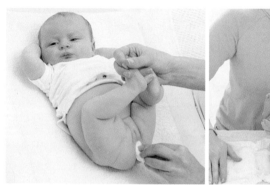

Clean your baby's bottom with a baby wipe or some wet cotton balls. Dry her carefully and apply barrier ointment (see right).

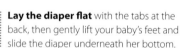

Lay the diaper flat with the tabs at the back, then gently lift your baby's feet and slide the diaper underneath her bottom.

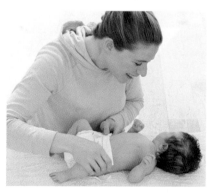

Bring the front of the diaper up between your baby's legs. The top of the diaper should align with her waist.

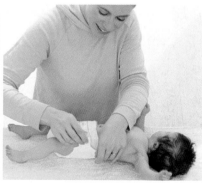

Unpeel the diaper's sticky tabs, one at a time, then pull each side firmly over the front of the diaper and press to fasten.

Diaper rash

If your baby has diaper rash, you'll know it. Some of the skin covered by the diaper—probably the genital area, the folds of the thighs and the buttocks—will appear red and inflamed. The affected areas can be either dry or moist and can sometimes look pimply.

The best remedy is to keep your baby clean and dry by changing her diaper frequently. When you're changing it, use just water and cotton balls or pads to clean the diaper area—this will probably clear up the problem if the diaper rash is allergy-based. Leave her diaper off for a while to allow the air to speed up the healing process. You can prevent diaper rash and protect irritated skin by coating your baby's bottom with a thin layer of barrier ointment after each diaper change.

A normal diaper rash should clear up after three or four days. If your baby's rash persists, spreads, or otherwise worsens or looks infected, talk to your doctor—he may prescribe a hydrocortisone or antibiotic cream.

Getting ready for pregnancy

Staying safe and healthy

Your pregnancy diary

Birth and beyond

Life as new parents

The state of your home brings new meaning to the word "disarray," and you're both totally exhausted. You've become an exhausted, downtrodden, overburdened mommy, while he may be feeling sidelined and deprived of attention. Welcome to parenthood!

Now's the time for you both to reach deep into your reserves of patience and understanding. Dads who return to work outside the home can start to see their partner and baby as a single unit that excludes them. After all, the parent who is out all day doesn't experience the intense bonding that comes with all those tedious-but-necessary tasks, as well as with the cuddling.

When you're both around, try to divvy up the baby care between you (including the less enjoyable parts). Perhaps bathtime could be dad's job before mom does the bedtime feeding. And be considerate if one of you has had more than their share of bottom-wiping or rush-hour traffic stress.

Not many things can soothe the tension of a hard day better than a meaningful and encouraging kind word. Don't underestimate the power of occasional reminders that you're both doing a great job. Being a parent really is the toughest, but most rewarding, thing you'll ever do. Try not to forget to remind each other how much you appreciate the effort you're both putting in.

Above all, keep communicating. Pay attention to each other, and make time to talk through things that are bothering you. You got together for a reason, so try not to lose sight of that.

80% of new moms say that the most surprising

thing they've learned about themselves since becoming a mom is that they didn't know they could be so selfless. Now that they have a baby, they always put his needs first.

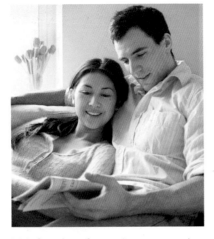

It's daunting when you're new parents but staying close and making sure you spend time together helps you both manage.

ParentsAsk...

When can we have sex again?

You can have sex again when you and your partner both feel that it's right for you. It's assumed that you should wait for your doctor to give you the go-ahead at your six-week postpartum checkup. But some people think it's a good idea to try making love before your checkup so you can discuss any problems you encounter.

New mothers can feel reluctant or uninterested in sex for a variety of reasons. The most obvious reason is soreness from an episiotomy and stitches. Fatigue is another overwhelming factor and, on top

of that, your body image might also hold you back—many women say that they just don't feel "sexy."

If your partner wants sex and you don't, it is important for you to talk about your feelings. Your partner may feel rejected, so it is up to you to explain the physical discomfort or anxieties that are holding you back. Words and cuddling can do much to convey affection and emotion, and you will both benefit from this closeness.

If sex is painful when you do get around to it, despite going carefully and gently, it is worth talking to your doctor about it.

How to manage

Daily life with a newborn can be chaos. Despite little or no previous experience, you are now responsible for the well-being, care, nourishment, and protection of a tiny new baby, 24 hours a day, seven days a week. No wonder you feel overwhelmed.

The good news is that things will become easier as you get to know your baby and discover what he likes and dislikes, and how he needs to be cared for. Until things settle into more of a routine, here are some ideas to help you get through:

● **Go for a walk** Planning a short walk every day, whatever the weather, may stop you from feeling like the walls are closing in on you.

● **Don't try to do too much** If you've always had high standards for housework, accepting that they may need to slip in the early weeks can take the pressure off. Just remember: your newborn doesn't mind if there are crumbs under the toaster. Alternatively, if you can afford one, hire a cleaner.

● **Find some company** Ask your doctor about mother-and-baby groups that meet in your area and make the effort to go to some.

● **Accept any offers of help** If you have visitors, don't make them coffee—ask them to make you coffee!

● **Set some time aside for yourself** Take a shower, put your feet up and read a magazine, or call a friend for a chat.

Dad's **Diary**

The first week of baby's life
"The first week of Leo's life was a blur. The three of us settled into something resembling a daily schedule. I would wake at night with him to change his diaper and hand him to Karen to be breast-fed. Then, my alarm would get me out of bed around seven o'clock. I would putter around the house, feeding the dog and making breakfast. Then, I'd wake Leo and Karen. After another feeding, Karen and I would spend time together with Leo. This was his early-morning full-of-milk cute phase of the day. It was prime-time baby as far as we were concerned. He'd lie on our bed and coo while Karen and I talked to him, sang songs, and just enjoyed ourselves as a new family."

"Things will become easier as you get to know your baby and his likes and dislikes."

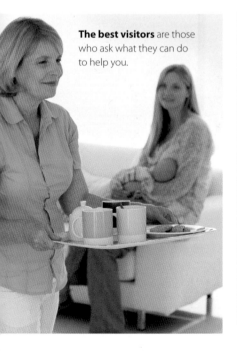

The best visitors are those who ask what they can do to help you.

Knowing when to call the doctor

Life as a new parent means you're on a steep leaning curve. You may worry that you need to call the doctor. Watch out for these warning signs:

● **Change in temperament** A baby who has a runny nose and a big smile is probably not as sick as a baby who has a runny nose and is lethargic.

● **Unusual crying** If your baby is crying more than usual and you can't comfort him, or if his cry is weak or unusually high pitched, he may be seriously ill.

● **Appetite** A baby who tires easily from sucking or loses interest in feeding is probably sick.

● **Abnormal bowel movements** Young babies, especially if breast-fed, may have very soft bowel movements. However, if he has watery stools, his stomach may be upset. If he is sleepy and has small, hard, or dry bowel movements, or if his stool is streaked with blood or mucus, or has the consistency of jelly, you should call your doctor.

● **Difficulty breathing** If your baby's breathing is labored or he's having trouble breathing, get help immediately.

● **Fever** If a baby under three months has a fever higher than 100.4º F (37.7º C), he should be examined by a doctor.

● **Vomiting for 12 hours or more** If this occurs or if he has other symptoms with it, such as fever or a rash, call your doctor.

Getting ready for pregnancy

Staying safe and healthy

Your pregnancy diary

Birth and beyond

Glossary

afterbirth The placenta is commonly called the afterbirth once it has been delivered.

alpha-fetoprotein This is a protein, produced by the fetus's liver, which can be detected in the mother's blood most accurately between 15 and 18 weeks of pregnancy. High levels of AFP may be associated with a neural-tube birth defect called spina bifida; low levels may be associated with Down syndrome.

amniocentesis An amniocentesis is a diagnostic test used to determine possible genetic abnormalities, usually performed between 15 and 20 weeks of pregnancy. Amniotic fluid is withdrawn from the amniotic sac by inserting a hollow needle through the abdominal wall.

amniotic fluid The clear straw-colored liquid in the amniotic sac in which the fetus grows. It cushions the baby against pressure and knocks, allows the baby to move around and grow without restriction, helps the lungs develop, keeps the baby at a constant temperature, and provides a barrier against infection.

Apgar score The Apgar scale is routinely used one and five minutes (and sometimes ten minutes) after birth to assess a newborn baby's health. It assesses five basic indicators of health: activity level, pulse, grimace (response to stimulation), appearance, and respiration.

bilirubin Bilirubin is a by-product of the normal breakdown of old red blood cells. Some newborn babies cannot metabolize it quickly enough, so it builds up under the skin to cause jaundice. If the bilirubin levels get too high it is stored in the brain and can cause brain damage, which is why some newborns are treated under phototherapy lamps to break down the bilirubin.

bloody show A "show" or "bloody show" is a discharge of mucus tinged with blood that results from the mucus plug dislodging from the cervix as labor approaches.

Braxton Hicks contractions The irregular "practice" contractions of the uterus that occur throughout pregnancy, but can be felt especially toward the end of pregnancy. They can sometimes be uncomfortable and intense, but they are not usually painful.

breech presentation A baby is said to be breech presentation, or in a breech position, when it is "bottom down" rather than "head down" in the uterus just before birth. Either the baby's bottom or feet would be born first.

cephalopelvic disproportion This is when a baby's head is too large to pass through the mother's pelvic opening. It is a common cause of obstructed labor and can result in delivery by cesarean section.

cervical stitch A cervical stitch is used to close a weak cervix to prevent miscarriage and premature labor. It is usually carried out between 14 and 16 weeks of pregnancy.

cervical weakness The condition in which the cervix painlessly opens before a pregnancy has reached full term. It can cause miscarriage in the

second trimester or premature labor in the third, but can sometimes be treated with a cervical stitch (see below left).

cervix The lower end or neck of the uterus which leads into the vagina, and which gradually opens during labor.

cesarean section A cesarean or c-section is when the baby is born through an incision in the mother's abdomen and uterus. It is used when a woman cannot give birth vaginally or if the baby is in distress or danger.

chorionic villus sampling (CVS) Chorionic villus sampling (CVS) is a diagnostic test done in early pregnancy, usually between 11 and 13 weeks of pregnancy. Some of the cells that line the placenta, the chorionic villi, are removed through the cervix or abdomen using a needle or catheter. The cells are tested to see whether the developing fetus has Down syndrome or other genetic abnormalities.

colostrum Colostrum is the first "milk" the breasts produce as a precursor to breast milk. It is rich in fats, protein, and antibodies, which protect the baby against infection and kick-start the immune system. It is gradually replaced by breast milk.

conception Conception or fertilization is the moment when sperm and egg meet, join, and form a single cell. It usually takes place in the fallopian tubes.

congenital problem Any problem with a baby that is present from birth or has developed during pregnancy and is not inherited.

contraction The tightening of a muscle. In labor, the strong, rhythmic contractions of the muscles of the uterus open up the cervix and push the baby out.

crowning During labor, when the baby's head can be seen at the opening of the vagina, it is said to "crown."

cyanosis A bluish coloration of the skin caused by lack of oxygen in the blood.

cytomegalovirus infection Cytomegalovirus (CMV) is a viral infection transmitted by saliva, breast milk, or urine. Relatively rare and mild, the infection does occasionally cause deafness, visual impairment, and neurological problems in a developing fetus.

diabetes Diabetes is a disorder in which the body does not produce enough insulin (the hormone that converts sugars into energy), resulting in too much sugar in the bloodstream. It can usually be controlled with appropriate treatment, diet, and exercise.

dilation Dilation, or dilatation, is the gradual opening (dilating) of the cervix during labor. At around 10 cm the cervix is fully dilated.

Doppler ultrasound Pocket-sized handheld device which can be used to listen to the baby's heartbeat during pregnancy.

doula A doula is a person who is specially trained to help during labor and after the birth of a baby. A doula might also help a new mother to breast-feed, or cook, clean, and care for older children.

dystocia This term means "difficult childbirth," usually when labor is not progressing. Uterine dystocia is when the contractions are not strong enough to deliver the baby. Shoulder dystocia is

when a baby's shoulders get stuck after the head has already been delivered.

eclampsia Eclampsia is a rare but serious condition which can affect women in late pregnancy. If preeclampsia (see opposite) is not treated, it can develop into eclampsia, which can cause convulsions and coma. It may require emergency birth of the baby.

ectopic pregnancy An ectopic pregnancy occurs when a fertilized egg implants outside the uterus, usually in a fallopian tube, but it can be anywhere in the abdominal cavity. There is not enough room for a baby to grow, so it must be surgically removed to prevent rupture and damage.

EDD The due date or estimated date of delivery (EDD) is the date when a baby's birth is expected. It is set by a doctor or midwife and is usually based on the first day of a woman's last menstrual period. An ultrasound "dating scan" may be used to give a more accurate estimate of the due date based on measurements of the baby's size.

edema Edema means swelling. It is caused by fluid retention in the body's tissues, and is very common during pregnancy.

effacement This is the thinning and shortening (sometimes called "ripening") of the cervix during early labor. During effacement, the cervix goes from more than an inch thick to paper thin.

electronic fetal monitor An electronic fetal monitor (EFM) is a device used to monitor the progress and vital signs of a baby during labor. It records the baby's heartbeat and the woman's contractions.

embryo The term for a developing baby during the first ten weeks of pregnancy; after that, it is called a fetus.

engagement Engagement, also called lightening or dropping, is when the fetus descends into the pelvic cavity. In first-time mothers, this usually happens two to four weeks before birth; babies of other women usually don't engage until labor begins.

episiotomy A surgical cut in the perineum (the area between the vagina and the anus), made to enlarge the vaginal opening and get the baby born more quickly, or to avoid a tear.

estrogen A hormone produced by the ovaries that plays many roles throughout the body, but is particularly influential, along with the hormone progesterone, in regulating the reproductive cycle.

external cephalic version (ECV) This is a procedure in which a doctor, using ultrasound images as a guide, attempts to massage a breech baby into a more favorable "head-down" position ready for birth.

fallopian tube There are two fallopian tubes, one on each side of the uterus, that lead from the area of the ovaries into the uterine cavity. When an ovary releases an egg, the closest fallopian tube draws it in and transports it down to the uterus.

fetal monitoring Tracking the heartbeat of a fetus and a woman's uterine contractions during labor.

fetus The name given to a growing baby after ten weeks of gestation; before ten weeks, the developing baby is called an embryo.

folic acid A B-complex vitamin that is essential for creating new blood cells, folic acid has been shown to reduce the incidence of neural tube defects such as spina bifida (incomplete closure of the spine) and anencephaly (partially or completely missing brain). It is recommended that all women trying to conceive should take a supplement of folic acid.

fontanelle Fontanelles are soft spots on a baby's head which, during birth, enable the soft bony plates of the skull to flex, allowing the head to pass through the birth canal. Fontanelles are usually completely hardened by a child's second birthday.

forceps birth A birth in which hinged, tonglike instruments (called forceps) are used to ease the baby's head through the birth canal.

fundal height The distance between the top of a pregnant woman's uterus (called the fundus) to her pubic bone. It is measured to determine fetal age.

gestation The period of time a baby is carried in the uterus; full-term gestation is between 38 and 42 weeks (counted from the first day of the last menstrual period).

gestational diabetes mellitus Gestational diabetes is a type of diabetes (when blood sugar levels become too high) that develops during pregnancy. It can be treated, and usually disappears after pregnancy.

gravida The medical term for a pregnant woman.

hemorrhoids Hemorrhoids are swollen blood vessels in the anus. They are caused by increased blood volume and pressure from the uterus on the veins in the legs and pelvis, and are common during pregnancy. Constipation can also cause (or compound) the problem.

hormone A chemical messenger from one cell (or group of cells) to another. Hormones are produced to stimulate or slow down various body functions. The levels of some hormones increase ten-fold during pregnancy.

human chorionic gonadotrophin This hormone is produced by the placenta and triggers the release of estrogen and progesterone. As it is excreted in urine, hCG is used in testing to detect pregnancy.

intrauterine growth restriction (IUGR) The slow growth of a fetus in the uterus, possibly resulting in a low-birthweight baby.

jaundice Jaundice can bring a yellow tinge to a newborn's skin; it is caused by too much bilirubin in the blood. Newborn jaundice usually begins on the second or third day of life. It may clear up on its own after a few days, or may be treated with special light treatment.

lanugo Downlike, fine hair on a baby. Lanugo can appear as early as 15 weeks, and typically begins to disappear sometime before birth.

lightening This occurs when the baby descends lower in the pelvic cavity during the last few weeks of pregnancy.

linea nigra A dark line which may develop during pregnancy, running from below the breasts, over the abdomen and the navel. It often fades after birth but doesn't always disappear entirely.

lochia This is the term used to refer to the vaginal discharge of mucus, blood, and tissue, which may continue for up to six weeks after birth.

meconium The dark, sticky substance released from a newborn's intestines into his first bowel movements. If visible in amniotic fluid prior to delivery, it can be a sign that the baby is in distress.

membranes The sac or "bag of water" filled with amniotic fluid in which the developing baby grows.

midwife A person who cares for women during pregnancy, labor, and birth.

miscarriage The loss of a baby before 24 weeks. After 24 weeks, the loss is called a stillbirth.

mucus plug The plug that blocks the cervix during pregnancy. It is often released with the onset of labor.

neonatal To do with the first four weeks after birth.

neonatal intensive care unit (NICU) An intensive care unit which specializes in the care of premature, low-weight babies and seriously ill babies.

obstetrician A doctor or surgeon who specializes in pregnancy, childbirth, and the immediate postpartum period.

ovaries A pair of gonads (sex glands) that produce key female hormones and eggs, and are found on either side of the uterus.

ovulation The moment at which a mature egg is released from the ovaries into the fallopian tubes—the time around when a woman is most likely to conceive.

oxytocin A hormone secreted by the pituitary gland that controls the contractions of the uterus and stimulates the flow of breast milk. Synthetic oxytocin may be used to induce labor.

palpitation An abnormal heartbeat, often strong and rapid, and often caused by stress.

pediatrician A doctor who specializes in treating babies and children.

pelvic floor The group of muscles at the base of the pelvis which help to support the bladder, uterus, urethra, vagina, and rectum.

perinatal Perinatal refers to the period just before, during, and immediately after birth.

perineum The perineum is the area between the vagina and anus. The perineal area often tears slightly during childbirth.

placenta An organ that develops in the uterus during pregnancy, providing nutrients for the fetus and eliminating its waste products. It is also referred to as the afterbirth because it's delivered after the baby.

placenta previa A pregnancy-related condition where the placenta is placed abnormally low in the uterus, possibly covering the cervix, usually necessitating a cesarean section.

postmature A postmature baby is a baby born at 42 weeks or more.

preeclampsia A condition a mother may develop in the second half of pregnancy, marked by sudden edema, high blood pressure, and protein in the urine. It can lead to complications such as eclampsia (see opposite), so prenatal care staff monitor women carefully for the warning signs.

pregnancy-induced hypertension A condition where a woman's blood pressure is temporarily elevated during pregnancy. It usually occurs during the last trimester.

premature baby A premature baby is one who is born before 37 weeks of gestation.

premature labor Labor that begins before 37 weeks.

progesterone A female hormone produced in the ovaries. It works with estrogen to regulate the reproductive cycle.

pudendal block Pain relief induced by anesthetizing the area around the vulva.

Rhesus incompatibility A condition in which a baby inherits a blood type from his father that is different from and incompatible with his mother's. It is usually not a problem in a first pregnancy but may cause problems with subsequent ones. Blood tests will usually determine if there is a problem before delivery.

sciatica Pain in the leg, lower back, and buttocks can be caused by pressure of the uterus on the sciatic nerve. Applied heat and rest may relieve the condition.

show A "show" or "bloody show" is the discharge of mucus tinged with blood that results from the mucus plug dislodging from the cervix as labor approaches.

stillbirth If a baby dies in the uterus before birth, at or from 24 weeks, it is called a stillbirth. The loss of a pregnancy before 24 weeks is called a miscarriage.

toxoplasmosis This is a parasitic infection carried by cats' feces and uncooked meat. It may cause stillbirth or miscarriage if a woman contracts it for the first time during pregnancy. To reduce the risk, pregnant women should avoid touching a cat's litter box and always wash their hands thoroughly after handling meat.

trimester A trimester is a period of three months. Pregnancy consists of three trimesters.

ultrasound In ultrasound procedures, high-frequency sound waves are used to create a moving image, or sonogram, on a television screen. Often done at various stages of pregnancy, ultrasound scans can help to identify multiple fetuses and detect anomalies.

umbilical cord The umbilical cord is the spongy, cordlike structure that connects a fetus to the placenta. It carries nourishment and removes waste via two arteries and a vein. The cord is cut after birth, and when the cord stump falls off, the baby's belly button is revealed.

uterus The uterus is the pear-shaped muscular organ in a woman's abdomen where an embryo will implant and develop throughout pregnancy.

vacuum A suction cup attached to a machine placed on the baby's head to help the baby through the vagina.

vagina The canal that leads from the outside world to the cervix (also called the birth canal).

vaginal birth after cesarean (VBAC) This term is used when a woman who has previously delivered a baby by cesarean section has a vaginal delivery for a subsequent baby.

vernix caseosa The vernix is a greasy, white substance that covers a baby in the uterus. It protects the baby's skin.

viable The term "viable" describes a baby who is considered capable of living.

zygote This is a medical term for a newly fertilized egg before it implants into the uterus.

Useful contacts and organizations

Fertility

American Fertility Association
www.theafa.org
(888) 917-3777

American Society for Reproductive Medicine
www.asrm.org
(205) 978-5000

Resolve
www.resolve.org
(703) 556-7172

Pregnancy

American College of Obstetricians and Gynecologists
www.acog.org
(202) 638-5577

Association of Women's Health, Obstetric and Neonatal Nurses
www.awhonn.org
(202) 261-2400, (800) 673-8499 (U.S.), (800) 245-0231 (Canada)

Centers for Disease Control and Prevention: Pregnancy
www.cdc.gov/ncbddd/pregnancy_gateway/index.html

Childbirth Connection
www.childbirthconnection.org
(212) 777-5000

March of Dimes
www.marchofdimes.com
(914) 997-4488

National Birth Defects Prevention Network
www.nbdpn.org

National Institute of Child Health and Human Development: Research on Pregnancy and Birth
www.nichd.nih.gov/womenshealth/research/pregbirth.cfm

National Women's Health Information Center: Healthy Pregnancy
www.womenshealth.gov/pregnancy
(800) 994-9662

Sidelines National Support Network
www.sidelines.org
(888) HI-RISK4 or (888) 447-4754

Labor and birth

American Academy of Husband-Coached Childbirth
www.bradleybirth.com
(800) 4-A-BIRTH, or (800) 422-4784, or (818) 788-6662

American Association of Birth Centers
www.birthcenters.org
(866) 54-BIRTH, (866) 542-4784, or (215) 234-8068

American Association of Nurse Anesthetists
www.aana.com
(847) 692-7050

American College of Nurse-Midwives
www.midwife.org
(240) 485-1800

American College of Obstetricians and Gynecologists
www.acog.org
(202) 638-5577

American Diabetes Association
www.diabetes.org
(800) DIABETES or (800) 342-2383

American Society of Anesthesiologists
www.asahq.org
(847) 825-5586

Association of Women's Health, Obstetric and Neonatal Nurses
www.awhonn.org
(202) 261-2400, (800) 673-8499 (U.S.), (800) 245-0231 (Canada)

Doulas of North America
www.dona.org
(888) 788-DONA or (888) 788-3662

International Childbirth Education Association
www.icea.org
(952) 854-8660

Lamaze International
www.lamaze.org
(800) 368-4404 or (202) 367-1128

Midwives Alliance of North America
http://mana.org/
(888) 923-MANA or (888) 923-6262

Breast-feeding

La Leche League International
www.llli.org
(800) LALECHE, (800) 525-3243, or (847) 519-7730

United States Breastfeeding Committee
www.usbreastfeeding.org
(202) 367-1132

Rights and benefits

Children's Health Insurance Program
www.cms.hhs.gov/home/chip.asp

IRS Adoption Credit
www.irs.gov/taxtopics/tc607.html

IRS Child and Dependent Care Credit
www.irs.gov/taxtopics/tc602.html

IRS Child Tax Credit
www.irs.gov/individuals/
article/0,,id=121434,00.html

IRS Tax Information for Parents
www.irs.gov/individuals/parents/index.html

Temporary Assistance for Needy Families
www.acf.hhs.gov/programs/ofa/tanf/index.html

U.S. Department of Agriculture's Women, Infants, and Children Program
www.fns.usda.gov/wic

U.S. Family and Medical Leave Act
www.dol.gov/whd/fmla/index.htm

Adoption

Joint Council on International Children's Services
www.jcics.org/International_Adoption.htm
(703) 535-8045

National Adoption Center
www.adopt.org
(800) TO-ADOPT, (800) 862-3678,
or (215) 735-9988

North American Council on Adoptable Children
www.nacac.org
(651) 644-3036

Support groups

Hope for Two: The Pregnant With Cancer Network
www.pregnantwithcancer.org
(800) 743-4471

La Leche League International
www.llli.org
(800) LALECHE, (800) 525-3243,
or (847) 519-7730

Resolve
www.resolve.org
(703) 556-7172

Sidelines National Support Network
www.sidelines.org
(888) HI-RISK4 or (888) 447-4754

For fathers

At Home Dad
www.angelfire.com/zine2/athomedad/

National Fatherhood Initiative
www.fatherhood.org
(301) 948-0599

Fathers' Forum
www.fathersforum.com
(510) 644-0300

The Fathers Network
www.fathersnetwork.org

General

Families and Work Institute
www.familiesandwork.org
(212) 465-2044

Family and Home Network
www.familyandhome.org
(703) 352-1072

MomsRising
www.momsrising.org

National Partnership for Women & Families
www.nationalpartnership.org
(202) 986-2600

9to5, National Association of Working Women
www.9to5.org
(414) 274-0925

Safety

National Institute for Occupational Safety and Health: The Effects of Workplace Hazards on Female Reproductive Health
www.cdc.gov/niosh/docs/99-104

Organization of Teratology Information Specialists
www.otispregnancy.org
(866) 626-OTIS or (866) 626-6847

U.S. Food and Drug Administration Food Safety for Moms-to-Be
www.fda.gov/Food/ResourcesForYou/HealthEducators/ucm081785

Index

Page numbers in *italic* refer to the illustrations

Acknowledgments

BabyCenter Acknowledgments:

BabyCenter would like to thank contributing editors Martine Gallie and Darienne Hosley Stewart for adapting content from our web pages to make it work on the printed page. Also Victoria Farrimond for her tireless work in managing this project.

Thank you to the BabyCenter team—Daphne Metland, Sasha Miller, Emma Woolfenden, Chess Thomas, Catherine Mendham, Rhianydd Thomas, Bernie Sheehan, Sam Wright, Jenny Leach, and Lynda Hale—for their expertise and contributions. All our health articles are checked and approved by the team of health professionals on our medical advisory board, but we'd like especially to thank consultant pediatrician and neonatologist Dr. Dwight Lindo and GP Dr. Philippa Kaye for their advice and assistance during this project..

And, finally, we'd like to thank Penny Warren, Glenda Fisher, Hilary Mandleberg, Emma Maule, Hannah Moore, Kevin Smith, Isabel de Cordova, and Saskia Janssen for their hard work in driving this project and for understanding and championing the BabyCenter ethos.

Publisher's Acknowledgments:

DK would like to thank Salima Hirani for proofreading; Hilary Bird for the index; Karen Sullivan for editorial consultancy; Carly Churchill and Sue Prescott for photographic assistance; Joanna Dingley for editorial assistance; Vicky Barnes, Roisin Donaghy, Nadine Wilkie, and Alli Williams for hair and makeup; Kate Simunek for designing the icons; Caron Bosler for Pilates advice; and all of our models: Adrian Bewsey; Heidi Carr; Rachel Chan and Niamh Chung; Carmen Ingrid Dillon; Katie, James, and Isabella Dockray; Francesca Elliott; Ava Freeman; Kavita Harrison; Carla and Alexa Haslock; Saskia Janssen; Sharmina Karim and Joshua Allen; Sian Lattimer Keller; Dorinda Kemp; Barbara Madley; Lesley Manalo; Zia Mattocks; Emma Maule; Susan Prescott; Nicola Richardson; Nicola Riley; Laura Roberts-Jensen and Quinn Jensen; Andrea Samayoa; Alberta Starr; Phillipa Strub and Molly Statham; Zai Swan.

Picture credits

The publisher would like to thank the following for their kind permission to reproduce their photographs:

(Key: a-above; b-below/bottom; c-center; f-far; l-left; r-right; t-top)

Alamy Images: Asia Images Group Pte Ltd 18; David J. Green—Lifestyle 219tl; Medical-on-Line 215tl; Paul Mogford 121tr; Picture Partners 275tl; Andres Rodriguez 17; Gary Roebuck 105; Chris Rout 264br; Trevor Smith 221bl; Alena Sudová 297cra; Liba Taylor 270; Andrew Twort 53; **Corbis:** Lisa B. 46–47; Rick Chapman 294; ER Productions 41; Michael A. Keller 123t; Daniel Kroells/Westend61 130; Johannes Mann 14; Marie-Reine Mattera 306bl; RK Studio/Blend Images 21; Andersen Ross/Brand X 253t; Norbert Schaefer 83; Alessandra Schellnegger 216; TH-Foto 183fbr; Bernd Vogel 42; Studio Wartenberg 92; Olix Wirtinger 96; **Getty Images:** altrendo images 15; Anthony-Masterson 306br; J.A. Bracchi 199; Roderick Chen 115; Sarah Cuttle 148; Peter Dazeley 188br; Marc Debnam 95tl; Digital Vision 155t; George Doyle 19, 87bc; Tracy Frankel 57; Eric Glenn 76; Robert Glenn 152; Jamie Grill 89; Dennis Hallinan 52; Noel Hendrickson 80tl; Frank Herholdt 99; Image Source 120bl; Jonathan Kantor 95tr, 125cr; Gavin Kingcome Photography 87br; David A Land 308; Bill Ling 38; Barbara Lutterbeck 183bl; LWA 12–13, 122br; Ericka McConnell 82; Paul Bradbury 117br; Hans Neleman 259t; Bernd Opitz 259bl; Lori Adamski Peek 129; Plush Studios/Bill Reitzel 112; Rayes 119; Andersen Ross 77, 169bl; Richard Ross 183bc (tomatoes); Sam Royds 175; rubberball 143; Stockbyte 25; Jerome Tisne 86; Betsie Van der Meer 20; VCL/Alistair Berg 156; Veer/Mark Adams 65; Visuals Unlimited 251t; Michael Wildsmith 103; Mel Yates 297tl; Yellow Dog Productions 302; David Young-Wolff 231; **iStockphoto.com:** Adrian Albritton 208; Ruth Black 155br; Matjaz Boncina 209; ranplett 144; Vivid Pixels 240–241; **Prof. J.E. Jirasek MD, DSc.:** 125br; **Mother & Baby Picture Library:** Dave J. Anthony 180, 184; Moose Azim 177; Ian Hooton 80tr, 84, 87bl, 90, 127b, 127t, 128, 171cl, 187cl, 223, 232, 243, 247, 274bl, 277; Ruth Jenkinson 181, 210, 245, 251b; Eddie Lawrence 273, 289; Paul Mitchell 101t; James Thomson 85; **Photolibrary:** FoodCollection 55cra; Vladimir Pcholkin 48; zoomphotographics 162; **Science Photo Library:** 137tr, 141br; AJ Photo 224, 304; Samuel Ashfield 280; Biophoto Associate 32; Neil Borden 157cb, 157clb; Neil Bromhall 33; BSIP, Astier 285t; BSIP, Laurent 263bl; CNRI 271; John Cole 171br; Christian Darkin 35cr; Adam Gault 222; Ian Hooton 22, 211, 212, 221t; La La 214; Eddie Lawrence 253b; Dr Najeeb Layyous 179; Living Art Enterprises, LLC 157bc, 157bl; Dr P. Marazzi 215tc; Dr Yorgos Nikas 35bc, 35bl, 35br; Lea Paterson 23; D. Phillips 27tc, 27tl; Antonia Reeve 279; P. Saada / Eurelios 137tl; Saturn Stills 101br; Mark Thomas 285bl; Anatomical Travelogue 117tr; **SuperStock:** age fotostock 183br

All other images © Dorling Kindersley

For further information see: www.dkimages.com

Answers to Dad's Diary Quiz, p. 145

Q1—a; Q2—c; Q3—b; Q4—d; Q5—a; Q6—c

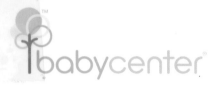

The ultimate guide to preconception, pregnancy, birth, and the first few weeks with a new baby, from BabyCenter—trusted by over 16 million parents around the world.

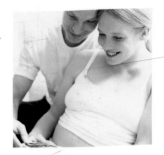

• *BabyCenter Pregnancy* is your best friend, mom, and doctor, all in one, providing both professional prenatal expertise and practical tips from parents who've been there and have the stretch marks to prove it!

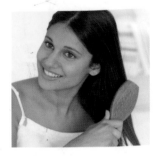

• We're with you every step of the way, week by week: with the information you need, when you need it, to help you make the best choices for you and your baby.

• What's safe? What can I eat? Why am I so tired and emotional? How will I know I'm in labor? *BabyCenter Pregnancy* has all the answers.

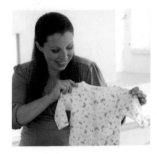

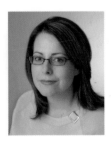

Linda J. Murray is the vice president of editorial and the global chief of BabyCenter. She jo fledgling site in 1998 and h build it into the leading online destination for new and expectant parents around the world.

Jacket images:
Front: Photolibrary: John Lund/Drew Kelly/
Blend Images
Back: Science Photo Library: Ian Hooton (top)
Editor portrait: Steve LaBadessa.
All other images © Dorling Kindersley
For further information see:
www.dkimages.com

Discover more at
www.dk.com

ISBN 978-0-7566-5040-7

51995

9 780756 650407